Practice Development in Nursing and Healthcare

SECOND EDITION

Edited by

Brendan McCormack

Director of the Institute of Nursing Research and Head of the Person-centred Practice Research
Centre, University of Ulster, Northern Ireland, UK
Professor II, Buskerud University College, Drammen, Norway
Adjunct Professor of Nursing, University of Technology, Sydney, Australia
Adjunct Professor of Nursing, Faculty of Medicine, Nursing and Health Care, Monash
University, Melbourne, Australia
Visiting Professor, School of Medicine and Dentistry, University of Aberdeen, UK

Kim Manley

Co-Director, England Centre for Practice Development, Canterbury Christ Church
University, UK
Associate Director, Practice Development, Transformational Research and Development, East
Kent Hospitals NHS Foundation Trust, UK
Visiting Professor, Canterbury Christ Church University; Visiting Professor, University of
Surrey, UK

Angie Titchen

Visiting Professor, University of Ulster, Northern Ireland, UK
Adjunct Professor, Charles Sturt University, Australia
Principle Investigator, Knowledge Centre for Evidence-Based Practice, Fontys University of
Applied Sciences, The Netherlands
Independent Practice Development and Research Consultant

WILEY-BLACKWELL

A John Wiley & Sons, Ltd., Publication

This edition first published 2013 © 2004, 2013 by John Wiley & Sons, Ltd

First edition published 2004 by Blackwell Publishing, Ltd

Wiley-Blackwell is an imprint of John Wiley & Sons, formed by the merger of Wiley's global Scientific, Technical and Medical business with Blackwell Publishing.

Registered office: John Wiley & Sons, Ltd, The Atrium, Southern Gate, Chichester, West Sussex, PO19 8SQ, UK

Editorial offices: 9600 Garsington Road, Oxford, OX4 2DQ, UK
The Atrium, Southern Gate, Chichester, West Sussex, PO19 8SQ, UK
2121 State Avenue, Ames, Iowa 50014-8300, USA

For details of our global editorial offices, for customer services and for information about how to apply for permission to reuse the copyright material in this book please see our website at www.wiley.com/wiley-blackwell.

Library of Congress Cataloging-in-Publication Data

Practice development in nursing and healthcare / edited by Brendan McCormack, Kim Manley, Angie Titchen. – 2nd ed.
     p.   cm.
   Includes bibliographical references and index.
   ISBN 978-0-470-67311-9 (pbk. : alk. paper)   1. Nursing.   2. Nurse practitioners.
I. McCormack, Brendan.   II. Manley, Kim, MN.   III. Titchen, Angie.
   RT82.8.P73 2013
   610.73–dc23

                                                                2012028350

A catalogue record for this book is available from the British Library.

Wiley also publishes its books in a variety of electronic formats. Some content that appears in print may not be available in electronic books.

Cover image: © iStockphoto / Mr-Spliberg
Cover design by Meaden Creative

Set in 10/12 pt Times by Aptara® Inc., New Delhi, India
Printed and bound in Malaysia by Vivar Printing Sdn Bhd

4   2016

Contents

Contributors

Jan Dewing
Head of Person-Centred Research and
   Practice Development Department of
   Nursing and Applied Clinical Studies
East Sussex Healthcare NHS Trust
Canterbury Christ Church University
Canterbury, UK

Co-Director
England Centre for Practice Development
Canterbury Christ Church University
Canterbury, UK

Visiting Professor
Institute of Nursing and Health Research
University of Ulster
Newtownabbey, UK

Visiting Professor
University of Wollongong
Wollongong, Australia

Jill Down
Lead Nurse Professional Development
Cambridge University Hospitals NHS
   Foundation Trust
Cambridge, UK

IrenaAnna Frei
Head of Practice Development in Nursing
Department of Nursing and Allied Health
   Professions
University Hospital Basel
Basel, Switzerland

Lecturer at the Institute of Nursing Science
University of Basel
Basel, Switzerland

Sally Hardy
Professor of Mental Health and Practice
   Innovation
School of Health Sciences
City University
London, UK

Carrie Jackson
Head of Department, Nursing and Applied
   Clinical Studies
Director, England Centre for Practice
   Development
Faculty of Health and Social Care
Canterbury Christ Church University
Canterbury, UK

Honorary Associate Professor
Faculty of Health and Behavioural Sciences
University of Wollongong
Wollongong, Australia

Honorary Clinical Academic Fellow
East Kent University Hospitals NHS
   Foundation Trust
Canterbury, UK

Jill Maben
Professor
King's College London
London, UK

Director
National Nursing Research Unit
Florence Nightingale School of Nursing
   and Midwifery
London, UK

Kim Manley
Visiting Professor and Co-Director
England Centre for Practice Development
Canterbury Christ Church University
Canterbury, UK

Visiting Professor
Surrey University
Guildford, UK

Tanya McCance
The Mona Grey Professor of Nursing
  Research and Development
Co-Director of Nursing Research and
  Development
Belfast Health and Social Caret Trust
Belfast, UK

Visiting Professor
England Centre for Practice Development
Faculty of Health and Social Care
Canterbury Christ Church University
Canterbury, UK

Brendan McCormack
Director, Institute of Nursing and Health
  Research and Head of the
  Person-Centred Practice Research
  Centre
University of Ulster
Newtownabbey, UK

Adjunct Professor of Nursing
University of Technology
Sydney, Australia

Visiting Professor
School of Medicine and Dentistry
University of Aberdeen
Aberdeen, UK

Professor II
Buskerud University College
Drammen, Norway

Ann McMahon
RCN Research and Innovation Adviser
Manager, RCN Research and Innovation
  Team
Royal College of Nursing
London, UK

Jo Odell
Practice Development Facilitator
Patients First Programme
Foundation of Nursing Studies
London, UK

Randal Parlour
Assistant Director
NMPDU HSE-West
CNME
St. Conal's Hospital
Letterkenny, Ireland

Jo Rycroft-Malone
Professor of Implementation Research
University Director of Research
Bangor University
Bangor, UK

Kate Sanders
Practice Development Facilitator
Foundation of Nursing Studies
London, UK

Theresa Shaw
Chief Executive, Foundation of Nursing
  Studies
Honorary Senior Research Fellow, Nursing
  and Applied Clinical Studies Faculty
  of Health and Social Care
Foundation of Nursing Studies, UK

Annette Solman
Director of Nursing
The Sydney Children's Hospitals Network
Sydney, Australia

Angie Titchen
Independent Practice Development and
    Research Consultant
Knowledge Centre for Evidence-Based
    Practice
Fontys University of Applied Sciences
Eindhoven, The Netherlands

Visiting Professor
University of Ulster
Newtownabbey, UK

Adjunct Professor
Charles Sturt University
Sydney, Australia

Associate Fellow
University of Warwick
Coventry, UK

Jonathan Webster
Director of Nursing and Quality
NHS North West London – Inner CCG
    Collaboration
London, UK

Val Wilson
Professor of Nursing Research and Practice
    Development
University of Technology
Sydney, Australia

Director of Nursing Research and Practice
    Development
The Sydney Children's Hospitals Network
    (Westmead)
Sydney, Australia

Joan Yalden
Practice Development Facilitator
Melbourne, Australia

Preface

Dancing with beauty rather than fighting ugliness.

(Marshall & Reason, 2008)

In the above quote, Marshall and Reason make the case for us to focus on the beauty of practice rather than the ugly parts. When reflecting on the evolution of practice development over the past 15–20 years, we can see the relevance of this quote for novices through to people with expertise in all health care professions. Practice development as a formalised movement for change has its origins in a nursing history that has strived to shake off a legacy of routine and ritual and embrace approaches to practise that privilege the individual in context. This is not to suggest that everything that went before was 'ugly' and that everything now is beautiful! But instead, what has been happening in nursing is reflective of general health care trends and indeed society as a whole, where individual experience, consumer rights and professional responsibility and accountability are paramount. The early days of practice development saw a significant focus on individualised patient-centred care and services and in particular a focus on improving particular practices (e.g. within nursing, pain management, incontinence management, continence promotion and pressure damage prevention). This pioneering and systematic work, whilst similar to what was happening in quality improvement, had a different focus in terms of the methods used, and also in the explicit contribution of nursing to quality of patient care. These explorations of the nursing contribution opened up many other opportunities for different questions about practice to be asked, and in particular, issues of leadership, culture and approaches to learning. Through the answering of questions such as these, systematic approaches to inquiry, informed by other traditions (such as action research and hermeneutic phenomenology), have enabled methodological progress in practice development that has continued and broadened to other health care professions ever since.

The evolution of practice development is underwritten by enormous commitment from passionate and determined individuals, by vision and leadership from people in positions of authority and by a drive among some academics to ensure that knowledge for and about practice is co-produced. In many ways, the landscape of contemporary practice development has changed significantly and it is increasingly integrated into other health care professions and organisational and strategic programmes of work, all with the common purposes of person-centredness, safety, accountability and quality of experience. None of these issues are mutually exclusive and so it makes sense that there has emerged a melding and blending of methods and a greater sense of the importance of collaborative and integrated approaches to improving services. Alongside this evolution, we have witnessed significant changes to the ways in which health and social care is delivered. The drive for services that are responsive to the needs of people and the recognition of the existential significance of persons retaining control over their own lives are paramount in contemporary health care models, frameworks and processes. Practice development with its focus on developing and sustaining workplaces that are evidence-informed and person-centred has made a significant contribution to the prioritisation of this agenda. As various chapters in this book contest, the methodology of practice development and methods of engagement that are collaborative, inclusive and participative have the potential to enable organisations to demonstrate commitment to person-centred services.

Our intention is to create a culture where emancipatory learning and transformational learning are central to the delivery of quality patient care. A laudable ideal indeed, but an idealism that we are not afraid of pursuing as practice developers. As the Irish Philosopher, John O'Donohue (1998: 148) says: "light has many faces – the dark has none!" There are many faces to the light we are pursuing, some of which are not welcoming, rather they are hostile. However, the alternative is to stay in the dark and pursue an agenda that we know does not achieve our vision for patient care. Paulo Freire, the Brazilian philosopher, believed that the ultimate purpose of adult education was the production of a strategically appropriate radicalism, based on humanistic ideals that focused on the unquestionable value of persons (see Freire, 1972). The reality of many of our practice cultures is that they are largely 'silent' in their critique of practice and the factors that hinder effectiveness in practice. Freire described this as the 'pedagogy of the oppressed'. Therefore, the purpose of emancipatory and transformational learning through practice development is to work with those who are oppressed to unveil this world of domination and commit to its transformation. Freire was idealistic, but he did recognise that such transformation was only possible through continuous and sustained development – something that is advocated by contributors to this book with a focus on participatory and active learning. What is important about Freire's philosophy is that he believed that educators and practitioners were culturally different, and therefore, the beginning of the process of transformation must include participant observation by educators 'tuning in' to the everyday experiences of the people. In the context of practice development, therefore, being alongside practitioners and other key stakeholders as co-learners is critical to understanding the contextualisation of learning. The reversal of the power-relationship between practice development facilitators and the people in a workplace creates a culture of shared learning that is 'the learning of equals', and thus, it reverses dominant power relationships. This form of learning is not focused on the learning of facts through technical-rational models of learning. It is instead focused on developing critical awareness or critical consciousness. In this way, as the work of Freire contests, changes in practice are sustained through critical consciousness that results in critical awareness of contextual and internal factors that need to be continuously addressed.

A key challenge for all of us, however, is that of creating the health care professional of the future, and therefore, professional development programmes must have an aim of helping staff to develop their ability to create such conditions for learning and development. Professional development programmes may help us to more easily grow into a niche that is created for us in an already established cultural system (i.e. learn how to work more effectively in an already established team), but it in itself will do little to help us become critical of the constraints that the structures of a health care system impose upon us or to change it. No amount of classroom-based learning will help us to feel less alienated from the organisations in which we work. And here lies a further irony – in order to play the recruitment game and compete with other employers, health care organisations increasingly use the lever of the quantity of professional development opportunities available to staff as a 'carrot'. However, empowering cultures are not created through such learning, but instead are created by an approach to cultural change that maximises opportunities to exercise autonomy, where decision-making is decentralised, where opportunities for professional development are available and where staff feel that they are valued and listened to. None of these characteristics are achievable through traditional approaches to learning, but yet, that is where staff development resources are targeted. Practice development with its focus on active, participatory and work-based learning has the potential to readdress this paradox and enable a more cost-effective and contextually appropriate professional to emerge.

So, whilst not wishing to overclaim the potential of practice development and the outcomes that are possible, we believe that this book demonstrates what is possible and how these possibilities might be achieved by a spectrum of readers from novice to expert within health care professions. The challenges of ensuring rigorous and creative approaches in an ever-changing health and social care landscape will prevail, but we believe that, more than ever, we are prepared for such challenges and have the tools and processes at our disposal. For in the words of Chardin (2008) '[t]he more one sees the better one knows where to look'.

Brendan McCormack
Kim Manley
Angie Titchen

REFERENCES

Freire P. (1985) *The Politics of Education: Culture, Power, and Liberation*. MacMillan, Basingstoke.
Marshall, J. & Reason, P. (2008) Taking an attitude of inquiry. In: *Towards Quality Improvement of Action Research: Developing Ethics and Standards* (eds B. Boog, J. Preece, M. Slagter & J. Zeelen), pp. 62–82. Sense Publishers, Rotterdam.
O'Donohue J. (1998) *Eternal Echoes: Exploring Our Hunger To Belong*. Bantam, New York.

Acknowledgements

The creation of this book has been a collaborative effort in its unfolding. We would therefore like to acknowledge the support of all the chapter authors who have drawn on their creative resources to push the boundaries of the text to develop chapters that are challenging, exciting and informed. The nature of practice development means that we are dependent on those with whom we collaborate to produce the evidence upon which we can build. Therefore, without colleagues in practice, leadership, management, research, policy and strategic roles, the evidence base for this book would be far more limited. Their commitment to the ongoing development of person-centred cultures that sustain individual and team growth and development is greatly appreciated. Our families, friends and colleagues have supported us throughout this project and we are very grateful to them. Finally, we are greatly appreciative of colleagues at Wiley Blackwell, who have gently encouraged us along the way, tolerated our missing of deadlines and applied systematic processes to ensuring the quality of the final product.

1 Introduction

Brendan McCormack[1], Kim Manley[2] and Angie Titchen[3]

[1]University of Ulster, Newtownabbey, UK
[2]Canterbury Christ Church University, Canterbury, UK
[3]Fontys University of Applied Sciences, Eindhoven, The Netherlands

WHY DEVELOP PRACTICE

Internationally, for the past 15 years, health care has been dominated by an agenda of reformation, modernisation and transformation. During this time, there has been a significant emphasis on person-centred care delivery in a strategic and political context that has been focused on cost containment and cost reduction. For many commentators this is indeed a paradox and one that is not 'healthy' in a health economy (Bechtel & Ness, 2010; Braithwaite, 2010). However, the challenges of delivering person-centred health care are not solely about economic resources, but are as much about the focus of staff and their priorities. Changing the model of care from one that is primarily hospital based, to one that is delivered as a partnership between service users, all care settings and public and private providers has resulted in major changes to the way care services are delivered and operationalised. These changes have been key features of the transformation agenda. Roles have needed to change among all professions, and professional boundaries have been increasingly blurred.

However, whilst there has been an emphasis in policy and strategy documents on the development of person-centred services, this has merely been, at worse, rhetoric, or at best, a simplistic idea based on providing service users and their families with more choices about how their health care is delivered. This view is reinforced by a continuous and sustained focus among patient advocacy groups and media commentators on the poor quality of care in hospitals, the poor treatment of vulnerable patients and a lack of respect and dignity in individual care practices (see, e.g., the UK Patients Association 'Care Campaign', http://patients-association.com/Default.aspx?tabid=237, and the recent 'I' newspaper series on poor nursing, http://www.independent.co.uk/life-style/health-and-families/features/nurses-do-not-wake-up-each-morning-intent-on-delivering-poor-care-7644061.html?origin=internalSearch). Most recently in the United Kingdom, a commission of inquiry into dignity in hospitals and nursing homes has been instigated by three major organisations – AgeUK, The Local Government Association and the NHS Confederation (http://www.ageuk.org.uk/home-and-care/improving-dignity-in-care-consultation/). The investigation has focused on understanding the contextual factors that, on the one hand, have resulted in some of the greatest

Practice Development in Nursing and Healthcare, Second Edition. Edited by Brendan McCormack, Kim Manley and Angie Titchen.
© 2013 John Wiley & Sons, Ltd. Published 2013 by John Wiley & Sons, Ltd.

advances in health care, whilst on the other, seem to have eroded the dignity of patient experience – particularly among older people. A key recommendation of the commission is:

> *Hospitals should introduce facilitated, practice-based development programmes – 'learning through doing' – to ensure staff caring for older people are given the confidence, support and skills to do the right thing for their patients.*

This recommendation by the Dignity Commission highlights the need for ongoing development of practice in clinical settings and reinforces the views of key commentators that widespread top-down organisational changes without concomitant bottom-up development programmes result in ineffective change processes and poor outcomes (Braithwaite et al., 2006). Indeed, Braithwaite and colleagues suggest that, without programmes of development at the micro level (clinical practice environment), the large-scale and top-down driven change has a negative impact. Drawing on their work that focused on introducing new information technology, they suggested that the imposing of reorganisations, restructuring and attempting to change corporate culture by senior management instigation frequently fell short and had the potential to create major patterns of dissension and resistance (Westbrook et al., 2007).

This evidence from Braithwaite et al. (2006), which confirms what has been known in the change literature for well over 30 years (see Ottaway, 1976; Beer, 1980), was recently reinforced by a personal story of a colleague who had had a recent hospital experience:

> *I don't think the <hospital name> nurses I encountered were uncaring. They were ill prepared for the tasks they faced, sometimes insensitive, unsupported by the structures and ethos of the service and very overwhelmed, but I wouldn't say they didn't care or that they didn't, for the most part, work hard. They reminded me of the adage 'the road to hell is paved with good intentions' and even if they had known more about dementia and mania, or at least have been aware of what they didn't know, they still couldn't have functioned adequately within the structures and systems (Personal Communication, 2011)*

Since its origins in the late 1970s, practice development has been aware of the pitfalls of top-down change alone, and so it pays attention to these local practices in clinical settings, whilst focusing on the need for a systems-wide focus on person-centredness and the development of person-centred cultures. In particular, practice development pays attention to what are increasingly acknowledged as 'the human factors' in health care – factors that focus on the relationship between staff's well-being, leadership, team relationships, morale, satisfaction and a sense of belonging among staff in the context of clinical effectiveness and patient outcome. For example, Maben et al. (2012) have identified that the quality of care for people in acute settings relies on resilience building and renewal for staff, leadership and support and teamwork. They also highlight the importance of adequate staffing. Whilst initiatives such as 'Transforming Care at the Bedside' (http://www.ihi.org/offerings/Initiatives/PastStrategicInitiatives/TCAB/Pages/default.aspx) address such contextual issues as these, others have commented that it should not be assumed that human factors in health care can be addressed by the transfer of quick-fix solutions (Cooke, cited in Feinmann, 2011). Whilst these initiatives and innovations do have an important role to play in changing practices and ensuring that systems are responsive to the needs of patients and families, developing evidence-informed and person-centred cultures of effectiveness needs a greater focus on understanding the motivation behind practices and working with these motivations to implement solutions as an integrated part of health care service delivery.

The development of person-centred cultures cannot be achieved through a focus on implementing solutions that address particular aspects of system ineffectiveness. Instead, sustained and integrated approaches to the creation of person-centred cultures systematically address embedded patterns in workplaces. To bring about fundamental change in complex systems requires the recognition of patterns that drive thinking and behaviour (Plsek, 2001). Patterns are often ignored or go unchallenged despite changes to structures and processes (Plsek, 2001). This is because patterns are associated with distinctive behavioural norms that manifest specific values, beliefs and assumptions within a workplace. These aspects together by definition are termed 'culture' (Schein, 2004), where implicit importance is placed on how things are done and what counts as important. Patterns describe problems that occur over and over again in an environment or operational context and they describe the core of a solution to that problem in such a way that it can be used an infinite number of times – without ever doing it the same way twice. As such, patterns can be much generalised at a conceptual level whilst they are absolutely unique at a local implementation level.

However, in their most recent work, McCance et al. (2012) have identified that despite what is known about the importance of person-centred care and the need for the development of person-centred cultures, the majority of service users only experience 'person-centred moments', that is, moments of time when care is person-centred set within an overarching care experience of routine. McCance et al. (2012) have concluded that person-centredness is a fragile concept and is dependent on a person-centred culture that has consistent care delivery, effective care coordination, good leadership, a knowledgeable and skilled care team, systems-wide support for person-centredness and a flexible model of care delivery. So, this would suggest that even within a stringent economic climate, principles of person-centredness can be maintained and quality systems enhanced if issues such as leadership, facilitation, teamwork and collective vision are held central in service development programmes. All of which are central concerns of practice development.

PRACTICE DEVELOPMENT – ITS ORIGINS

In 2004 *Practice Development in Nursing* was published (McCormack et al., 2004) and its publication was a political act and landmark in making visible significant work that had previously been undertaken in establishing practice development as a movement in the development of nursing practice. Prior to its publication, practice development had been evolving through a range of projects that had each focused on different approaches to improving patient care in different settings, but which had also focused on articulating the contribution of nurses to effective patient care. The term 'practice development' was at that time widely but inconsistently used in British nursing. It was used to address a broad range of educational (McKenna, 1995), research (Rolfe, 1996) and audit (NHSE, 1996) activity. In much of the literature, there was an emphasis on the use of research evidence in practice (e.g. Kitson et al., 1996). Practice development was underdeveloped as a methodology, and whilst there was a lot of enthusiasm for the methods because they resonated with the increased emphasis on quality improvement, clinical audit and using research in practice, there was no coordinated approach, nor indeed common understanding of the most effective methodologies.

In 2002, Garbett and McCormack published the first concept analysis of practice development, and this analysis brought together what had been until then a disparate body of work that used different methods, but all of which had the shared intention of developing patient care and nursing practice. The principles that underpinned this body of work included:

- an emphasis on improving patient care;
- an emphasis on transforming the contexts and cultures in which nursing care took place;
- the importance of employing a systematic approach to effect changes in practice;
- the continuous nature of practice development activity;
- the nature of the facilitation required for change to take place.

(Garbett & McCormack, 2002)

The concept analysis highlighted that there were clear areas of congruity between work being undertaken by practice developers and the kinds of practice being promoted in the national health care policy at that time. For example, the then England's Chief Nursing Officer launched a publication in the wake of the NHS Plan (Mullally, 2001) that emphasised the importance of learning from practice, being responsive to patients and developing adaptability to change. Clearly, these themes resonated with the principles underpinning practice development, and so the importance of the contribution of staff working in the many and varied practice development roles across the United Kingdom were clearly central to the wholesale cultural shift that was being demanded of the NHS. Networks such as 'The UK Developing Practice Network' were focused on that agenda and did much to advance understanding of the role of the Practice Development Nurse in the United Kingdom.

The publication of *Practice Development in Nursing* in 2004 added to a growing body of conceptual, theoretical and methodological advances in the development of frameworks to guide practice development, including workplace culture (Manley, 2004), person-centredness (Binnie & Titchen, 1999; Dewing, 2004; McCormack, 2004; Nolan et al., 2004), practice context (McCormack et al., 2002), evidence (Rycroft-Malone et al., 2004), evidence implementation (Rycroft-Malone et al., 2004), values (Warfield & Manley, 1990; Manley, 2000a, 2000b; Manley, 2004; Wilson, 2005; Wilson et al., 2005) and approaches to learning for sustainable practice (Dewar, 2002; Titchen, 2003; Titchen & McGinley, 2003; Wilson et al., 2005; Hardy et al., 2006; Wilson et al., 2006).

Practice development was defined as:

A continuous process of improvement towards increased effectiveness in patient centred care. This is brought about by enabling health care teams to develop their knowledge and skills and to transform the culture and context of care. It is enabled and supported by facilitators committed to systematic, rigorous continuous processes of emancipatory change that reflect the perspectives of both service users and service providers. (McCormack et al., 2004, 316)

This definition has been widely used internationally in shaping practice development programmes. The specific focus on the culture and context of care was one of the unique characteristics of practice development compared with other quality improvement methods, but even more significant was the emphasis on 'emancipatory change'. Previously, Binnie & Titchen (1999) and Manley (2001) had illustrated the impact of change processes that had as a central focus the emancipation of individual staff to take control of their own practice and the practice context, and develop knowledge and skill in freeing themselves from perceived and real barriers to effectiveness. Processes such as developing shared values among team members, having a shared vision for ideal practice, developing team relationships, using work-based reflective learning strategies, engaging in critical questioning and adopting a systematic approach to changing everyday practice were developed into facilitation strategies that set out to help individuals become empowered with the knowledge, skills and expertise to develop practice. This approach was also different to action research as the emphasis was not on the answering of particular research questions through the taking of action and its evaluation, but instead the focus was on enabling practitioners to answer their own questions that they had about their practice. Whilst the development of transferable knowledge is the primary purpose of participatory action research, this is a secondary purpose of practice development.

PRACTICE DEVELOPMENT NOW

It is clear that, as practice development methodology has evolved and matured, there is greater consistency among the methods used, set within a shared understanding of methodology (as multiple authors in this book will testify). The work of *The International Practice Development Collaborative (IPDC)* – a collaboration between practice developers in Europe, North America and Australia – has added a significant body of knowledge to the field and enabled greater understanding of methodological perspectives, systematic approaches to evaluation, formal programmes of facilitation development and international collaboration on practice development programmes. The evaluation of these activities and the evidence derived has resulted in the identification of common 'transferable principles' that underpin all practice development activities. These principles were first published in *Practice Development in Nursing: International Perspectives* (Manley et al., 2008a). These principles continue to guide contemporary practice development activities, including much of the work presented in this book:

Principle 1: Practice development aims to achieve person-centred and evidence-based care that is manifested through human flourishing and a workplace culture of effectiveness in all health care settings and situations.

The aim of practice development is to develop effective workplace cultures that have embedded within them person-centred processes, systems and ways of working.

Principle 2: Practice development directs its attention at the micro-systems level – the level at which most health care is experienced and provided, but requires coherent support from interrelated mezzo and macro-systems levels.

Whilst many approaches to developing quality services emphasise organisational approaches to achieving change and development, practice development has as its primary focus, the settings themselves (wards, departments, clinics, etc.) in which health care practice is experienced by service users. It is at this level that service users most closely interact with practitioners, practice teams and patient pathways, and in which their experience of health care systems is directly influenced.

Principle 3: Practice development integrates work-based learning with its focus on active learning and formal systems for enabling learning in the workplace to transform care.

Practice development uses approaches to learning in and from practice as a key strategy for transforming practice. Skilled facilitation and formal systems for enabling learning as well as its assessment, implementation and evaluation in the workplace are instrumental to effective practice development. Engaging in these activities goes some way towards generating learning cultures that sustain developments in practice and individual, team and organisational effectiveness.

Principle 4: Practice development integrates and enables both the development of evidence from practice and the use of evidence in practice.

Practice development is one methodology for the systematic implementation of practice change and innovation as well as providing a person-centred approach.

Principle 5: Practice development integrates creativity with cognition in order to blend mind, heart and soul energies, enabling practitioners to free their thinking and allow opportunities for human flourishing to emerge.

Contemporary practice development has embraced creativity with much enthusiasm and indeed some of the exciting advances in practice development relate to the way creative and cognitive processes are integrated in development strategies. McCormack & Titchen (2006) have led the development of the methodology of 'critical creativity', which blends the creative art forms used in practice development with reflexivity located in the critical paradigm. This is facilitated through the blending and weaving that is evident in skilled facilitation in order to achieve the outcome of human flourishing.

Principle 6: Practice development is a complex methodology that can be used across health care teams and interfaces to involve all internal and external stakeholders.

Whilst the purpose and impetus for practice development is simple, namely improving care for the users of health care in a way that enables all to flourish by working with practitioners and health care teams, its methodology is complex. The complexity stems from working with a number of complementary methodologies and a set of associated methods in a systematic and intentional way. The complexity arises because practice development is not a single intervention but a collection of interventions based on specific philosophical principles drawn from a number of methodologies that inform it, with a particular stance about how people change, develop, learn and transform their practice in a way that is sustainable and continues to be effective.

Principle 7: Practice development uses key methods that are utilised according to the methodological principles being operationalised and the contextual characteristics of the programme of work.

Previous work (McCormack et al., 2006) has identified key methods used in practice development (Box 1.1).

Principle 8: Practice development is associated with a set of processes including skilled facilitation that can be translated into a specific skill set required as near to the interface of care as possible.

Whilst practice development is now associated with the specific set of methods identified in Box 1.1, practitioners and practice teams require help in developing their expertise in the use of these methods in practice (Manley & Webster, 2006). Once this expertise is developed, practitioners and practice teams become self-sufficient in their ongoing use of practice development methods. This is because methods integrate the self-sustaining skills of learning in and from practice or learning as inquiry (Manley et al., 2009), evidence use, evidence development and systematic evaluation of practice change and innovation necessary for a changing health care context.

Box 1.1: Practice development methods

- Agreeing ethical processes
- Analysing stakeholder roles and ways of engaging stakeholders
- Being person-centred
- Clarifying the development focus
- Clarifying values
- Clarifying workplace culture
- Collaborative working relationships
- Continuous reflective learning
- Developing a shared vision
- Developing critical intent
- Developing participatory engagement
- Developing a reward system
- Evaluation
- Facilitating transitions
- Giving space for ideas to flourish
- Good communication strategies
- Implementing processes for sharing and disseminating
- High challenge and high support
- Knowing 'self' and participants

Principle 9: Practice development integrates evaluation approaches that are always inclusive, participative and collaborative.

Being systematic in practice development work differentiates it from ad hoc ways of changing practice and emphasises the need for evaluation. The principles of participation, collaboration and inclusivity always underpin evaluation activity in practice development (McCormack et al., 2006).

WHAT THIS BOOK HAS TO OFFER

If you are interested in developing your knowledge and skills about practice development, then this is the book for you. We see this book as 'foundational', as it addresses the building blocks of effective practice development, that is, key concepts and frameworks that bring those concepts to life, applied theories that can be used to make sense of the experience of practice development and a range of practical experiences shared through case studies, metaphors, images and reflective accounts. In doing this through a diversity of writing styles, the book is relevant to everyone who is interested in practice development – undergraduate students studying evidence-informed practice (for example), registered practitioners who are developing their facilitation skills, people in formal practice development facilitation roles who want to advance their expertise, managers who want to understand the need to support practice development in their service(s) and researchers who are engaged in the co-production of knowledge with all key stakeholders.

This book builds upon the practice development foundations already established and extends and further develops many of the conceptual and theoretical perspectives, methodological approaches, methods, tools and processes of the previous work undertaken in the evolution of practice development. We use the definition of practice development that arose from the work presented in Manley et al. (2008b) (Box 1.2).

Box 1.2: Practice development definition

Practice development is a continuous process of developing person-centred cultures. It is enabled by facilitators who authentically engage with individuals and teams to blend personal qualities and creative imagination with practice skills and practice wisdom. The learning that occurs brings about transformations of individual and team practices. This is sustained by embedding both processes and outcomes in corporate strategy. (Manley et al., 2008b, 9)

Each chapter of this book picks up various dimensions of this definition and brings it to life conceptually, theoretically, creatively, reflexively and practically. In doing this, the book is guided by three frameworks:

1. Practice development conceptual framework.
2. Person-centred practice theoretical framework.
3. A framework for holding on to the whole practice development journey.

Practice development conceptual framework

The conceptual framework of Garbett and McCormack (2002) (Figure 1.1) has been developed and adapted as our knowledge of practice development has evolved and grown. This framework identifies the key components of practice development and provides a visual representation of the key components and their interconnections.

On the outside of the figure are 'shared values and vision', representing the importance of practice development activity being built upon a collective vision for ideal practice and the values underpinning this vision. At the centre is the ideal situation of having a 'person-centred culture'. However, we know that this is something that is always in transition and is rarely achieved as an ideal state. However, having a shared vision for what this could look like begins the process of identifying 'where we are now' in terms of the reality of that vision and the existence of a person-centred culture. So the part of the figure that focuses on 'transforming individuals and contexts of care' addresses the methodologies, methods, processes and tools that can be used to help teams to move closer to the vision of a person-centred culture and respond to issues that need to be changed to do so. The two 'arrows' in the figure represent the key facilitation strategies used – 'authentic engagement' as a facilitator and the adoption of 'facilitated active learning' processes. You will see in this book that the issue of authenticity as a facilitator is critical, and facilitators need to know themselves in order to develop authentic relationships with teams. Authentic engagement also encompasses the importance of using evaluation strategies that are consistent with the values of the practice development programme and the principles of collaboration, inclusion and participation. Active learning embraces different learning styles and the use of the whole

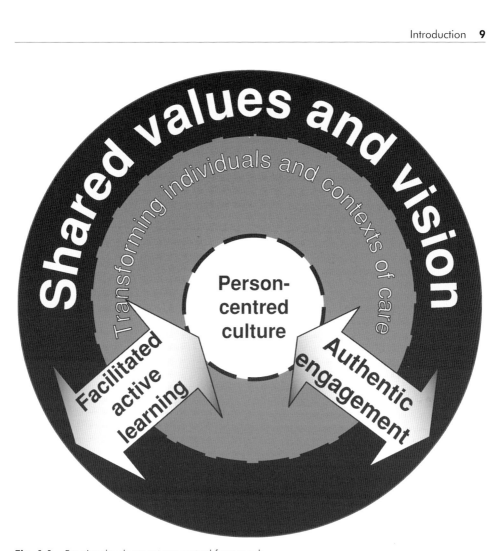

Fig. 1.1   Practice development conceptual framework.

self and not only the mind in learning. Throughout this book, you will see reference to this framework and its use illustrated in a variety of ways.

Person-centred practice theoretical framework

The definition of person-centredness below, adapted from McCormack et al. (2010), identifies the essential characteristics of person-centredness, whilst also highlighting the importance of the development of culture to support person-centredness:

> *Person-centeredness is an approach to practice established through the formation and fostering of healthful relationships between all care providers, older people and others significant to them in their lives. It is underpinned by values of respect for persons, individual right to self-determination, mutual respect and understanding. It is enabled by cultures of empowerment that foster continuous approaches to practice development.*

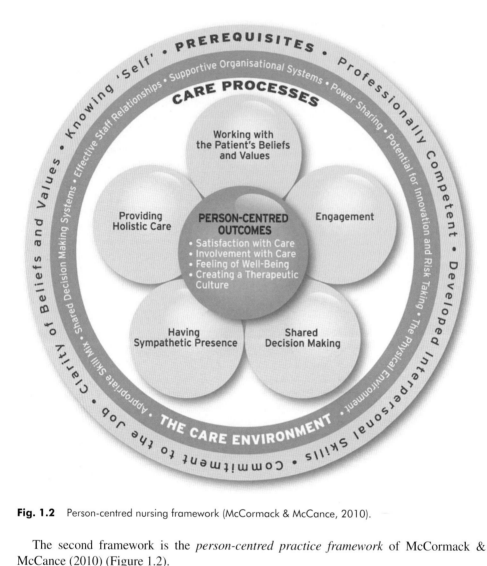

Fig. 1.2   Person-centred nursing framework (McCormack & McCance, 2010).

The second framework is the *person-centred practice framework* of McCormack & McCance (2010) (Figure 1.2).

The person-centred practice framework was first developed in 2006 (McCormack & McCance, 2006) and then further developed in 2010 (McCormack & McCance, 2010). It was derived from previous empirical research focusing on person-centred practice with older people (McCormack, 2001) and the experience of caring in nursing (McCance, 2003). In summary, the framework comprises the following four constructs:

1. **Prerequisites,** which focus on the attributes of the practitioner and include the following: being professionally competent; having developed interpersonal skills; being committed to the job; being able to demonstrate clarity of beliefs and values; knowing self.
2. **Care environment,** which focuses on the context in which care is delivered and includes the following: appropriate skill mix; systems that facilitate shared decision-making; effective staff relationships; organisational systems that are supportive; the sharing of power; the potential for innovation and risk taking; the physical environment.

3. ***Person-centred processes,*** which focus on delivering care through a range of activities and include the following: working with patient's beliefs and values; engagement; having sympathetic presence; sharing decision-making; providing holistic care.
4. ***Outcomes,*** the central component of the framework, are the results of effective person-centred practice and include the following: satisfaction with care (in particular 'experience of good care'); involvement in care; feeling of well-being; creating a therapeutic environment.

The relationship between the constructs suggest that, in order to deliver positive outcomes for both patients and staff, account must be taken of the prerequisites and the care environment, which are necessary for providing effective care through person-centred processes.

A framework for holding on to the whole practice development journey

We know from experience that 'holding' on to the whole practice development journey is a challenging thing to do, and for a novice practice developer, it can seem like an overwhelming task, due to the variety of activities, issues and relationships involved all the way along. Further, as you engage with this book you will come to see that practice development is not a linear approach to change but instead requires cycles of action and reflection with multiple and key stakeholders all of whom have a particular perspective to offer. Thus, some activities get repeated time and time again and sometimes it is necessary to 'go backwards in order to move forwards!' This can feel frustrating at times, but holding on to an overall plan for the journey and accepting that small steps are necessary will help to maintain motivation. This theme is picked up more substantially in Chapter 3.

Figure 1.3 sets out a representation of the practice development journey as a *continuous process* and we offer it as a metaphorical representation of practice development and a support mechanism for aiding reflection on progress. It also helps to reinforce the significance of each stage of the journey and the connections between each as a systematic approach is adopted. The key stages of the practice development journey are:

- Knowing and demonstrating values and beliefs about person-centred care.
- Developing a shared vision for person-centred care.
- Getting started together: measuring and evaluating at each stage.
- Creating a practice development plan.
- Ongoing and integrated action, evaluation, learning and planning.
- Learning in the workplace.
- Sharing and celebrating.

Each chapter of this book works with these frameworks in a variety of ways. We begin in Chapter 2 with a focus on learning. In order to begin the practice development journey and enjoy the unfolding and unfurling of practice development and all its intricacies, it is good to be equipped with key foundational knowledge, skills and processes. In this chapter, Kate Sanders and Jo Odell from the Foundation of Nursing Studies (an organisation dedicated to the advancement of practice development; http://www.fons.org/) work with Jonathan Webster (an experienced health service manager and practice developer) and share their journeys of learning to be a practice developer. They illustrate through their own reflexive experiences

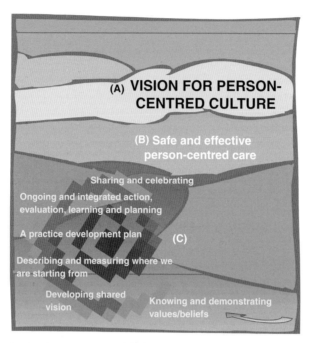

Fig. 1.3 The practice development journey. (A) Ultimate outcome; (B) outcome; (C) elements of a practice development journey; spiral: symbolising multiple starting points (but always keeping the outcomes in mind) and re-iterative movement between the elements of the journey.

each of the practice development stages presented in the book and show how learning to be a practice developer never ends and is indeed a lifelong process.

Having considered the learning needed to be an effective practice developer, we apply this to the fundamental elements of practice development. Chapter 3 explicates the essences of practice development in contemporary health and social care, explaining how practice development can be operationalised in the context of shared governance, safe and effective care and patient pathways. Since Edition 1 of this book, there is no doubt that the health and social care context has changed significantly and health and social care practice exists in highly pressurised environments.

Theresa Shaw picks up this issue in Chapter 4 when she addresses the issue of 'methodology'. In Edition 1 of *Practice Development in Nursing*, we put forward two distinct but complementary methodologies (technical and emancipatory practice development), and this representation of methodology has had a significant impact on shaping practice development programmes. Since then, we have learned a lot more about methodological principles that guide practice development activity, and so, this technical and emancipatory distinction is less helpful. Theresa addresses this issue and shows how different methodological perspectives can be helpfully applied in different contexts and cultures.

The big challenge for many, however, is 'getting a feel' for practice development, and our experience in our development programmes is that many novice (and indeed some experienced!) practice developers struggle to understand the practice development journey and what a complete journey might look like. The 'framework for holding on to the whole practice development journey' offered in this book should help to some extent with this issue, and Chapter 5 has been deliberately positioned early in the book so as to show a complete journey over a 3-year period. Whilst the case study presented is a large national programme of work, the essential practice development ingredients are all there and can be extrapolated to any project, no matter how big or how small.

The case study set out in Chapter 5 requires consistent and effective facilitation at a variety of levels, due to its complexity as a programme of work. However, it is now widely accepted that facilitation is key to all practice development. In Chapter 6, Angie Titchen, Jan Dewing and Kim Manley take the reader through a journey of understanding particular tools that are used in practice development work. Remember that in the conceptual framework for practice development, 'active learning' and 'authentic engagement' are key strategies. Having a repertoire of tools and processes to enable effective action and reflection on action is important. Whilst the tools and processes are not the 'be all' in themselves as they need to be used intentionally within the particular methodological perspective adopted, they provide a useful resource to enhance our real 'self' as facilitators. You will probably notice that this chapter is written in a different style – that of a 'novelette'. This style of writing enables the reader to enter the experience of the facilitators in the chapter and to go on the journey with them.

Chapter 7 revisits one of the frameworks presented in Edition 1 of *Practice Development in Nursing* and gives it a modern twist! The *promoting action on research implementation in health services* (PARIHS) framework has influenced practice development work internationally and is one of the most often cited frameworks in use in knowledge utilisation, knowledge translation and research implementation activities. Jo Rycroft-Malone is a leading player in these knowledge fields and has also been instrumental in the development of the PARIHS framework. In this chapter, she provides an overview of the PARIHS framework and how it is being used currently. In practice development, working with different forms of evidence, in different contexts, requires different and adaptable facilitation approaches, and this is a key focus of this chapter.

In Chapter 8, Kim Manley and Carrie Jackson, members and leaders of the 'England Centre for Practice Development' (http://www.canterbury.ac.uk/health/EnglandCentreforPracticeDevelopment/Home.aspx) join with Annette Solman (an experienced Director of Nursing) to explore the issue of culture. They draw on the original conceptual framework of an effective workplace culture by Manley et al. (2011) and unpack it in the context of what an effective culture looks like, feels like and is experienced, and how it is facilitated. An effective workplace culture is also a person-centred culture – one that values the humanity of all and as such is a key consideration in practice development work.

A key issue in exploring workplace culture is being clear about how to evaluate developments in the effectiveness of the culture of person-centredness – the main focus of Chapters 9 and 10. In Chapter 9, Sally Hardy, Val Wilson and Tanya McCance explore how evaluation methodologies can be integrated into practice development programmes and show the importance of considering evaluation methods at each stage of the practice development journey. Chapter 10 continues the evaluation theme, but this time with a particular focus on evaluating outcomes associated with person-centred practice. 'The conceptual framework for practice development' has as its central focus, the development of person-centred cultures. However, as yet there are few frameworks available for evaluating person-centred outcomes. The framework offered by the authors not only builds on the previous work of Brendan McCormack and Tanya McCance but also includes the innovative work of Jill Maben and colleagues who have a focus on nurses' work-life and how practice cultures sustain and nurture excellence in practice. This is one of the first times that these perspectives have been combined, and we believe that it offers a unique opportunity to combine different development approaches with a focus on person-centred cultures.

Practice developers pay particular attention to 'process', and the saying 'trust the process' is often the key mantra of practice development facilitators – particularly when they are being challenged about not focusing on outcomes enough! Chapter 11 is process orientated, but with a particular focus on challenging how we engage in facilitation work, that is, the challenge of being creative in our facilitation practice in order to create space for alternative and novel experiences and solutions. When practice developers think about being creative in their work, it is likely that they will source the work of Angie Titchen as one of the key informants and creative thinkers in the field. Angie has worked for over 20 years with creative and artistic approaches that ease people (or sometimes even push them!!) out of usual ways of thinking and being. In Chapter 11, Angie works with Ann McMahon (an experienced practice developer and researcher) to show how creative processes can be brought to facilitation processes. The idea of the 'radical gardener' is an inspirational idea that is lived through the chapter, and so the reader can get a real feel for not only creativity itself but also its enactment as part of a practice development process. However, all good gardeners need to take stock of what they have done and need to stand back and admire or critique their work and what has been achieved. Most gardeners will tell you that this should happen as we go along rather than waiting until the end and deciding that the design was all wrong!

Chapters 12 and 13 place practice development in the different contexts in which it operates. Whilst practice development focuses on the 'micro' level in organisations (i.e. the clinical setting or the place where practitioners work and patients receive care), it cannot ignore the organisational, strategic and policy context. Contemporary health and social care practice is a political activity and it would be naïve to assume that these can be ignored in practice development activities. So in Chapter 12, Jan Dewing, Jill Down and IrenaAnna Frei consider the organisational context and approaches we can use to locate practice development within an organisational context. Of particular interest is the way strategic development is seen as a dynamic, creative process of weaving connections that enable shared meanings between people and working with complexity and chaos. In Chapter 13, Randal Parlour and Joan Yalden (both experienced practice developers) worked with Kim Manley to synthesise their different approaches to practice development in different contexts (teams and organisations). They show how the outcomes arising can be blended into a single unified approach that extrapolates the methodological essences of their studies into a single set of evaluation 'triggers' that transcend particular settings/contexts, and strategies that can be transferred to achieve specific outcomes. Their work was informed by 'action hypotheses' – a particular approach used in action research and their use here shows how these kinds of 'tools' can enable the development of an outcomes and impact framework from multiple case studies that blends individual, team and organisational perspectives.

In the final chapter, we (hopefully) provide some informed commentary on the overall book. We use a framework derived from our work in 'Critical Creativity' (Titchen & McCormack, 2010) to frame our commentary and provide some reflection on where we are now as practice developers and a potential direction of travel.

We hope that this book provides you with support, insight and, more than anything else, inspiration to engage with practice development processes and work towards creating cultures that are genuinely person-centred and respectful of individual humanity. We have provided a text that is rich with resources, tools, processes, reflections, insights and personal sharing. However, no matter what tool or process you draw upon, never forget that it is the passion and determination that *you* have for effective and person-centred health and social care practice that will be your key resource. For as John O'Donohue reminds us:

> *All the possibilities of your human destiny are asleep in your soul. You are here to realize and honour these possibilities . . . Possibility is the secret heart of time . . . In its deepest heart, time is transfiguration. Time minds possibility and makes sure that nothing is lost or forgotten . . . Possibility is the secret heart of creativity . . . (O'Donohue, 1998, pp. 30–31)*

REFERENCES

Bechtel, C. & Ness, D. (2010) If you build it, will they come? Designing truly patient-centered health care. *Health Affairs*, **29**, 914–920.

Beer, M. (1980) *Organization Change and Development*. Goodyear Publishing Company, Santa Monica, CA.

Binnie, A. & Titchen, A. (1999) *Freedom to Practise: The Development of Patient-Centred Nursing*. Butterworth Heinemann, Oxford.

Braithwaite, J. (2010) Restructuring is not the answer: healthcare reform. 23 October. The Australian.

Braithwaite, J., Westbrook, M.T., Hindle, D., Iedema, R.A. & Black, D.A. (2006) Does restructuring hospitals result in greater efficiency? An empirical test using diachronic data. *Health Services Management Research*, **19**, 1–12.

Dewar, B. (2002) Evaluation of work-based learning in a community nursing health degree programme: the students' perspective on the impact of practice. *New Capability*, **5** (1), 10–15.

Dewing, J. (2004) Concerns relating to the application of frameworks to promote person-centredness in nursing with older people. *International Journal of Older People Nursing*, **13** (3a), 39–44.

Feinmann, J. (2011) Safer healthcare depends on in-depth investigation, not quick fixes, says expert. http://www.bmj.com/content/342/bmj.d2685 (Accessed 8 October 2012).

Garbett, R. & McCormack, B. (2002) A concept analysis of practice development. *NT Research*, **7** (2), 87–100.

Hardy, S., Titchen, A., Manley, K. & McCormack, B. (2006) Re-defining nursing expertise in the United Kingdom. *Nursing Science Quarterly*, **19** (3), 260–264.

Kitson, A., Ahmed, L.B., Harvey, G., Seers, K. & Thompson, D.R. (1996) From research to practice: one organizational model for promoting research-based practice. *Journal of Advanced Nursing*, **23** (3), 430–440.

Maben, J., Peccei, R., Adams, M., Robert, G., Richardson, A. & Murrells, T. (2012) Patients' experiences of care and the influence of staff motivation, affect and wellbeing. Final report, NIHR Service Delivery and Organisation programme, Southampton.

Manley, K. (2000a) Organisational culture and consultant nurse outcomes: Part 1. Organisational culture. *Nursing Standard*, **14**, 34–38.

Manley, K. (2000b) Organisational culture and consultant nurse outcomes: Part 2. Consultant nurse outcomes. *Nursing Standard*, **14**, 34–39.

Manley, K. (2001) Consultant nurse: concept, processes, outcome. Unpublished PhD thesis, RCN Institute/ Manchester University.

Manley, K. (2004) Transformational culture: a culture of effectiveness. In: *Practice Development in Nursing* (eds B. McCormack, K. Manley & R. Garbett), pp. 51–82. Blackwell Publishing Ltd., Oxford.

Manley, K. & Webster, J. (2006) Can we keep quality alive? *Nursing Standard*, **21** (3), 12–15.

Manley, K., McCormack, B. & Wilson, V. (eds.) (2008a) *Practice Development in Nursing: International Perspectives*. Blackwell Publishing Ltd., Oxford.

Manley, K., McCormack, B. & Wilson, V. (2008b) Introduction. In: *Practice Development in Nursing: International Perspectives*, (eds K. Manley, B. McCormack & V. Wilson), pp. 1–16. Blackwell Publishing Ltd., Oxford.

Manley, K., Sanders, K., Cardiff, S. & Webster, J. (2011) Effective workplace culture: the attributes, enabling factors and consequences of a new concept. *International Practice Development Journal*, **1** (2), Article 1. http://www.fons.org/library/journal/volume1-issue2/article1 (Accessed 5 October 2012).

Manley, K., Titchen, A. & Hardy, S. (2009) Work based learning in the context of contemporary health-care education and practice: a concept analysis. *Practice Development in Healthcare*, **8** (2), 87–127.

McCance, T., Gribben, B., Mitchell, E. & McCormack, B. (2012) *Improving the Patient Experience by Exploring Person-centred Care*. The Belfast Health and Social Care Trust (BHSCT) Person-centred Care Programme. Final report, BHSCT, Belfast.

McCance, T.V. (2003) Caring in nursing practice: the development of a conceptual framework. *Research and Theory for Nursing Practice: An International Journal*, **17** (2), 101–116.

McCormack, B. (2001) *Negotiating Partnerships with Older People – A Person-Centred Approach*. Ashgate, Basingstoke.

McCormack, B. (2004). Person-centredness in gerontological nursing: an overview of the literature. *Journal of Clinical Nursing*, **13** (3A), 31–38.

McCormack, B., Dewar, B., Wright, J., Garbett, R., Harvey, G. & Ballantine, K. (2006) *A realist synthesis of evidence relating to practice development*. Final report to NHS Education for Scotland and NHS Quality Improvement Scotland. http://www.healthcareimprovementscotland.org/previous_resources/policy_and_strategy/a_realist_synthesis_of_evidenc.aspx (Accessed May 2012).

McCormack, B., Dewing, J., Breslin, L., Tobin, C., Manning, M., Coyne-Nevin, A., Kennedy, K. & Peelo-Kilroe, L. (2010) *The Implementation of a Model of Person-Centred Practice in Older Person Settings*. Final report, Office of the Nursing Services Director, Health Services Executive, Dublin.

McCormack, B., Garbett, R. & Manley, K. (2004) A clearer vision of practice development. In: *Practice Development in Nursing* (eds B. McCormack, K. Manley & R. Garbett), pp. 315–329. Blackwell Publishing Ltd., Oxford.

McCormack, B., Kitson, A., Harvey, G., Rycroft-Malone, J., Titchen, A. & Seers, K. (2002) Getting evidence into practice: the meaning of 'context'. *Journal of Advanced Nursing*, **38** (1), 94–104.

McCormack, B. & McCance, T. (2006) Development of a framework for person-centred nursing. *Journal of Advanced Nursing*, **56** (5), 1–8.

McCormack, B. & McCance, T. (2010) *Person-centred Nursing: Theory, Models and Methods*. Blackwell Publishing Ltd., Oxford.

McCormack, B. & Titchen, A. (2006) Critical creativity: melding, exploding, blending. *Educational Action Research*, **14** (2), 239–266.

McKenna, H. (1995) Skill mix substitutions and quality of care: an exploration of assumptions from research. *Journal of Advanced Nursing*, **21** (3), 452–459.

Mullally, S. (2001) *The NHS Plan – An Action Guide for Nurses, Midwives and Health Visitors*. Department of Health, London.

NHSE (1996) *Promoting Clinical Effectiveness: A Framework for Action*. NHS Executive, Leeds.

Nolan, M., Davies, S., Brown, J., Keady, J. & Nolan, J. (2004) Beyond 'person-centred' care: a new vision for gerontological nursing. *International Journal of Older People Nursing* (*in association with the Journal of Clinical Nursing*), **13** (3a), 45–53.

O'Donohue, J. (1998) *Anam Cara: Spiritual Wisdom from the Celtic world*. Bantam Press, London.

Ottaway, R.N. (1976) A change strategy to implement new norms, new style and new environment in the work organization. *Personnel Review*, **5** (1), 13–18.

Plsek, P.E. (2001) Redesigning health care with insights from the science of complex adaptive systems. In: *Crossing the Chasm: A New Health System for the 21st Century*, pp. 309–322. National Academy Press, Washington.

Rolfe, G. (1996) *Closing the Theory-Practice Gap: A New Paradigm for Nursing*. Butterworth-Heinemann, London.

Rycroft-Malone, J., Seers, K., Titchen, A., Harvey, G., Kitson, A. & McCormack, B. (2004) What counts as evidence in evidence-based practice. *Journal of Advanced Nursing*, **47** (1), 81–90.

Schein, E.H. (2004) *Organizational Culture and Leadership*, 3rd edn. John Wiley & Sons, San Franscisco, CA.

Titchen, A. (2003) Critical companionship: part 1. *Nursing Standard*, **18** (9), 33–40.

Titchen, A. & McCormack, B. (2010) Dancing with stones: critical creativity as methodology for human flourishing. *Educational Action Research: An International Journal*, **18** (4), 531–554.

Titchen, A. & McGinley, M. (2003) Facilitating practitioner-research through critical companionship. *NTResearch*, **8** (2), 115–131.

Warfield, C. & Manley, K. (1990) Developing a new philosophy in the NDU. *Nursing Standard*, **4** (41), 27–30.

Westbrook, J.I., Braithwaite, J., Georgiou, A., Ampt, A., Creswick, N., Coiera, E. & Iedema, R. (2007) Multi-method evaluation of information and communication technologies in health in the context of wicked problems and socio-technical theory. *Journal of the American Medical Informatics Association*, **14**, 746–755.

Wilson, V. (2005) Developing a vision for teamwork. *Practice Development in Healthcare*, **4** (1), 40–48.

Wilson, V., McCormack, B. & Ives, G. (2005) Understanding the workplace culture of a special care nursery. *Journal of Advanced Nursing*, **50** (1), 27–38.

Wilson, V, McCormack, B. & Ives, G. (2006) Replacing the 'self' in learning. *Learning in Health and Social Care*, **5** (2), 90–105.

2 Learning to be a Practice Developer

Kate Sanders[1], Jo Odell[1] and Jonathan Webster[2]

[1] Foundation of Nursing Studies, London, UK
[2] NHS North West London – Inner CCG Collaboration, London, UK

INTRODUCTION

I (Kate) was invited to write this chapter following on from a chapter that I wrote about my first insights into being a practice developer (Sanders, 2004). To help me unearth and share how I have continued to learn to be a practice developer, I have invited two colleagues, Jo and Jonathan, to co-write the chapter with me. By reflecting on and capturing our own individual experiences, and then sharing them to stimulate critical dialogue with each other, we have been able to identify influences and enablers that have and continue to shape the way in which we work as practice developers.

Over the last 10 years, I have been working for the Foundation of Nursing Studies (FoNS) primarily as an external facilitator of practice development, helping individuals and teams to develop new ways of working, thereby enabling them to provide care that is high quality, evidence based and is centred on the needs of patients. Prior to this, I worked clinically in a variety of acute and community settings, most latterly as a health visitor. Jo has recently joined the team at FoNS, but prior to this, over the last decade she has worked in clinical practice in a variety of roles that have enabled her to work as an internal facilitator of practice development. These roles have included A&E (Accident & Emergency) sister, clinical supervision lead, project lead for older people and most recently a facilitator of the NHS Institute for Innovation and Improvement Productive Series. Jonathan has always been clinically based, and whilst he has never had a 'formal' practice development role, the desire to place the patient and person at the centre of care has been a key influence to the way in which he has worked as an individual, a clinical leader and now in an NHS commissioning role. Jonathan and I have worked together on a number of occasions, as internal/external facilitators to enhance dignity in care in acute health care settings and as facilitators at international practice development schools.

The chapter starts by outlining our shared understanding of practice development and describing what we believe a practice developer is and the skills that they require. We then share individual narratives that capture the different paths/journeys that we have taken to become practice developers. Through these narratives we aim to:

- share our learning and development as practice developers;

Practice Development in Nursing and Healthcare, Second Edition. Edited by Brendan McCormack, Kim Manley and Angie Titchen.
© 2013 John Wiley & Sons, Ltd. Published 2013 by John Wiley & Sons, Ltd.

- identify key themes about the 'what' and 'how' of our ongoing path/journey of development; and
- translate our learning, making it 'real' to contemporary practice.

A discussion of the key themes arising from the narratives follows, before introducing and reflecting upon a framework for understanding and supporting the development of expertise relating to facilitating practice development. We conclude with some suggestions for enabling development.

WHAT IS PRACTICE DEVELOPMENT? OUR UNDERSTANDING

Practice development has become a widely used phrase to describe activities that health care professionals use to develop practice and improve patient care (Titchen & Higgs, 2001; Garbett & McCormack, 2002; McCormack & Garbett, 2003; Manley & McCormack, 2004; McCormack et al., 2006). It includes both nursing (Manley, 1997; McCormack et al., 1999) and the broader multi-professional team (Walsh, 2000) across the range of health services and health care settings (Dewing, 2008). Unsworth (2000) suggests that whilst the term has been widely used, the concept historically has remained nebulous and poorly articulated, in which there has been a greater concentration on describing the process rather than investigating the conceptual frameworks that support practice development. This is demonstrated by the term being used interchangeably with others such as 'research into practice' (Mallett et al., 1997) and also to describe a broad range of educational (McKenna, 1995), continual professional development (Aggergaard et al., 2005; Walsgrove & Fulbrook, 2005), research (Rolfe, 1996) and audit (NHSE, 1996) activity. Recent years, however, have seen an increased understanding about the key underlying principles and methodological perspectives (McCormack et al., 2004; Manley et al., 2008), further strengthened by growing international collaboration.

Practice development has on occasions been presented as a 'linear' or 'task/project-based' process, sometimes known as technical practice development (Dewing, 2008). Whilst this approach may be effective in achieving the development of a new assessment process, for example, it may not achieve sustainable implementation of the assessment as there is increasing recognition that achieving sustainable change in the culture of care is much more 'complex' and 'multifaceted' (Dewing & Wright, 2003). This complexity is articulated in 'emancipatory' practice development (Manley & McCormack, 2004) that uses the concepts of critical social theory and emphasises the development of individual practitioners and the cultures and contexts within which they work to achieve sustainable changes in practice. According to Garbett and McCormack (2002), practice development is easier to understand and characterise in terms of its purpose, attributes and consequences. Page and Hamer (2002) identify a number of key characteristics of practice development:

- Patient focus
- Actively engaging practitioners
- Interprofessional activity
- Evolutionary
- Transferable rather than generalisable

What becomes clear from these characteristics is that whilst practice development is diverse by definition, it is however clearly focused on its anticipated outcome, which is to improve patient care through emancipatory approaches to transform individuals, the context of care and the culture in which practitioners work (Garbett & McCormack, 2002). These approaches usually require facilitation, to enable health care practitioners to develop an awareness of the reality of practice, to identify differences between what practitioners believe is happening and what is observed and experienced and to stimulate the desire to change. The facilitator creates the conditions for reflection, critique, collaboration, high challenge and high support and active learning (Dewing, 2008); and recent literature is encouraging the use of creative and imaginative approaches to enable meaningful engagement, transformation and human flourishing, informed by a new methodology, transformational practice development (Titchen & McCormack, 2010).

Manley and McCormack (2004), argue that if practice developers are to be effective, there is a need for them to be aware of and understand the worldview that they are working from, as this will underpin the methods and processes that they use and impact on the outcomes for practice and the people they are working with. For this reason, when writing this chapter about how we have learnt to become practice developers, we thought that it was important to articulate the worldview that we are working from, as we believe that this has and will continue to influence our ways of learning.

We believe that we are all working from an emancipatory worldview, and as such, we embrace the definition of practice development as articulated in Chapter 1 (Box 1.2). That we share this worldview has not just been taken for granted. For example although we (Kate and Jo) have only recently started working together as part of the same team at FoNS, individually we are conscious of working from an emancipatory worldview. We are also aware that FoNS uses emancipatory practice development to underpin its ways of working. Working with the same worldview has contributed to Kate working for the organisation for more than 10 years, and was also a reason for Jo recently joining the organisation. However, that we (FoNS, Kate and Jo) share the same worldview is not just assumed; FoNS' values form an essential part of its strategy as an organisation and are spoken about, regularly reviewed and used to shape the work that we do. Similarly, exploring values and beliefs about practice development formed an important part of the interview process when Jo joined the organisation, and the ways in which we work individually and as a team are shared and discussed on a regular basis, both formally and informally.

WHAT IS A PRACTICE DEVELOPER?

As well as identifying the worldview of practice development that we are working from, we felt that it was also important to share our understanding of what a practice developer 'is'.

McCormack et al. (1999) identify that with the greater 'acceptance' of person-centred nursing, practice development has been able to focus on clinical effectiveness, patient outcomes and evidence-based practice. They assert that with this 'drive', a plethora of roles concerned with practice development have emerged, but with little sense of an overall person-centred purpose or strategic context. There is, however, a dearth of literature about the roles of those involved in practice development. In the early 2000s, Garbett and McCormack (2002) undertook a concept analysis of practice development, and from this data (literature review, focus group discussions and telephone interviews), it was possible for them to explore the characteristics, qualities and skills of practice developers. In this work,

McCormack and Garbett (2003, p. 317) identified 'practice developers' as 'professionals who have formal responsibility for developing practice in organisations'. Whilst six role functions were identified in the literature, the practice developers involved in the focus groups talked primarily about two of these functions: promoting and facilitating change; and translation and communication. A number of attributes required by practice developers were also identified (see Box 2.1).

Box 2.1: Attributes required by a practice developer

- Values and beliefs, commitment to improving patient care, enabling not telling
- Facilitative skills
- Energy and tenacity
- Flexibility, sensitivity and reflexivity
- Knowledge
- Creativity
- Political awareness 'being in the middle'
- Credibility

Adapted from McCormack and Garbett (2003, p. 324)

However, despite this clarification of role and attributes, McCormack and Garbett acknowledge the complexity of the activities that practice developers were involved in, also suggesting an overlap between these activities and those of clinical leaders. Likewise, they argue that the attributes identified were similar to those required by senior clinicians or managers.

Since the publication of this work, there have been many changes within health care in the United Kingdom, particularly within the NHS. The mid-2000s saw the loss of many formal practice development roles within Trusts as a result of 'cutbacks' (Manley & Webster, 2006), but in recent years, there has been an emergence of new roles; for example practice educators whose aim is to enhance learning in practice and Productive Series facilitators whose aims are to deliver defined practice or service improvement 'projects' within specific timescales that have been characterised by fixed- or short-term contracts of employment. Such roles tend to have a narrow focus rather than the development of individuals and teams to achieve sustainable, long-term cultural change.

A realist synthesis of practice development by McCormack et al. (2006) identified that role ambiguity still existed for 'practice developers' and that there was still a lack of understanding about the expertise that was needed to facilitate practice development. Instead of focusing on practice development roles, they advocate for the development of 'transferable principles' based on 18 practice development methods that would enable the facilitation of practice development within and across organisations (see Chapter 1, Section 'Practice Development Now', 'Principle 7').

The move away from a view that there is a need for specific practice developer roles to one that embraces the notion that any health care practitioner could be a facilitator of practice development fits with our view of our role within the emancipatory practice development worldview, and our experience of supporting a wide variety of practitioners and practice developments in the workplace. However, within this worldview, we acknowledge that the facilitation of practice development is complex and multifaceted (Manley, 2004; Simmons,

2004). It requires facilitators with the skills to enable health care teams to transform the cultures and contexts of care (McCormack et al., 2010), using reflection to help practitioners to understand what needs to change (i.e. the difference between what people say is done and what happens in reality) and identify actions to achieve practice change. The skills required are summarised by Manley (2001) and include:

- working with values, beliefs and assumptions;
- challenging contradictions;
- developing critical intent of individuals and groups;
- developing moral intent;
- focusing on the impact of the context/system on practice as well as practice itself;
- using self-reflection and fostering reflection in others;
- enabling others to 'see the possibilities';
- fostering widening participation and collaboration by all involved.

Van der Zijpp and Dewing (2009, p. 203) argue that to be effective at enabling others requires commitment to 'continuous transitions of growth and development'. Similarly, Manley and Titchen (2012) suggest that practitioners need help to explore their own effectiveness and become skilled facilitators before they can assist others to become more effective in their work. With this in mind, we will now focus on how we have and continue to learn to be practice developers or facilitators of practice development.

UNDERSTANDING HOW WE ARE LEARNING TO BE PRACTICE DEVELOPERS: CREATING NARRATIVES

We have used the process of writing narratives or stories to enable us to make sense of how we are learning to become practice developers. We started this process individually, using a variety of creative approaches to help us to explore our learning. This included using the body, creative imagination and expression through picture cards, reflective walks, writing poetry and prose, and led to each of us beginning to tell our individual stories. In addition to using these approaches, we also engaged in reflection and critical dialogue; firstly with ourselves, but as we continued to write, then also with each other; to share and challenge ideas, thereby enabling us to deepen understanding of our experience and discover meaning (Horsfall & Titchen, 2007; Holloway & Wheeler, 2010).

Bolton (2006) argues that an effective mode of reflective practice and reflexivity can be achieved through professional narrative and story exploration. She continues that all professional and personal experience is naturally storied and that telling or writing stories are human ways of understanding, communicating and remembering. Narratives about vital or key areas of professional experience can be communicated and explored directly and simply through expressive writing, allowing the taken for granted everyday day practice to become something that can be 'pulled and pushed' to see what happens (Bolton, 2006). Boje (2001) makes a distinction between storytelling and narrative, noting that traditionally narrative has been viewed as an elite method that stands above storytelling. Whilst he acknowledges the 'organising' process of narrative, which adds 'plot' and 'coherence', he also advocates the concept of ante-narrative. An ante-narrative is essentially a story, but what Boje is saying, is that in the telling of the story, the storyteller necessarily organises his/her story in a way, which for them makes sense (Fulbrook, 2003). This pre-narrative stage is part of the process of narrative, but at this point it is told as an account of incidents or events without proper plot sequence or coherence. Once the ante-narrative has been organised into a beginning, middle and an end, giving it coherence, it becomes a narrative (Boje, 2001). In the process of deconstruction/reconstruction, the writer moves from ante-narrative to narrative. This act of engagement and refinement, through reflection on events, is referred to as active inquiry (Vezeau, 1994). It is a retrospective 'sense making' activity in which many meanings may be synthesised (Weick, 1995).

NARRATIVE 1: JO

The picture – a journey

When I look back now over my career and journey to date, I guess the first thing to say is that in the early days I didn't realise I was a practice developer, I instinctively knew I had a passion to develop and change, both personally and in my clinical practice, and to challenge and not to accept the 'status quo'. My journey started by taking a degree in nursing from the Southbank University; at the time this was one of the first degree nursing courses, and I can remember being something of an oddity to my fellow Registered General Nursing students. I believe that this approach to learning gave me a well-grounded education and more importantly, the opportunity and encouragement to constantly question 'why'.

I have continued to develop this questioning approach by seeking varied clinical roles and learning opportunities within them. These opportunities have been many and varied, some I have sought out and some have apparently sought me out. For example I have actively sought out different roles to enable me to work in a variety of clinical areas and settings including surgical, orthopaedics, care of older people, community hospitals and accident and emergency. This has enabled me not only to learn a wide variety of clinical assessment skills, but has also enabled me to gain different perspectives on cultures and contexts that impact on clinical care.

Traditional influences, such as 'taught' post-registration clinical courses, where my experience has been as the passive recipient of information, relayed by the teacher, have also contributed to my personal learning over time. But also along the way I have had the opportunity to get involved in local practice development and quality initiatives, where external facilitators have enabled me to learn from my practice and from within myself, by using a range of enabling strategies such as critical companionship (a helping relationship in which an experienced facilitator accompanies another on an experiential learning journey) (Titchen, 2004; Odell et al., 2006; Brown & Harrison, 2009), critical dialogue and structured reflection using reflective models such as Gibbs (1988) and Johns (1997). These approaches to learning have aided my development in greater ways than any traditional course, as this learning has been personal and relevant and I have been able to transfer my learning directly into my everyday practice. An example of this was when an external facilitator enabled me to develop a personal awareness of the level of challenge and support I was offering to nurses in an action learning group I was facilitating. The facilitator sat in on the group as an observer and then fed back to me during a period of one-to-one critical dialogue, that my questions were very challenging. This enabled an awareness of the high challenge/high support model and because of this I was able to develop strategies to enable me to balance my approach and put this into action when next facilitating the group.

To achieve greater learning for myself, I have learnt that I need to create space and time for reflection and critical dialogue for myself to consider and develop understanding of the effect that these initiatives may have had in practice and whether they worked or not. I recognised early on that I reflect better when I am in critical dialogue with another person or a group of people; I don't do well on my own as I tend to go into 'a downward spiral' and am much less objective. Therefore, whatever role I have taken, I have negotiated a regular and structured reflective space for myself with another person that I knew and trusted. To recognise a trusted person, I have looked for people who work in similar ways to myself and value reflection as a way of learning. This was often on a one-to-one basis, structured by the use of ground rules and a reflective model, where I was able to talk about an issue I was facing in practice with the facilitator, who would offer me 'challenge and support' in the form of the questions they used, to enable me to make sense of my situation and as such, find a way forward or a solution to whatever practice issue I was facing at the time.

In recognition of the benefit of this way of learning for myself, I sought out a master's in practice development, from the University of Bournemouth. This master's degree is quite unusual in academic circles as there are no lectures and the modules are based on reflective critical dialogue narrative and are focused around one's own practice situation at the time. So, for example for my dissertation, I was able to use the older person's project I was working on at the time, rather than create another project to satisfy the academic requirements. I really loved writing my dissertation as this approach to learning offered me the reflective space to understand what I was doing using frameworks and theories to enable me to use the principles of emancipatory practice development (Manley et al., 2008), by developing understanding as opposed to copying others, which I would have previously done.

The biggest influences for me have come from the opportunities that 'apparently have landed at my feet'. With hindsight, I now appreciate that others had seen the potential in me or as one person described me as a 'mover and shaker', and that I was seen as someone who would come through with the 'goods on top of the day job'; but equally, I recognise now that I embraced these opportunities as something exciting and new. So, as I have progressed in my career, I have learnt to be very open to new opportunities and grab these with both hands, wherever they may take you.

One such opportunity was to take part in a development programme run by the Royal College of Nursing (RCN). My service manager at that time, signed our teams up to take part in this programme with myself as an internal facilitator along with three other colleagues. I had no idea what would be involved or even what an internal facilitator was at the time! However, I trusted and respected my manager as she had demonstrated to me, over our time of working together, great skills in being able to see the potential in people and situations. I saw her as something of a visionary. The following 1-year journey involved me taking part in development workshops, where we were exposed to creative ways of learning, inspirational people and reflective learning in groups. In turn, I had the opportunity to develop and refine my skills as a facilitator by facilitating action learning sets for clinical staff, supported by an external facilitator who exposed me to practice development models, tools and techniques. This culminated in me co-presenting at a conference with the external facilitator from the RCN and publishing a small reflective article (Odell, 2004). Wow what a year!

When I went on to lead my own projects within subsequent roles, I always used some methods and approaches that had particularly impacted on me, which I now had the confidence to experiment with and recreate in my own practice. One such area was using patient narrative to understand experiences and needs of care. I was asked as a requirement of the RCN programme to ask one patient to tell me about their life, their hopes and fears for the future.

Despite my initial reaction, which was 'I can't ask that', I was encouraged by the external facilitator to persevere and 'give it a go'. What I discovered by asking those questions was that my perspective of the patient I was caring for changed from the dimension of seeing a patient who was poorly in bed, to seeing a person who had a life, with family and relationships, who on top of that also happened to be unwell. The person I was caring for emerged through the narrative. Knowing the person meant I was able to care for them more effectively as I now knew what was important to them. As a result of having my own perspective changed so much, I have had the confidence to introduce this at every opportunity – either with students I was mentoring or when working with clinical teams on a large practice development project.

The picture – light at the end of the tunnel

When reflecting back on my journey, it hasn't always gone in ways I thought was ideal, but this has provided valuable insights and learning, particularly about the values and beliefs I hold as a practice developer.

In a previous role, I was expected to deliver 'traditional' training on a regular basis, on a subject I knew inside out and backwards, and yet each time I was reduced to a nervous wreck. Prior to this, as someone who had presented at many national and international conferences, I thought of myself as a confident person, so what was wrong? After seeking out a reflective space with a colleague, it occurred to me that I didn't really believe that attending a training lecture to purely increase knowledge in an area facilitates changes in practice or behaviour. I recognised that the physical reaction I was experiencing was a result of working against one of my core beliefs.

In another role, I was managing a project as an external facilitator. The ethos of the project was to work with clinical teams to facilitate a change of ward processes where the team identified duplication of effort; however, I felt that the project didn't take account of the importance of the culture and context of care, only of the processes of care. Because of my worldview of emancipatory practice development, when I was working with the teams, I used various practice development tools, such as the values clarification exercise (Manley, 1997), and encouraged them to reflect on how the culture and context of care would help or hinder any changes they wanted to implement. However, my experience was that at a corporate level, there was no recognition of the value of facilitation roles or working with staff to develop their practice; instead, a technical practice development approach was emphasised. My learning from this experience is the recognition of the values that drive the organisation and the culture at different levels of the organisation and the ways that one can work to influence these.

The picture – mother and baby – nurturing others

When I think back to all the people who have inspired or encouraged me to try something new or to follow in their footsteps, I wonder what it is about those people that have really inspired me to action. They are small in number but great in passion. I think it was their way of being, their value set that was lived through their actions, that they demonstrated that they really cared about nursing and person-centred practice and that they really cared about me (graceful care). In reverse, along the way, I hope that I have touched or inspired people in a similar fashion and in summary I have learnt from working with these inspirational people that through developing an awareness of my own values and beliefs, caring for self and others and being true to one's self is very important.

In knowing self, I have also learnt that this requires an awareness of my own strengths and weaknesses. During a 3-day leadership development programme, I was keen and open to take part in role-play with actors, as I was comfortable with creative ways of learning. However, after a day when all went well, I was in a situation where I felt extremely unsafe surrounded by a group of people who I felt hadn't demonstrated a value set similar to mine. I went to pieces and felt totally unable to perform the role-play I was being asked to do by the facilitators. Through reflection I recognised the importance of feeling safe within a group. This experience therefore highlighted for me the importance of working with shared values and how important the role of the facilitator is in enabling this to happen.

Conclusion

In writing my narrative, I realise that I have been on a journey as I learn about practice development, changing practice and myself. As I learn through critical dialogue with myself and with others, I am touched or inspired by people along the way. I realise I will continue to be on a journey, as continuous learning is a part of life and learning about who we are. What is important to me are my values and beliefs, and in turn, what I can offer to others I work with in terms of developing the skills and knowledge of facilitation and practice development.

NARRATIVE 2: KATE

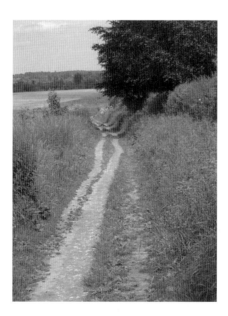

Fig. 2.1 My praxis path.

The path stretched out ahead
Well-worn in places
Sometimes it is bound by vigorously growing hedgerows and grassy banks

But at other times, it opens onto fields with the changing landscape reaching
out into the distance
Sometimes the path is in shade
Sometimes it is in bright sunlight

This image (Figure 2.1), poem and subsequent entry I wrote in my journal are a personal reflection on the process of learning to be a facilitator of practice development. It is a continuous process. There are people, theories, models and frameworks that guide me, to help me to understand what a facilitator of practice development is and what it isn't; but there are also different routes and new ground that I can discover. Sometimes I progress alone, and sometimes with others. The process enables the growth and transformation of self, others and cultures. The process involves highs and lows, confusion and clarity.

Learning from and with others

At the beginning of my path, I was conscious of *learning from others*, people who I considered to be experienced facilitators of practice development, role models. For example when reflecting on an experience of being a participant at a 5-day practice development school in 2000, I remember watching the facilitators, feeling intrigued and curious, but also uncomfortable and confused. And yet, although there was much I couldn't make sense of, I felt absorbed, compelled – hooked. Something was telling me that what I was seeing and hearing made sense and was worth sticking with. At the time I couldn't explain why I felt like this, but in retrospect I think that I was experiencing people working in ways that were congruent with how I believed I should and wanted to work.

Over the next couple of years, I was given opportunities to work as a co-facilitator; working alongside experienced practice development facilitators to facilitate action learning groups and also practice development workshop activities with larger groups. I can remember observing the other facilitators and asking questions to myself; thinking what are they doing, why are they doing it like that and how would I do it? I was searching for patterns (or looking for footprints); something that I could copy or follow and gradually, I found that I began to recognise some. I was able to ask the facilitators questions and also given opportunities to practice.

Confused Discomfort
Moments of Stillness and Movement
Then Revelation

At times, I felt out of my comfort zone – anxious that I was attempting to do things that I may not yet have the skills to achieve or were not my preferred ways of working, uncertain about how I would respond to the unknown and unexpected, or when I perceived that things didn't go well; but it helped to work with others who supported me and provided guidance when I asked for it rather than trying to rescue me or take over; and each time I learnt more and grew in confidence.

As I began to facilitate individuals and groups on my own, I followed the patterns (or footsteps) that I had noticed, but later I began to create my own patterns (or chart my own route along the path). At first, I did this in a conscious and planned way. For example on an occasion when I had to facilitate a meeting with a group of people amongst which there was a lot of tension, I sought advice from someone who I considered to be very skilled and experienced. She was able to help me plan how I would help the group to agree with a structure for the meeting that would ensure everyone's views could be heard, and issues could be identified and prioritised before discussion. Establishing the structure in this way gave me confidence to challenge group members when they did not follow the agreed structure, for example interrupting when someone was sharing their perspective, and therefore, enabled the meeting to progress effectively with positive outcomes for all. As my experience grew, I discovered that at times I instinctively knew what to do. When visiting a clinical area that was under a lot of scrutiny from external review processes due to a critical incident, an unexpected opportunity arose and I was asked if I could facilitate a workshop with a group of staff on the same day. I discovered that I was able to work with the group, using a combination of creative and cognitive approaches to enable them to explore and verbalise their views about patient care on the unit; identify the different stakeholder groups involved in patient care and to consider how their perspectives could be sought; and finally, to begin to participate in decision-making about development opportunities.

The patterns are not fixed and unchanging, through creativity, *reflection* and *critical dialogue* with myself and with others, there is always the opportunity to recognise that there is more to discover.

Random Unforeseen
Learn about Self from Others
Insightful Beauty

Another way in which I have learnt from others has been through *feedback*, both formal and informal. Feedback has enabled me to develop a deeper understanding of myself as I learn to become a practice developer, often stimulating the need to reflect firstly alone, and then to engage in dialogue with others to develop new insights and actions to enhance my learning further. For example a comment from another practice developer made me realise that others may hold different views than me on the skills and confidence that I have as a facilitator. Consequently, my consciousness was raised to the need for me to be aware of my learning needs and to ask for support from others when I needed it. Similarly, formal feedback from a participant in a group that I had been working with offered a new perspective on my attributes as a facilitator. I was able to use this perspective on another occasion to give myself confidence to try working in a different way rather than using a familiar approach, to present myself with a new learning opportunity.

As I progress along the path, I appreciate that whilst I continue to learn from others, I am now able to *learn with others*. At first, when working with other facilitators I was happy to facilitate workshops, as they had planned or suggested, for example, but as my experience and confidence has grown, I am now able to contribute to discussions and share ideas when planning ways of working. This confidence has also impacted upon how I work with people. When reading through my reflective journals, I recognise that initially I felt a sense of 'having to get it all right' and needing to have answers, but later being able to work in a much more cooperative and collaborative way with individuals and groups, more able to work alongside people, to listen to and understand their practice reality, to enable rather than direct their learning and practice change by asking questions such as 'how can we?' or 'how shall we?'

Engaging with theory

My involvement in a project to develop and implement a family health assessment in my role as a health visitor was a pivotal moment on my path, as it provided an opportunity for personal learning arising from a crisis in the project. I realised that up until this point, the ways in which I had worked to develop practice were not underpinned by theory, but based on assumptions or what 'felt right'.

The initial module of my master's degree and the subsequent writing of a book chapter enabled me to reflect on my experience of developing practice to this point, immerse myself in practice development theory, explore my own values and beliefs about practice development and develop personal theories about how I wanted to work in the future as a practice developer. This was a springboard for me.

Frameworks and Models
Guiding Lights Reference Points
Recognise Patterns

The haiku (a Zen poem) reflects my personal learning process from this point, starting with familiarising myself with theories and models, seeing them being used by others, talking about them and then using them myself in a planned way in my role as a practice developer, before moving on to being able to draw upon them more 'in the moment'. Movement along the path was reflected in some of my journal entries. One entry identified that I wanted to be able to make connections between the different concepts of practice development. At this point, I was aware that I was becoming familiar with individual concepts; for example I understood the importance of enabling others to explore their values and beliefs and felt confident about facilitating this process with individuals and teams. Similarly, I was developing a deeper understanding of workplace culture through my involvement in some theoretical work with others to clarify this concept and could enable teams to explore their own workplace cultures using creative approaches. A later entry captures a moment when I recognised 'movement' along the path. When working with a team to develop an evaluation strategy, I experienced a real sense of the concepts coming together. For example I could see how their vision statement could be used to inform their evaluation questions; when considering the stakeholders, the opportunities to enable their inclusion and participation became clear; and I recognised how the processes of data collection and analysis could become learning opportunities for staff. This enabled me to consider how I could most effectively facilitate this programme of work with the team.

Walking, standing, running – my praxis path

At first I thought that the path represented the process of learning to become a practice developer, but then I realised that I could not separate this from my role as a facilitator of practice development; the two seem intertwined. In my day-to-day work as a practice developer, I am learning all the time. Despite my growing expertise, new experiences always present new challenges and new learning opportunities. By reflecting on and talking with others about these experiences, I am able to gain new insights and understandings about my practice and myself, which I am then able to use to inform the ways in which I work. And so I experience moving along the path as a continuous process of practising, reflecting, realising, understanding, and practising again – as in *praxis*.

NARRATIVE 3: JONATHAN

My ongoing pathway as a practice developer has been influenced by many different elements, both related to my professional practice and development as a nurse working with older people, and for me as a person. Very early on into my role as a student nurse, I saw practice and worked with clinical leaders that I aspired to; practice and clinical leaders that ensured that 'patients' were central to care through role-modelling supported by articulation:

> *I was in my second year as a student nurse; the ward was very busy, and we were caring for a lot of very sick patients. One afternoon I was caring for a man who suddenly collapsed. It was the first time I had experienced this type of situation, I felt stressed and anxious. Whilst the team attempted resuscitation, the Senior Sister from the neighbouring ward took me to the back of the screened area and talked through what was happening and what people were doing. Following this, we went and sat with the man's wife where I saw the Senior Sister talk with the lady. As I watched (and was part of) the context, I saw, sensed and felt skilled, compassionate care. The following day, the Senior Sister came and found me, she wanted to check if I was OK and we reflected on what had happened the day before. In that brief time I learnt so much about skilled, compassionate nursing, suddenly I felt that I understood what skilled, compassionate care looked like and recognised what type of nurse I wanted to be.*

Similarly, I saw and experienced ways of working that I questioned because what I was experiencing was at 'odds' with my own sense of what I felt to be 'right'; at the time I knew that what I was experiencing wasn't right, I was unable (at that time) to articulate why, instead I relied on technical rather than tacit knowledge (i.e. knowledge that is known but cannot be easily expressed verbally but can be uncovered through reflection both 'in' and 'on' action) to support my understanding and thinking:

> *At the end of my first year, I had a placement on a long term care ward for older people. Ways of working were focussed on getting the jobs done – a bath book, toilet rounds and an expectation that all patients would be up and in the dining room for breakfast at 8.30 am was the norm. I knew that task centred practice wasn't right, it didn't feel right and I rebelled, however at the time I was unable to articulate how task-centred practice dehumanises the person (care activities become a task to be completed) and the negative impact on expert therapeutic care.*

As a practice developer and learning to become a practice developer, my pathway of learning is ongoing. I have never held a post in which 'practice development' has been in the job title, instead practice development has been integral to the roles I have held (because of the value I place on practice development), in which I have shaped and crafted these posts based on the principles and underpinning values of emancipatory practice development. Each time I have worked with, or have been part of a team, I have learnt something new, as I reflect upon what worked well and what I could do differently in the future. As I became more experienced as a nurse, and latterly holding operational and strategic leadership posts in practice and commissioning, my understanding of the importance of 'who I am', both as a nurse and person, has become more defined through facilitated reflection and critique of my practice working with others, so that I have felt more comfortable with myself and authentic in my values, recognising the synthesis between the 'professional' and the 'person', that is 'this is who I am' and 'this is how I try to live the values I embody both in my professional and personal life'. Such understanding and insight has worked alongside the development of theoretical knowledge and understanding of practice development gained through study in which knowledge is key; however, integral to this, is the application of knowledge (from learning) to practice and the subsequent development of knowledge from practice, the core aim being to improve care for patients (people).

As a charge nurse in the late 1990s, I didn't use the terms 'practice development' or 'person-centred care'; instead, I articulated the way in which we worked as a team as 'practice that kept the patient central to care'. Reflecting upon my learning and development at that time, I now know that both 'practice development' and 'person-centredness' were central to how we worked as a team (leading to emancipatory transformation) and my role as a charge nurse. In subsequent posts, through greater understanding of both theoretical and tacit knowledge embedded within practice gained from: facilitated reflection, role-modelling (supported by articulation), learning both in and from practice through critique, academic study and critical dialogue with self and others, I started to reach-up from practice, to stretch my arms and look upward to the light, and in doing so, I recognise that I was experiencing Fay's (1987) three stages of development (enlightenment, empowerment, emancipation) leading to 'emancipation'.

At times as a practice developer, I have felt constrained by traditional (non-creative) thinking and ways of working and frustrated by what I perceive to be a lack of authenticity and person-centredness. My pathway as a practice developer has drawn me to the natural world that at times of feeling lost has helped centre my sense of perspective, well-being and inner energy (who I am, what's important to me and what steps I should take next) through reflection and dialogue with self and, at times, others:

'Walking with Angie – Oxfordshire'

Sleep, dormancy, rest,
I sense peace and rejuvenation.
I hear sound, but no noise,
I see light, but no brightness,
I feel strength, resting, re-energising.

I look down, Wood Anemones shine light,
Snow drops bow their heads in respect for the season,
unassuming but strong, giving hope.
Lichen encapsulates sleeping trees and moss carpets walls.
Trees reach-up to the sky in celebration of sleep, of life.
The light is fading, but I look-up,
I rejoice at the peace, the silent strength the forthcoming light.

(Webster, 2009)

Learning to become a practice developer has required a number of skills and attributes that I have learnt and developed through collaborative working and critiquing my own practice through critical companionship, which has been underpinned by reflection both 'in' and 'on' action. Skills and attributes developed have included the ability to seek and collaboratively agree on different solutions; to think and work 'out side of the box', which constrains creative thinking and working with patients and teams; to be creative and flexible; to be opportunistic and politically aware; to be outcome focused; to be authentic to self and others (but not naïve) and to have a clear vision (based on collaborative working) and understanding of the pathway in which the 'person' is central to all activity. Frequently, the context has not been perfect – competing or lack of control over operational and practice agendas, not enough staff, pressure to deliver and demonstrate for the here and now, constantly changing priorities, traditional professional hierarchies and lack of value of emancipatory change compared to technical change. Having worked within and been part of a number of different organisations and teams, these themes have emerged to a greater or lesser extent and are (in my view) the 'real' world. As a practice developer, what comes to the fore is the need to work with the 'real world' context that will never be perfect or ideal:

> *I recognised early on into a post that there was a very strong technical approach to developing practice in the Trust – training, competencies and policies (the place and influence of context and culture played no part). I knew (through experience of working with both teams and individuals as a practice developer) that such approaches would not deliver the transformation that was required to improve care and develop practice; however I felt also that the context and culture would not be welcoming to any different approaches. I knew that there were key objectives that needed delivering and that there was little time. I therefore introduced subtle changes to the work that I was leading that added greater collaboration and creativity such as, seeking out, engaging and collaborating with others; using picture cards along with claims, concerns and issues at meetings that I chaired. When asked to review a service we i.e. the team I was working with, used observations of care and developed a protocol for using patient stories to evaluate care. These were small changes in the organisation, but significant, that delivered the timely outcomes that were expected.*

Finding and welcoming back creativity (which I felt became lost at one stage in time) has helped me to explore and make sense of my learning as a practice developer. At times, in a world that has felt so technically centred and driven, creativity has enabled me to explore through reflection and critique my own thoughts and values (that would have been difficult to capture in words alone). Similarly, using creative approaches with teams and individuals has at times 'unlocked' a deeper understanding for me and those practitioners I have worked with, which would have been lost or missed in more 'traditional' methods of learning, that is, 'teaching'. Working and learning with like-minded people has supported and enabled my development as a practice developer through critical companionship, it has also reduced a sense of isolation and enabled learning with and from others.

My ongoing pathway as a practice developer has taken many twists and turns in direction (Figure 2.2). At times, I have felt immensely frustrated by workplace cultures that inhibit

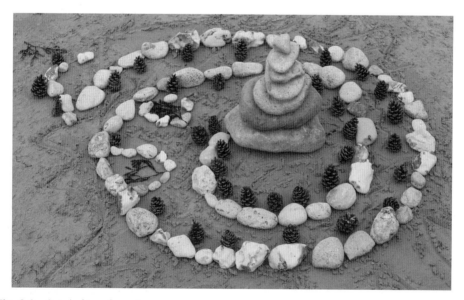

Fig. 2.2 Spiral of transformation.

or sabotage practice development and contexts that appear to be counter to innovation and development in person-centred care. Similarly, I have shared the jubilation and enjoyment with others when programmes of emancipatory change, development and practice transformation have brought about positive changes to patient care that are owned and driven forward by teams and individuals. Being grounded in the real-world context; having the ability to apply and generate both technical and tacit knowledge to and from the setting in which one works; being credible and person-centred; determined; authentic and professionally passionate about developing practice, practitioners and therapeutic care are all key elements in my view in learning to become a practice developer.

LEARNING TO BE A PRACTICE DEVELOPER: MAKING SENSE

Holloway and Wheeler (2010) suggest that narratives will often prioritise the experiences that are most important to the individual. Although our paths/journeys have been very different, it is possible to draw out some common themes from our narratives that illustrate firstly what we have learnt, and secondly, how we have learnt to become practice developers, and also to illustrate how this process continues for us all.

ATTRIBUTES

The narratives suggest that initially, we did not necessarily see ourselves as 'practice developers' but we were aware of an inherent interest in developing or changing practice; for each of us, this surfaced in different ways and at different stages of our development as nurses. As a consequence of this interest, we have assumed this purpose as part of our roles, whatever these may be, that is clinical, leadership, development or strategic. This interest is based upon the assumptions that there is always more to learn and that care can always be improved. It has been enabled by being curious and questioning (at times, even challenging the culture and context) and has focused on putting patients (people) at the centre of care.

We have been open to, actively sought and embraced opportunities to develop ourselves and our practice, even though at times this has meant that we have been out of our 'comfort zones'. This has included recognising opportunities such as learning in and from our own clinical practice (both on our own or with others), or when leading clinical teams; and formal opportunities arising from practice development roles, involvement in practice development programmes or programmes of education, for example master's degrees.

BECOMING AWARE

We recognise that initially, the ways in which we worked to develop practice, both individually and with others, may have been based upon the assumptions identified earlier and/or what did or did not 'feel right', rather than an ability to verbalise and therefore share the values and beliefs that we held about person-centred practice and enabling change in both the context and culture of care. This reflects the use of pre-cognitive knowing (Higgs & Titchen, 2007), such that at this time, our practice was guided by our intuition, for example, rather than an ability to think about and/or verbalise the ways in which we wanted to practice, thereby being intentional. However, we realise that we are on a journey that enables us to be increasingly aware of our values and beliefs and how they influence the ways in which we work as individuals, with others and to develop person-centred practice, contexts and cultures (as in cognitive knowing; Higgs & Titchen, 2007). Consciousness-raising is a practice development process that relates to 'enlightenment' within critical social science (Fay, 1987) and is a key starting point for the development of practice (Manley & McCormack, 2004).

This path or journey is never-ending; for example, even through the writing of this chapter, we have become aware that we are beginning to work within a transformational practice development worldview (Titchen & McCormack, 2010). Not that we have left emancipatory practice development behind; on the contrary, we are beginning to realise that we are adding to it through new ways of knowing, doing, being and becoming as a practice developer that fit within the worldview of critical creativity. When we look back on our narratives, we can see now how we are combining creative with cognitive approaches in our practice development work.

Nevertheless, in this chapter, we continue with our intention to make sense of and promote emancipatory practice development, as we believe that that is the best place to start as a novice practice developer.

ENABLED BY OTHERS

We are aware that we have been influenced by others, not only people who have inspired and encouraged us, people who have acted as role models enabling us to learn about ourselves and to develop practice know how, but also who have demonstrated person-centred ways of working. In critiquing our pathways/journey to becoming practice developers, skilled facilitation has been a recurrent theme as learning 'in' and 'on' practice does not happen in a haphazard way – facilitation and collaboration can be seen as being intrinsically linked and are integral to emancipatory approaches.

Our narratives identify that we have been influenced by people who could be described as transformational leaders. Key works, including Bass (1985), Kouzes and Posner (1987), Sashkin and Burke (1990) and Manley (2001), identify six processes of transformational leadership:

1. Developing a shared vision
2. Inspiring and communicating
3. Valuing others
4. Challenging and stimulating
5. Developing trust
6. Enabling

Transformational leaders share some similarities with skilled facilitators, and both act with moral intent, using sociological, psychological and learning theories, multiple intelligences and teaching/learning skills that enable individuals and teams to change themselves and their contexts for the better (Manley et al., 2011). Transformational leadership is also one of the enabling factors to the development of an effective workplace culture (Manley et al., 2011; see Chapter 8).

Similarly, we have had opportunities to work with facilitators who demonstrate the attributes of enabling facilitation (Shaw et al., 2008) (see Box 2.2).

Box 2.2: Attributes of enabling facilitation

Self

- Knowing own beliefs and values
- Authenticity

Working with clear principles

- Philosophy
- Frameworks/models

Knowing and skill set

- Building person-centred relationships, one to one and groups
- Establishing vision and ownership
- PD methods and processes
- Working effectively in differing context and cultures
- Accessing and using different types of evidence and resources

Adapted from Shaw et al. (2008, p. 152).

Working with such people has enabled us to 'see' inspirational and authentic ways of working, to initially copy and practice their ways of working ('do'), 'think' about the principles and theories underpinning this way of working, towards developing authentic ways of 'being' (adapted from Crisp & Wilson, 2011). In this way, we can move from being enabled to enabling others.

ENGAGING IN CRITICAL REFLECTION AND FEEDBACK

Engaging in critical reflection has been an essential means of learning for us all; enabling us to learn about ourselves and our practice as facilitators. This includes informal approaches to reflection, for example not only reflecting (thinking) opportunistically in practice, but also formal approaches to reflection including clinical supervision, working with critical companions (Titchen, 2004) and inviting feedback from others. We have enabled reflection in different ways, including; reflective models, reflective writing, dialogue with others and creativity such as walks in nature, painting, photography and poetry.

Critical reflection is a means of looking 'systematically and rigorously at our own practice' (Rolfe et al., 2001, p. xi), to enable learning and deepen understanding about our actions, and practical and theoretical knowledge, with the ultimate purpose of using this to improve our practice (Rolfe et al., 2001). The use of structured approaches to enable reflection helps individuals to explore and reveal tacit knowledge from their experiences (Schön, 1983). This process requires the ability to think (cognitive ability) and the ability to think about thinking (metacognitive ability) (Titchen, 2009). Rolfe (1996) uses the term 'Nurse Technician' to describe a nursing role that focuses on 'passively implementing' theories into practice compared to the 'Nurse Practitioner' who generates informal theory that is ongoing, from their own practice, based on reflection 'in' and 'on' action. In learning to become practice developers, we would argue that critical reflection and dialogue with self, based upon reflection 'in' and 'on' action has been integral to our continued growth and ongoing development.

As the focus of emancipatory practice development extends beyond the implementation of a specific change in practice to the transformation of individuals, teams enabling the development of person-centred cultures, this requires facilitators who can help to create the conditions in which teams can question current practice and develop new understandings that stimulates action (Dewing, 2008; McCormack & McCance, 2010).

We believe that facilitators of practice development should work authentically as authenticity is a core concept of person-centredness (McCormack & McCance, 2010). For us, authenticity means living and being true to the values that one espouses (talks about). It is embedded in who we are, what we believe and how we behave/act. McCormack and McCance (2010) argue that being authentic requires us to draw upon four perspectives of personhood – the attributes, reflective, moral and embodied perspectives – not only to enable effective decision-making for ourselves, but also to enable us to help others to be authentic, for example supporting practitioners to challenge or question poor practice.

Authenticity is identified as one of the attributes of enabling facilitation (Shaw et al., 2008). This is described in terms of 'personal integrity, honesty and transparency . . . trust and mutual respect' (Shaw et al., 2008, p. 160).

Engaging in critical reflection and receiving feedback is essential to being authentic and is not something that can be assumed. Crisp and Wilson (2011, p. 175) believe that the more 'authentic and systematic' the reflections, the more beneficial it will be for our ongoing development. As facilitators of practice development, we need to continuously reflect on our understanding and use ourselves (knowing self), to become aware and to address contradictions in our practice. Additionally, if we are working in ways that enable personal and holistic development of others, being authentic requires that we commit to this process ourselves. McCormack and McCance (2006, p. 475) argue that 'before we can help others, we need to have insight into how we function as a person' (see Chapter 10).

This process is ongoing and we continue to develop our 'knowledge of self' as a prerequisite to enabling person-centred care (McCormack & McCance, 2010), and an element of holistic practice knowledge which facilitators draw upon (RCN, 2006).

As well as engaging with critical reflection, we also developed knowledge about self by receiving feedback from others. Giving and receiving feedback is a core skill in emancipatory practice development. This can be done on an informal basis, such as in one-to-one encounters, or asking participants in a meeting, workshop or action learning set, for example, to provide feedback about the effectiveness of our facilitation; or more formally, using an approach such as 360-degree feedback. Garbett et al. (2007, p. 343) suggest that 360-degree feedback is a 'means of critically examining practice and fostering deeper and more productive professional relationships'.

Inherent in the concept of feedback is 'disclosure'. Over time, both critical reflection and feedback can increase self-disclosure. This process can be supported by the use of Johari's Window, a model of awareness named after Joseph Luft and Harrington Ingham (Joe and Harri) and first introduced in 1955. This model provides a means of looking at how self-exploration, together with feedback from others, can increase awareness of self and new potential. It can be used as a framework to obtain feedback on performance and can increase self-awareness about the known and unknown self, skills and abilities. The aim of using the window, a box divided into four quadrants (open, blind, hidden and unknown), is to enlarge the public (open) domain and to reduce the unknown and hidden knowledge areas of personal, professional and specialist practice (see RCN, 2007).

Driscoll (2007), based on the work of Johns (2000) and Johns and Freshwater (2005), suggests a number of ways in which reflection can be effective. We have used these to illustrate ways in which we have used critical reflection to develop our knowledge and understanding about ourselves as people and practice developers (see Table 2.1).

DEVELOPING AND USING KNOWLEDGE TO INFORM PRACTICE

We have all committed to developing and using knowledge to inform our ways of working. This was not something that initially we did consciously, but all of us have been stimulated by events in practice to develop a deeper understanding about our ways of working. This has been achieved by engaging with theoretical knowledge, then applying this knowledge to practice, reflecting on this practice, and developing new knowledge about self, about practice and about theory (as in metacognition and reflexivity; Higgs & Titchen, 2007) and experiential (and personal) theoretical knowledge (Rolfe & Fulbrook, 1998).

Higgs et al. (2001) argue that three forms of knowledge are needed to inform professional practice: (1) knowledge derived from science or theory, (2) professional experience and (3) personal experience. They further discuss that expertise in professions, such as nursing, is found in practice wisdom and practice artistry, both of which require the integration or blending of these three forms of knowledge (Higgs et al., 2001). We recognise from our own narratives the blending and interchange between the three forms of knowledge at different times in our own journeys, and with different origins and priorities, depending on the context and influences on us at various times.

At times, we have used our personal knowledge to guide our practice, for example leading teams based upon a personal belief that patients should be placed at the centre of care. Similarly, we have used professional knowledge, developed through initially observing other's practice and then starting to copy their actions, before adapting them to fit the contexts that we were working in, supported by critique and knowledge transfer (Bellman et al., 2010). Different incidents or triggers have stimulated our intellectual curiosity about practice development and other related theories. Primarily, these triggers have been based in practice, but have led us all to undertake more formal but practice-based programmes of learning (master's and PhD). This curiosity facilitated our exposure to and willingness to engage with theoretical knowledge about practice development, facilitation, adult learning, reflection, and much more.

Although we can identify different forms of knowledge and suggest how we may have used these as we learn to become practice developers, it is likely that we are often using more than one form of knowledge, although unaware of this. As we have developed our expertise, however, we have become more conscious of and increasingly intentional about the use of and blending of the different forms of knowledge. For example, Jo, Kate and another colleague were recently developing a workshop programme for participants who were leading practice development projects in a variety of health care settings. The focus of the day was on enabling the participation of both staff and service users in the projects. Table 2.2 identifies the forms of knowledge that they used to develop the programme.

An integral part of professional practice can be understood as the ability to innovate and to be able to 'question' traditional ways of working based on empirical evidence. Academic study in isolation will not automatically ensure subsequent application to practice. However, enabled by a workplace culture that supports learning and development, practitioners with support to apply their acquired knowledge and skills to practice will 'make sense' of the

Table 2.1   Examples of how we have used reflection to enable our learning and development.

Outcomes of reflection	Examples of effective reflection
To voice the contradictions of practice	Having reflected on a situation in practice that did not go as I had expected, I (Kate) became aware that I had assumed that the team I was working with shared my values and beliefs about working in partnership with families. I learnt about the value of undertaking a values clarification exercise as a way of recognising contradictions between the values and beliefs that are talked about and the ways in which we actually practice.
To understand the factors that have limited the ability to achieve one's vision	I (Jonathan) was working with a nursing team on developing a plan for older persons care. I had spent much time working with the ward nurses in helping them own and take forward the work. The charge nurse who had espoused support and ownership, however, was 'horrified' and 'angry' when he saw the outcome from the values clarification and observations of care. I recognised through reflection that I should have spent more time in supporting him through the process and should have been more aware of the local 'political' tensions.
To expose and confront distorted understandings and beliefs about self	I (Jonathan) was on a ward where a man was very disorientated and agitated. The ward team looked to me as a clinical 'expert' for advice and I provided technical direction rather than support, based on facilitation, in helping them work with and care for him more effectively. Through reflection, I recognised dissatisfaction with myself, as the approach taken had not been enabling or facilitative. I identified how I would act differently in the future as the approach taken was at odds with my own values and beliefs and what was needed at the time was to support the team more effectively.In a reflective conversation with a colleague, I (Jo) was able to reflect on why I had been unsuccessful in an interview for a role as a facilitator. Following this, I was able to balance my belief that I wasn't good enough for the job with a heightened awareness that the interviewer's concept of facilitation was very different from my own.
To look at situations in different ways	Following a reflection on a facilitated creative walk with others, my (Kate's) consciousness was raised about intentional action in facilitation. Initially, I had felt confused about my experience as I felt like I had been 'led' rather than 'facilitated' and this felt uncomfortable; however, by sharing my reflections with others, I was able to recognise how facilitators may lead others to enable them to take risks to facilitate opportunities for transformational learning.
To gain new insights and discover alternative methods of responding in practice	Instead of directing a situation that I (Jonathan) was being challenged over, I stopped and reflected. I approached the nurse involved and asked her to describe what had happened by drawing on questions from Gibb's (1988) reflective cycle. From the interaction I saw positive change and learning.
To nurture a commitment to practice that may have become 'numbed' through working in unsympathetic work environments	As part of a reflective walk, I (Jo) was able to identify that I felt like I was working in the 'dark', where those I was working with did not appear to value my own worldview of practice development. This enabled me to realise the limited effect that I had as a facilitator on enabling change in an unsympathetic work environment or culture.
To support ourselves and others to become empowered to take action in practice	Feedback to the Trust highlighted concerns in relation to food and nutrition on one ward. I (Jonathan) was under pressure to carry out an audit and report the findings. I reflected on my learning as a practice developer and chose to work collaboratively with the ward team. Working with the Junior Sister and Practice Development Facilitator, we evaluated practice based on the 'Seven Steps to End Malnutrition in Hospital' (Age Concern, 2006). Having used an observations of care framework and reviewed the records, the team took ownership of the work and developed a plan for development and change focused upon improving the patient's experience of food and nutrition on the ward.

Source: Adapted from Driscoll (2007, p. 41).

Table 2.2 The forms of knowledge used when planning a workshop.

Forms of knowledge	Knowledge used
Theories	Principles of practice development – in particular, participation of all stakeholders; integrating creativity and cognition; practice development as a facilitated process
	Facilitation theory
	Adult learning theories, including preferred learning styles, transformational learning processes and the use of multiple intelligences
	Group dynamics and processes
	Models of participation
Professional experience	Knowledge of project teams, the focus of their work and their practice context
	Experience of facilitating similar workshops
	Experience of working with each other as co-facilitators
Personal experience	Awareness of values and beliefs about practice development and the facilitation of learning
	Knowledge about selves as people and facilitators

complexities of health care and the unique nature of human interaction. Therefore, generating a greater understanding from professional practice, based on the synthesis between knowledge gained from both academic and practice-centred critical enquiry, is the key.

MOVING ALONG THE PATH: CHECKING OUR PROGRESS AND PLANNING THE ONGOING JOURNEY

Through narratives, we have been able to unearth the ways in which we have learnt and continue to learn to become practice developers. Although our journeys are individual, it has been possible to find areas of commonality and to share these with you. A framework to help practice developers think 'through self-development and possible strategies for enhancing progress' has been developed by Crisp and Wilson (2011, p. 174). Influenced by the Piagetian concepts of assimilation and accommodation, the framework proposes that there are three stages of development: (1) preliminary, (2) progressive and (3) propositional (see Table 2.3).

Table 2.3 Facilitating practice development: stages of development.

Preliminary	Essentially an egocentric stage, when practice developers will copy or imitate others as they are making sense of practice development methodology and its facilitation in relation to themselves and their practice.
Progressive	Generally a lengthy stage with three phases (early, middle, and latter), which is largely activity based, whereby practice developers learn by repeating 'rule'-based actions until they feel able to translate their learning and adopt more flexible ways of working.
Propositional	This stage is characterised by flexibility of thought and action as the practice developer has a deep understanding of the principles, theories, actions and outcomes of practice development.

Source: Adapted from Crisp and Wilson (2011).

Table 2.4 Moving through the stages of the framework.

Preliminary	When I (Kate) was first introduced to practice development, I felt intrigued but also uncomfortable and confused. I felt that I needed time to start to 'digest' some of the new theories and ideas that were being introduced to me. I believe that I was egocentric in terms of trying to make sense in relation to my own experiences of developing practice, but I felt that I took a relatively considered approach when thinking about how I would use 'new' approaches when working with others. I believe that my learning during this stage was enabled by: • having a critical companion to facilitate learning from practice; • undertaking a master's programme that provided an opportunity to engage with theory and develop my skills of critical reflection; • having opportunities to work with and learn from skilled facilitators; • being exposed to practice development activities in multiple contexts in my role as an external facilitator of practice development as these provided opportunities to see 'how' or 'if' theories and processes 'fit', and to challenge the assumption that practice development can 'fix' everything.
Progressive	As my knowledge developed, I began to develop a clearer understanding of what practice development is and what it is not – however, this presented challenges as an external facilitator, when working with others who may not have shared the same perspectives, for example the importance of engaging staff to enable learning rather than focusing on achieving a task. At this stage, my actions were more activity based, partly because of my level of expertise, but also due to the limitations of my external role. These were activities that I had seen being facilitated, had experienced myself and therefore, felt able to facilitate for others. Initially, I did follow the 'rules', but then gradually started to recognise when to become flexible or creative, for example in discussion with a group, I introduced a different model of group clinical supervision. My development was enabled by: • continuous and varied opportunities to facilitate practice development; • ongoing access to a critical companion; • working with others who were more experienced or maybe had different perspectives, as this provided opportunities to challenge my own thinking; • being introduced to and encouraged to use theory to inform my practice, for example Heron's (1999) facilitation theory; • exposing myself to creative learning opportunities, as these enabled me to gain new perspective on theories and concepts; and to learn more about myself as a person and as a facilitator.
Propositional	Movement into this phase came with increased confidence in my knowledge about practice development and my skills as a facilitator. I recognise that I draw on this knowledge not only when planning, but also 'in the moment', and can verbalise my thinking and decision-making for others. Whilst I experience increased confidence in my ways of working, this is not the same as certainty, as I continue to question myself, the theories that I draw upon and the processes that I use. I do this through working with others, reading, practising and using creative and cognitive approaches to reflecting with myself and with others.

The development of expertise occurs as knowledge, skills and theory is interpreted by our internal 'schemas', or mental frameworks, which in turn change over time in response to our developing knowledge, skills and theories. Whilst schemes are useful, as they can help us to quickly interpret large amounts of information, they can also hold back development if they cause us to exclude or ignore information or ideas that do not fit with our existing mental frameworks in favour of information that confirms our existing beliefs and ideas.

Crisp and Wilson (2011, p. 175) argue that a fundamental difference between Piaget's staged approach to development in infants and this framework lies in the practice developer's ability to 'critically examine their thinking and responses'. Our experiences would confirm this view, as engagement in critical reflection has been and will continue to be the key process underpinning our development; this view is reflected in Table 2.4, which provides an example of how Kate has progressed through the stages of the framework.

To further explore and understand the stages of development, Crisp and Wilson (2011) identify four domains – (1) seeing, (2) doing, (3) thinking and (4) being – and the characteristics of 'thinking/actions' within each of these domains at each stage of the framework. Through our discussions when writing this chapter, we were personally able to identify the significance of each of these domains in our development (examples of these are reflected in Kate's progression outlined in Table 2.4); but we were also able to acknowledge the differences between us in relation to our preferred styles of learning, for example Jo acknowledges that she prefers to 'see' something before she tries it herself, and to recognise the opportunities for being flexible within these domains and taking on new challenges to promote learning.

CONCLUSION

Our pathway/journey to become practice developers has been different for each of us. However, having worked together, we have recognised that we have a shared understanding of practice development and the underpinning values and beliefs needed for the potential of emancipatory practice development to transform cultures and contexts of care, the ultimate aim being to improve care for patients (people). At different times of our ongoing development, frameworks (Gibbs, 1988; Crisp & Wilson, 2011), conceptual models (Fay, 1987) and competences (RCN, 2006) (as an illustration) have supported and shaped both our thinking and practice as practice developers. Irrespective of the roles we have held, we recognise the importance of seeking out opportunities for reflective dialogue with self and others along with the need to critique our assumptions, beliefs and actions. Our learning and understanding has been underpinned by clinical academic study, however, fundamental to this has been the application of knowledge to practice and the development of knowledge, learning and understanding from our practice.

Working collaboratively with individuals and teams in constantly changing settings requires much skill and flexibility (and at times tenacity) within contexts and cultures that may not always be ideal. However, we recognise that there will always be opportunities for learning (no matter how small), and that as facilitators of practice development working with and understanding the real world is key to helping individuals transform both the culture and context of care. At times, this may mean 'taking risks' and trying a different approach in which we step outside of what we may feel comfortable with, however, central to this is the ability to work with and 'hold' the potential outcome through skilled facilitation.

In this chapter, we have aimed to share our ongoing learning to become practice developers. What becomes clear is that although career pathways may take individuals in different directions, at the core of our practice (irrespective of the post or job title) is a belief in the values underpinning emancipatory practice development, and the ability to work with teams and individuals in a collaborative, authentic, person-centred way, one in which learning, understanding and development is embedded within practice.

REFERENCES

Age Concern (2006) *Hungry to be Heard. The Scandal of Malnourished Older People in Hospital.* Age Concern, London.

Aggergaard, L.J., Maundrill, R., Morgan, J. & Mouland, L. (2005) Practice development facilitation: an integrated strategic and clinical approach. *Practice Development in Health Care*, **4** (3), 142–149.

Bass, B.M. (1985) *Leadership and Performance Beyond Expectations.* Free Press, New York.

Bellman, L., Webster, J. & Jeans, A. (2010) Knowledge transfer and the integration of research, policy and practice for patient benefit. *Journal of Research in Nursing*, **16** (3), 254–270.

Boje, D.M. (2001) *Narrative Methods for Organisational and Communication Research.* Sage Publications, London.

Bolton, G. (2006) Narrative writing: reflective enquiry into professional practice. *Educational Action Research*, **14** (2), 203–218.

Brown, A. & Harrison, K. (2009) Working with critical companionship. In: *Revealing Nursing Expertise through Practitioner Inquiry* (eds S. Hardy, A. Titchen, B. McCormack & K. Manley), pp. 93–109. Wiley-Blackwell, Oxford.

Crisp, J. & Wilson, V. (2011) How do facilitators of practice development gain the expertise required to support vital transformation of practice and workplace cultures? *Nurse Education in Practice*, **11** (3), 173–178.

Dewing, J. (2008) Implications for nursing managers from the systematic review of practice development. *Journal of Nursing Management*, **16** (2), 134–140.

Dewing, J. & Wright, J. (2003) A practice development project for nurses working with older people. *Practice Development in Health Care*, **2** (1), 13–28.

Driscoll, J. (2007) Supported reflective learning: the essence of clinical supervision? In: *Practising Clinical Supervision: A Reflective Approach for Healthcare Professionals* (ed. J. Driscoll), 2nd edn, pp. 27–52. Elsevier Limited, London.

Fay, B. (1987) *Critical Social Science: Liberation and Its Limits.* Polity Press, Cambridge.

Fulbrook, P. (2003) *The Nature of Evidence to Inform Critical Care Nursing Practice.* Unpublished PhD thesis, Bournemouth University.

Garbett, R., Hardy, S., Manley, K., Titchen, A. & McCormack, B. (2007) Developing a qualitative approach to 360-degree feedback to aid understanding and development of clinical expertise. *Journal of Nursing Management*, **15** (3), 342–347.

Garbett, R. & McCormack, B. (2002) A concept analysis of practice development. *Nursing Times Research*, **7** (2), 87–100.

Gibbs, G. (1988) *Learning by Doing: A Guide to Teaching and Learning Methods.* Further Education Unit, Oxford Polytechnic, Oxford.

Heron, J. (1999) *The Complete Facilitator's Handbook.* Kogan Page Limited, London.

Higgs, J. & Titchen, A. (2007) Qualitative research: journeys of meaning-making through transformation, illumination, shared action and liberation. In: *Being Critical and Creative in Qualitative Research* (eds J. Higgs, A. Titchen, D. Horsfall & H.B. Armstrong), pp. 11–21. Hampden Press, Sydney.

Higgs, J., Titchen, A. & Neville, V. (2001) Professional practice and knowledge. In: *Practice Knowledge and Expertise in the Health Professionals* (eds J. Higgs & A. Titchen), pp. 3–9. Butterworth Heinemann, Oxford.

Holloway, I. & Wheeler, S. (2010) *Qualitative Research in Nursing.* Wiley-Blackwell, Oxford.

Horsfall, D. & Titchen, A. (2007) Telling participant's stories. In: *Being Critical and Creative in Qualitative Research* (eds J. Higgs, A. Titchen & D. Horsfall), Hampden Press, Sydney.

Johns, C. (1997) *Becoming an Effective Practitioner through Guided Reflection.* Unpublished PhD thesis. Milton Keynes, Open University.

Johns, C. (2000) *Becoming a Reflective Practitioner.* Blackwell Science, Oxford.

Johns, C. & Freshwater, D. (eds) (2005) *Transforming Nursing through Reflective Practice*, 2nd edn. Blackwell Science, Oxford.

Kouzes, J.M. & Posner, B.Z. (1987) *The Leadership Challenge.* Jossey-Bass, San Francisco, CA.

Luft, J. & Ingham, H. (1955) The Johari window: a graphic model of interpersonal awareness. *Proceedings of the Western Training Laboratory in Group Development.* UCLA Extension Office, Western Training Lab, University of California.

Mallett, J., Cathmoir, D., Hughes, P. & Whitby, E. (1997) Forging new roles: professional and practice development. *Nursing Times*, **93** (18), 38–39.

Manley, K. (1997) A conceptual framework for advanced practice: an action research project operationalising an advanced practitioner/consultant nurse role. *Journal of Clinical Nursing*, **6** (3), 179–190.

Manley, K. (2001) *Consultant Nurse: Concept, Process, Outcome.* PhD thesis, University of Manchester/RCN Institute.

Manley, K. (2004) On workplace culture: is your workplace effective? How would you know? *Nursing in Critical Care*, **9** (1), 1–3.

Manley, K. & McCormack, B. (2004) Practice development: purpose, methodology, facilitation and evaluation. In: *Practice Development in Nursing* (eds B. McCormack, K. Manley & R. Garbett), pp. 33–50. Blackwell Publishing Ltd., Oxford.

Manley, K., McCormack, B. & Wilson, V. (2008) Introduction. In: *International Practice Development in Nursing and Healthcare* (eds K. Manley, B. McCormack & V. Wilson), pp. 1–16. Blackwell Publishing Ltd., Oxford.

Manley, K., Sanders, K., Cardiff, J. & Webster, J. (2011) Effective workplace culture: the attributes, enabling factors and consequences of a new concept. *International Practice Development Journal*, **1** (2), Article 1. http://www.fons.org/Resources/Documents/Journal/Vol1No2/IPDJ_0102_01.pdf (Accessed 22 February 2012).

Manley, K. & Titchen, A. (2012) *Being and Becoming a Consultant Nurse: Towards Greater Effectiveness through a Programme of Support.* RCN, London.

Manley, K. & Webster, J. (2006) Can we keep quality care alive? *Nursing Standard*, **12** (3), 12–15.

McCormack, B., Dewar, B., Wright, J., Harvey, G. & Ballantine, K. (2006) *A Realist Synthesis of Evidence Relating to Practice Development: Final Report to the NHS Education for Scotland and NHS Quality Improvement Scotland.* NHS Quality Improvement Scotland, Edinburgh.

McCormack, B., Dewing, J., Breslin, L., Coyne-Nevin, A., Kennedy, K., Manning, M., Peelo-Kilroe, L., Tobin, C. & Slater, P. (2010) Developing person-centred practice: nursing outcomes arising from changes to a care environment in residential settings for older people. *International Journal of Older People Nursing*, **5** (2), 93–107.

McCormack, B. & Garbett, R. (2003) The meaning of practice development: evidence from the field. *Collegian*, **10** (3), 13–16.

McCormack, B., Manley, K. & Garbett, R. (eds) (2004) *Practice Development in Nursing.* Blackwell Publishing Ltd., Oxford.

McCormack, B., Manley, K., Kitson, A. & Harvey, G. (1999) Towards practice development – a vision in reality or reality without vision. *Journal of Nursing Management*, **7** (5), 255–264.

McCormack, B. & McCance, T. (2006) Developing a conceptual framework for person-centred nursing. *Journal of Advanced Nursing*, **56** (5), 472–479.

McCormack, B. & McCance, T. (2010) *Person-Centred Nursing: Theory and Practice.* Wiley-Blackwell, Oxford.

McKenna, H. (1995) Nursing skill mix substitutions and quality of care: an exploration of assumptions from research literature. *Journal of Advanced Nursing*, **21** (3), 452–459.

National Health Service Executive (1996) *Clinical Guidelines: Using Clinical Guidelines to Improve Patient Care within the NHS.* HMSO, London.

Odell, J. (2004) Listen to my story. *Nursing Older People*, **16** (3), 39.

Odell, J., Holbrook, J. & Sander, R. (2006) Improving the hospital experience for older people. *Nursing Times*, **102** (2), 23–24.

Page, S. & Hamer, S. (2002) Practice development – time to realize the potential. *Practice Development in Health Care*, **1** (1), 2–17.

Rolfe, G. (1996) *Closing the Theory-Practice Gap: A New Paradigm for Nursing.* Butterworth-Heinemann, Oxford.

Rolfe, G., Freshwater, D. & Jasper, M. (2001) *Critical Reflection for Nursing and the Helping Professions: A Users Guide.* Palsgrave, Basingstoke.

Rolfe, G. & Fulbrook, P. (1998) *Advanced Nursing Practice*, p. 225. Butterworth Heinemann, Oxford .

Royal College of Nursing (2007) *RCN Workplace Resources for Practice Development.* Section 2.8.

Royal College of Nursing (2006) *Facilitation Standards.* http://www.rcn.org.uk/_data/assets/pdf_file/0005/64517/RCN_Facilitation_Standards_V1.pdf (Accessed 22 February 2012).

Sanders, K. (2004) Developing and implementing a family health assessment: from project worker to practice developer. In: *Practice Development in Nursing* (eds B. McCormack, K. Manley & R. Garbett), pp. 291–314. Blackwell Publishing Ltd., Oxford.

Sashkin, M. & Burke, W.W. (1990) Understanding and assessing organisational leadership. In: *Measures of Leadership* (eds K.E. Clark & M.B. Clark), pp. 297–326. Leadership Library of America, West Orange, NJ.

Schön, D. (1983) *The Reflective Practitioner*. Temple Smith, London.

Shaw, T., Dewing, J., Young, R., Devlin, M., Boomer, C. & Legius, M (2008) Enabling practice development: delving into the concept of facilitation from a practitioner perspective. In: *International Practice Development in Nursing and Healthcare* (eds K. Manley, B. McCormack & V. Wilson), pp. 147–169. Wiley-Blackwell, Oxford.

Simmons, M. (2004) Facilitation of practice development: a concept analysis. *Practice Development in Health Care*, **3** (1), 36–52.

Titchen, A. (2004) Helping relationships for practice development: critical companionship. In: *Practice Development in Nursing* (eds B. McCormack, K. Manley & R. Garbett), pp. 148–174. Blackwell Publishing Ltd., Oxford.

Titchen, A. (2009) Developing expertise through nurturing professional artistry in the workplace. In: *Revealing Nursing Expertise through Practitioner Inquiry* (eds S. Hardy, A. Titchen, B. McCormack & K. Manley), pp. 219–243. Wiley-Blackwell, Oxford.

Titchen, A. & Higgs, J. (2001) A dynamic framework for the enhancement of health professional practice in an uncertain world: the practice-knowledge interface. In: *Practice Knowledge and Expertise in the Health Professions* (eds J. Higgs & A. Titchen), pp. 215–225. Butterworth Heinemann, Oxford.

Titchen, A. & McCormack, B. (2010) Dancing with stones: critical creativity as methodology for human flourishing. *Educational Action Research*, **8** (4), 531–554.

Unsworth, J. (2000) Practice development: a concept analysis. *Journal of Nursing Management*, **8** (6), 317–326.

Vezeau, T.M. (1994) Narrative Inquiry in Nursing. In: *Art and Aesthetics in Nursing* (eds P.L. Chinn & J. Watson), pp. 41–66. National League for Nursing Press, New York.

Walsgrove, H. & Fulbrook, P. (2005) Advancing the clinical perspective: a practice development project to develop the nurse practitioner role in an acute hospital trust. *Journal of Clinical Nursing*, **14** (4), 444–455.

Walsh, M. (2000) Chaos, complexity and nursing. *Nursing Standard*, **14** (32) 39–42.

Weick, K.E. (1995) *Sense Making in Organisations*. Sage Publications, London.

van der Zijpp, T.J. & Dewing, J. (2009) A case study of learning to become a PD facilitator: 'climbing the tree'. *Practice Development in Health Care*, **8** (4), 200–215.

3 What Is Practice Development and What Are the Starting Points?

Kim Manley[1], Angie Titchen[2] and Brendan McCormack[3]

[1]Canterbury Christ Church University, Canterbury, UK
[2]Fontys University of Applied Sciences, Eindhoven, The Netherlands
[3]University of Ulster, Newtownabbey, UK

INTRODUCTION

The purpose of this chapter is to provide a contemporary explanation and illustration of practice development as a complex intervention relevant to health care practice, drawing on key insights to illustrate how different aspects of practice development have evolved. The chapter aims to help the reader to develop a thorough understanding about practice development's principles, processes and outcomes linked to getting started as a practice developer. It also helps the reader to think about current policies or initiatives in their workplace that practice development can address.

The chapter will help novice practice developers to work towards:

- assessing and developing their own skills in relation to facilitating practice development journeys;
- developing a greater appreciation about what practice development is and the criteria that need to be fulfilled if using practice development as a complex intervention;
- thinking about projects and initiatives in their own workplace suitable for using practice development as an approach.

In Chapter 1, today's health care context and the challenges we face have been identified. Practice development is an approach that can positively address this context, although more work is required to demonstrate this to external agencies (Manley et al., 2011a; Commission on improving dignity in care for older people, 2012). To understand how practice development achieves its outcomes, it is necessary to develop insight into how people learn and act in the workplace and to focus on the role of both clinical leadership and facilitation of learning, development, effectiveness and innovation. Although the nine principles of practice development (Manley et al., 2008), introduced in Chapter 1, encompass all that practice development is, for the novice it is often very difficult to know where to start as its facets appear complex. Over the past 20 years, practice development has developed its methodological and theoretical foundations extensively and can be defined today as 'a complex intervention' recognised by the presence of a combination of criteria that can be applied to any context or health care issue. The chapter intends to help the reader not only to understand where practice development has come from in parallel with developing practical insights

Practice Development in Nursing and Healthcare, Second Edition. Edited by Brendan McCormack, Kim Manley and Angie Titchen.
© 2013 John Wiley & Sons, Ltd. Published 2013 by John Wiley & Sons, Ltd.

within the context of the practice development journey but also to embrace different starting points. But first, consideration is given to how practice development has become associated with a specific approach.

DEVELOPING PRACTICE OR PRACTICE DEVELOPMENT?

Many practitioners have included within their job descriptions the expectation that they will continue to develop their practice within their professional role. This very general understanding has been linked with the expectation that all practitioners will keep up to date by participating in continuous professional development that improves their knowledge and skills in relation to changing roles and contexts. This expectation is the cornerstone of human resource management theory and practice that has been influential in health care organisations and their management over past decades. Whilst recognising that it is always important to keep up to date through journal reading, attending conferences and participating in higher education, there is an assumption underpinning this general approach, that is, by developing knowledge and skills, we will use these new-found skills and knowledge within our everyday practice and our practice and services will be developed to meet the needs of our patients and service users. The reality though is very different in that:

- practitioners may become enthused about new ideas and initiatives as well as the best evidence when engaging with external events, but when returning to their workplace, they experience constrains that work against implementing their ideas into practice, 'it just becomes too difficult to swim against the tide', especially as an individual;
- practitioners are so busy on 'their hamster wheel of busyness' 'getting the work done' in a way that they always have that there is no time to get off the wheel and reflect with others on how they are working and whether they are using their time in the most effective way;
- the ideas/research and policies practitioners are expected to implement take little account of what this means for different contexts or how practitioners engage with the ideas so that they develop ownership and become self-directing through internalisation. To comply with the influence of others is not an effective strategy for sustaining change in the workplace (Kelman, 1961; Kelman & Hamilton, 1989);
- practitioners often tend to work individually rather than collectively when implementing new approaches/evidence or ideas. This works against the idea that 'my idea' becomes 'our idea'.

A second assumption often held is that it is usually necessary to leave the workplace to attend external events to develop practice rather than use the workplace as the main resource for learning through work-based and workplace learning (Manley et al., 2009). For workplace leaning to become a reality, both a learning culture and the availability of facilitators of learning who can capitalise on any learning opportunity are required.

The landscape painted above in relation to developing practice and continuous professional development has existed since the 1970s and is still present today, although the challenges are different in terms of the pace of change, the greater focus on quality and its measurement, patient experience, innovation and productivity. Commonly in the 1990s, practice development described ad hoc single projects usually undertaken by motivated individuals around 'good ideas' implemented within the workplace without a clear systematic approach and evaluation plan to demonstrate outcome (Garbett & McCormack, 2002). Without a systematic approach, it was very difficult to evidence impact, influence policy or those holding the purse strings. Practice developments that did use systematic approaches to action, evaluation and research did, however, influence policy and practice in the late 1990s, but this was short-lived and died away when key players at the Department of Health or government level moved on.

Within the above context, a concept analysis of practice development was undertaken (Garbett & McCormack, 2002) that marked the beginning of how practice development began to be defined more specifically as an approach identified by a number of attributes. One of the outcomes of this theoretical development was that it became a search term in the British Nursing Index, the British equivalent of CINAHL database, whereas previously it was necessary to search on the terms 'practice' and then 'development' to identify literature and research in this area.

Practice development today is not, therefore, the same as either continuous professional development or ad hoc projects in practice, but it is a specific intervention characterised by particular features that became formalised in the Garbett and McCormack (2002) concept analysis, as outlined in Figure 1.1 in Chapter 1. The use of concept analysis, the approach used by Garbett and McCormack to develop a common understanding of practice development and its attributes, is also a useful tool in practice development work. It is often used at the beginning to develop frameworks that capture a shared understanding about a particular concept in practice and how it can be implemented and evaluated, for example safeguarding, practice learning, patient care, the role of the link practitioner for areas such as infection prevention and control, pain management and so on. The concept analysis framework involves identifying the characteristics of a concept, the enabling factors and the consequences and outcomes. An example of such an application is the framework developed to describe the supervisory role of the ward manager (RCN, 2011). This framework enables ward managers to think about how they maintain consistent standards of care in their own areas, which includes enabling opportunities for learning and development in the workplace. Another example is the framework for a person-centred culture of effectiveness that is used in Chapter 8 of this book.

PRACTICE DEVELOPMENT FROM CONCEPT ANALYSIS TO DEFINITION AS A COMPLEX INTERVENTION

The 1990s saw the beginning of practice development's theoretical journey, for example the theorised principles for action within Alison Binnie's practice development diamond (Binnie & Titchen, 1999). Building on this and other work, the concept analysis referred to above (Figure 1.1, Chapter 1) (Garbett & McCormack, 2002) helps to identify the foundation skills required by those involved in practice development. We suggest that this is a good place to start for the novice practice developer.

Five themes encompass the concept of practice development within a continuous process including the purpose of person-centred care through transforming the contexts and cultures in which care takes place. This purpose is achieved through 'learning in and from practice' particularly linked to growing reflective ability, employing a systematic approach to change and working with shared values and beliefs – all of which are recognised as requiring skills in facilitation.

Questions that will help you begin to reflect on your own values and beliefs, as well as, your own knowledge and skills in relation to these key components of practice development are identified in Table 3.1. Reflecting on these questions and clarifying your own values and

Table 3.1 Questions to help reflect on values and beliefs, knowledge and skills in relation to the key components of practice development.

Component of practice development framework	Questions to ask yourself and guide your reflection	Specific chapters that help with exploring these questions
Person-centred care	• What does person-centred care mean to you? • What does person-centred care mean to others in your team? • How do you know if you and your team are providing person-centred care? • What do your patients and service users think about the care your team provide? • How do you develop a shared vision about person-centred care across your team and with your stakeholders?	• Person-centred care and human flourishing (Chapter 10) • A practice development journey (Chapter 5) • Evaluating person-centred care (Chapter 9) • Enabling creativity and innovation (Chapter 11, Vignettes 1–3)
Transforming contexts and cultures	• How does context and cultures influence person-centred care and other outcomes? • What is an effective context and culture? • What is your leadership approach and how does it impact on your workplace culture? • What is the culture of your workplace? • How can you improve the culture of your workplace? • What are your agreed ways of working with each other? • What is your shared purpose and vision?	• Person-centred care and human flourishing (Chapter 10) • A culture of effectiveness (Chapter 8) • A practice development journey (Chapter 5) • PARIHS (Chapter 7) • Action Hypothesis (Chapter 13) • Strategic approaches (Chapter 12)
Values and Beliefs	• What are your core values and beliefs? • What are the values and beliefs of your team members and stakeholders? • Which values and beliefs are important to attend to? • How do you develop shared values and beliefs? • How do we know if you are implementing these shared values and beliefs? • What values and beliefs are experienced by you and your team?	• Person-centred care and human flourishing (Chapter 10) • A culture of effectiveness (Chapter 8) • Practice development methodology (Chapter 4) • A practice development journey (Chapter 5) • Action Hypothesis (Chapter 13) • Enabling creativity and innovation (Chapter 11, Vignette 1)

Table 3.1 *(Continued)*

Component of practice development framework	Questions to ask yourself and guide your reflection	Specific chapters that help with exploring these questions
Learning in and from practice	• What does learning in and from practice mean to you and your team members? • How do you help others to learn in and from practice? • How do you help others to be creative and innovative? • How do you help others to be effective in the workplace as individuals and teams? • How do you use reflection in your practice and with others to help them with learning?	• Learning to become a practice developer (Chapter 2) • Facilitating learning and development (Chapter 6) • A practice development journey (Chapter 5) • Harnessing creativity and innovation (Chapter 11)
Systematic approaches to change	• What does being systematic mean? • What evidence do you have about your workplace that can act as a baseline for change? • What tools can you use to evaluate your teams practice and effectiveness as well as improvement? • What are your patients and service users experience of your service?	• PARIHS (Chapter 7) • A practice development journey (Chapter 5) • Evaluating person-centred care (Chapter 9) • Strategic approaches (Chapter 12)
Facilitation skills	• What skills do you have to facilitate learning, development, effectiveness and innovation in the workplace rather than the classroom? • How do you help others to learn in the moment of practice? • How do you help your team to learn and reflect as a team? • How do you obtain feedback on the way you support and challenge others with their learning? • How do you facilitate continuous development and inquiry?	• Learning to be a practice developer (Chapter 2) • Facilitating learning and development (Chapter 6) • A practice development journey (Chapter 5)

beliefs are important first steps to knowing yourself and being authentic (see Chapter 2) as well as providing the basis for developing your own personal development plan to develop the skills and knowledge you require for practice development.

Reflecting on these questions will help you assess and prioritise the areas that you need to develop, and this may also guide how you use this book through the signposts provided to specific chapters that will help you address your identified priorities.

The early theoretical work on clarifying the purpose, attributes and enabling factors of practice development is, therefore, helpful for novices when identifying the skill set required to be a practice developer regardless of whether your role is as a practitioner, team leader, specialist, designated practice developer, researcher or clinical educator. This early work has outlined a broad framework and key criteria for what constitutes practice development.

EMBELLISHING THE CONCEPT OF PRACTICE DEVELOPMENT WITH EXPLICIT METHODS, WAYS OF WORKING AND CREATIVITY

Building on the initial framework, further theoretical work has been undertaken around the concepts related to practice development in areas such as context (McCormack et al., 2002), culture (Manley, 2004; Manley et al., 2011b), person-centred care (Dewing, 2004; McCormack, 2004; Nolan et al., 2004), facilitation and enablement (Shaw et al., 2008) including critical companionship (Titchen, 2000), latterly active learning (i.e. learning that involves mind, imagination, body, heart and soul) (Dewing, 2008) and praxis evaluation (i.e. a form of stakeholder evaluation that pays particular attention to reflexivity and being intentional) (Wilson et al., 2008). The insights resulting from this programme of theoretical development help us: refine the way we help others to provide person-centred care; establish cultures of effectiveness; be systematic and evaluate our practice development initiatives; and facilitate and enable others more effectively in the workplace. However, three major methodological and theoretical developments have enhanced our understanding of practice development to embellish the original foundation framework. These insights are touched on here so as to build our understanding about what this means for practice development practically.

The first relates to our methodological understanding associated with the terms, technical, emancipatory (Manley & McCormack, 2004) and transformational (Titchen & McCormack, 2010) approaches to practice development. Each of these terms has a fundamental impact on how practice development is facilitated and how it overlaps with aspects of project management and service improvement, informed by methodological considerations. These insights and implications for facilitation are explained and developed in detail in Chapter 4 by Theresa Shaw.

The second methodological and theoretical insight is derived from the NHS Education for Scotland study (McCormack et al., 2006), which used 'realistic synthesis' (see Chapter 9) to examine evidence derived from practice development projects, interviewing experts and analysing the literature. This study enabled two key aspects of practice development activities to be identified and made more explicit. The first included the methods used in practice development, and the second included the ways of working that characterise a practice development approach. Nineteen different methods used in practice development work were broadly identified and comprise practice development principle 7, outlined in Chapter 1. These methods alone do not constitute practice development as fundamental to their use is *how* the methods are used within the workplace. These ways of working are defined as the 'CIP principles' to reflect a way of being that is Collaborative, Inclusive and Participative and thus provide a simple guide to how practice development work is undertaken. Although simple to remember, they often require a real change in our everyday behaviour to enact. As individuals, we will have our own visions and aspirations for what we may want to achieve in practice, but in practice development work, everyone's voice is important. So, any project to be distinguished as practice development would always involve using the three CIP principles to co-construct direction and spirals of action planning as stakeholders touched by the focus of the work are engaged. Story 3.1 shows what this means for a novice practice developer.

Story 3.1: Learning to recognise when a common vision is absent and what it means to use the CIP principles in practice

Alice was a new ward manager and within a critical companionship relationship she identified that she was having a challenging time with her team. Whenever she tried to encourage her team to behave in different ways so as to achieve improved documentation of care or support patients with eating and drinking, they would make an initial effort but would then stop, saying that it was too busy and they needed to prioritise patient care. When asked by her critical companion what staff had meant by 'patient care', there appeared to be no common understanding. Alice thought that maybe the staff meant physical care, but she was unsure. This challenge from the critical companion enabled Alice to reflect and develop insights into two areas. First, she realised that everyone was using the term 'patient care' in different ways and there was no shared vision about what this meant, and what the shared priorities should be from a team perspective. Second, it helped her to reflect on how she could address this issue as she realised that she had done all the 'telling' and 'directing' and that she needed to listen to her staff and provide opportunities where they could construct together an action plan for going forward. Therefore, the next questions Alice asked herself were 'how was she going to develop this common understanding about the term patient care?' and 'how was she going to develop an action plan that was collaborative, inclusive and participative?' Normally, she would have just developed her own action plan and presented this to her team to adopt – with discussion of course!

The third methodological and theoretical development that has refined our understanding of emancipatory practice development is the notion of a new worldview called critical creativity (McCormack & Titchen, 2006). The underpinning worldview (philosophical approach) that explains how emancipatory practice development achieves its outcomes is critical social science. However, McCormack and Titchen argue that critical social science is no longer enough to support the way they and others are developing and refining practice development ways of working and being. Fundamentally, these new ways are concerned with human flourishing and with juxtapositioning the wisdom of the body and creative expression and imagination with cognitive ways of knowing (see Chapter 11; Titchen & Horsfall, 2011; Manley et al., 2011a, 2011b). Critical creativity has become an integral part both theoretically and practically to practice development as both a process and outcome manifesting itself in the concept of human flourishing (Titchen & McCormack, 2008). Practically, this will be recognised in the actions of facilitators who can 'authentically engage with individuals and teams to blend personal qualities and creative imagination with practice skills and practice wisdom' (McCormack et al., 2008, p. 9).

So, our understanding of practice development as an approach now encompasses the development of cultures of effectiveness, provision of person-centred care and achievement of human flourishing for all involved, and is achieved through working in a way that is collaborative, inclusive and participative, combining criticality and creativity, drawing on the nineteen different methods through systematic inquiry, learning in and from practice and working with shared values and beliefs as part of a continuous process. Story 3.2 illustrates this enhanced approach.

Story 3.2: Integrating the development of a shared vision and the CIP principles within the critical creativity worldview to establish creative spaces within a health care organisation

A number of practice development facilitators employed by a health organisation had just returned enthused and excited from an international practice development school where they clearly flourished as budding practice developers. They had been exposed to creative ways of expressing ideas and visions whilst at the school and were keen to develop a regular creative space that anyone could attend in the health organisation. In the first meeting, they used the CIP principles, picture cards and creative expression to facilitate and build a set of ground rules to enable a safe environment for the creative space, and also a vision based on agreed values and beliefs. At a subsequent meeting, they built on this to produce a flyer, so that others would know what to expect and would feel welcomed, involved and included. Participants identified collaboratively a way of using the creative space–time in an inclusive and equitable way as an approach for systematically evaluating the value of the creative space over a period of time. Gradually, new and different people began to attend. These people embraced the opportunity to use the space for creative thinking (thinking outside of the box), creative expression and imagination and coming to know and trust the innate wisdom carried in their bodies. The evaluations at the end of each session illustrated a positive sense of well-being from attending the sessions and endorsed the value of an opportunity to consider more holistically the issues that they faced in everyday practice.

Reviewing the following definition of practice development, readers are challenged to identify the concepts that they recognise from the evolution of practice development covered so far in this chapter:

> *Practice development is a continuous process of developing person-centred cultures. It is enabled by facilitators who authentically engage with individuals and teams to blend personal qualities and creative imagination with practice skills and practice wisdom. The learning that occurs brings about transformations of individual and team practices. This is sustained by embedding both processes and outcomes in corporate strategy. (McCormack et al., 2008, p. 9)*

One aspect, not yet covered, but explicit in the definition is the importance of sustaining practice development by embedding both processes and outcomes in corporate strategy. An illustration of this is provided in Chapter 13, where a health care organisation commissioned the development of a framework using practice development as an approach. Developed initially with some stakeholder groups, the framework was subsequently integrated into the organisation's quality and organisational development strategies. Then, through full sign up from the organisations executive board, it was possible to begin to embed the framework across the organisation as 'a shared purpose' framework. Through using the CIP principles to engage other organisational groups not previously involved, a single shared purpose framework for the organisation could be established around the four outcomes of person-centred care, effective care, safe care and a workplace culture that can sustain these outcomes. You will note that these organisational purposes are very similar to the purposes of practice development. Whilst, this example may be something that a novice practice developer would not embark on it is important to have a vision about what is possible as a clinical leader (Manley, 2000). Story 3.3 illustrates how thinking about embedding your practice development work within corporate policy makes a difference to the success of your project or initiative.

Story 3.3: Learning to put forward a case to achieve organisational support

Within action learning a senior clinical nurse was reflecting on her application for funding to undertake a PhD because research and development had been considered an essential aspect of her role by her organisation. She had completed an internal study application form and submitted this to the organisation for the purpose of seeking funding. To her surprise, the funding request was rejected but she could not understand why, particularly as R&D expertise was required by her organisation. Challenging and supportive questions provided by peers within action learning focused on teasing out what she was trying to achieve in her application, how she had presented the need for the funding, and how she had used the organisation's corporate objectives to structure the application. The senior nurse developed self-awareness from this process, realising that she did not actually know what the organisation's objectives were. She concluded that she had not presented a case to show how funding the PhD would deliver on organisational objectives. Her request was seen as not associated with the business of the organisation and the organisation could not see the benefit of supporting the request. Her priority action point was to find out what her organisation's strategic objectives were, and to rewrite her funding application around these to include the benefits that would be expected for both the organisation and the patient's experience. On re-submitting the application, she was successful.

CURRENT CHALLENGES FOR PRACTICE DEVELOPMENT

Practice development has developed an internal integrity and credibility for those who have been exposed to it and use it. However, there are challenges with convincing external agencies that practice development as an approach is worth investing in (Manley et al., 2011a). So, just as the individual in the story presented in Story 3.3 had to put up an explicit case for support, practice development needs to provide a parallel case about its value as an intervention with evidence of its impact in a form that will influence policy, research commissioners and funders. Whilst practice development can now be clearly explained in terms of its purpose, methodology, methods and outcomes through the principles outlined in Chapter 1, it is still a complex phenomenon. Our challenge then is to enable practice development to be understood by external funders, policy makers and researchers as a powerful approach for delivering on today's health agendas, in a way that it will be seriously considered as an intervention that deserves to be researched and supported further. To this end, presenting practice development as 'a complex intervention' is one approach because complex interventions are recognised by the research community as a specific type of intervention (MRC, 2008).

PRACTICE DEVELOPMENT AS A COMPLEX INTERVENTION

Complex interventions are usually described as interventions that contain several interacting components. There are, however, several dimensions of complexity: it may be to do with the range of possible outcomes, or their variability in the target population, rather than with the number of elements in the intervention package itself. (MRC, 2008, p. 7)

On the surface and from the journey we have undertaken in this chapter to understand the pivotal aspects of practice development, it seems from analysing the definition of a complex intervention above that practice development would lend itself to being considered as such. Some of the dimensions of complexity that make an intervention complex are identified by the Medical Research Council (MRC) in the degree of flexibility or tailoring of the intervention permitted. The dimensions include:

- the number of interactions between components within the experimental and control interventions;
- the difficulty of behaviours required by those delivering or receiving the intervention;
- the groups or organisational levels targeted by the intervention;
- the variability of outcomes.

(MRC, 2008)

It is recognised that the development of a complex intervention is a lengthy process of developing, piloting, evaluating, reporting and implementing and that all stages are important and to neglect adequate development work *or*:

proper consideration of the practical issues of implementation, will result in weaker interventions, that are harder to evaluate, less likely to be implemented and less likely to be worth implementing. (MRC, 2008, p. 4)

Whilst practice development can be considered to have passed through all the phases outlined by the MRC and be ready for more formal evaluation as a complex intervention the test comes from answering the questions posed by the MRC. Table 3.2 addresses these questions in relation to practice development.

From populating Table 3.2, it is apparent that with regard to practice development appropriate answers can be demonstrated to all the questions required to argue that it is a complex intervention. In addition, practice development can be used at all the levels identified by the MRC, namely by:

- individuals, e.g. members of the public, patients, health or other practitioners, or policy makers;
- community units, e.g. hospitals, schools or workplaces
- whole populations;
- more than one of these levels.

Table 3.2 Assessment of practice development as a complex intervention.

MRC question	Answer with regard to practice development
What you are trying to do: what outcome you are aiming for?	• Person-centred care • Contexts and cultures of effectiveness • Human flourishing
How will you bring about change?	Using the CIP principles to facilitate: • identification and implementation of shared values and beliefs with stakeholders; • learning in and from practice about a specific/generic issue using reflective practice, creative imagination and expression and active learning to generate self-awareness that then motivates implementation of shared values; • systematic change using multiple evidence sources.
Does your intervention have a coherent theoretical basis?	• Underpinned by critical social science and critical creativity. • Realistic synthesis identifies the methods and CIP principles. • Participative and critical action research approaches and stakeholder evaluation provides research approaches that demonstrate principles in action.
Have you used this theory systematically to develop the intervention?	Yes, from initial concept analysis of the intervention through to realistic synthesis and concept analysis of related concepts.
Can you describe the intervention fully so that it can be implemented properly for the purposes of your evaluation, and replicated by others?	Specific criteria can be used to identify the presence of the intervention these are being developed through an impact framework that have inclusion criteria for practice development, its processes and outcomes as well as its impact (see Table 3.3).
Does the existing evidence – ideally collated in a systematic review – suggest that it is likely to be effective or cost effective?	Effective in: • person-centred care; • achieving knowledge transfer; • increasing individual effectiveness and others' effectiveness; • other areas of research impact.
Can it be implemented in a research setting, and is it likely to be widely implementable if the results are favourable?	Yes, it can be implemented in any research setting.Results have already been favourable across different settings (see Chapters 4, 5, 9 and 13).

A salient point though is made by the MRC:

[I]f an intervention is seeking to achieve change at more than one level, e.g. influencing prescribing behaviour and patient outcomes, then processes and outcomes also need to be measured at each level. (MRC, 2008, p. 14)

This point endorses the need, recognised by Manley et al. (2011a), for developing a framework that includes criteria for recognising the presence of practice development, its processes and outcomes as well as its impact. Such a framework would enable data to be collected from every practice development project/initiative globally to demonstrate more powerfully the contribution and impact of practice development.

To summarise this section of the chapter, it is fitting to share some of the criteria questions in this emerging framework that would need to be demonstrated in any project that stated that

Table 3.3 An emerging impact framework for practice development.

Criteria questions to ascertain the use of practice development as a complex intervention and its processes. Options for these criteria questions have not been included here, neither have the outcome and impact questions (Manley & Hardy, 2012).

1. **Inclusion criteria: identifying practice development projects/initiatives**
   (a) *Collaboration, inclusion, participation (CIP principles)*
       (i) Which stakeholders were represented in your project/study?
       (ii) How were stakeholders engaged in your project/study?
   (b) *Ethics*
       (i) What ethical processes were used with stakeholders/participants in your project/study?
   (c) *Shared ownership/vision*
       (i) How did you develop shared ownership and a shared vision for your project/study?
   (d) *Facilitation*
       (i) Who were the project facilitators?
       (ii) What approach to facilitation was used?
   (e) *Evaluation*
       (i) How was the project/study evaluated?
2. **Starting points to your practice development project/study**
   What was the starting point (purpose) for the project/study?
   (a) *Values*
       (i) Which values were focused on in your project/study?
   (b) *Workplace culture*
       (i) How was workplace culture assessed implicitly or explicitly in your project/study?
3. **Methodology/methods**
   (a) What methods were used to facilitate critical reflection and learning?
   (b) What methods were used to promote and enable critical creativity?
   (c) What methods were used to help participants become practitioner–researchers/inquirers into their own practice?
   (d) How was feedback and critical learning utilised?

practice development was the approach used (Table 3.3). As a novice practice developer, these criteria can be used at any level of project complexity to guide the use of practice development in any setting and to challenge yourself to demonstrate both your understanding and use of this complex intervention.

Having developed an appreciation of what practice development is and its key characteristics from considering how it has evolved over the past 20 years, novice practice developers will be thinking about when to use practice development and how to get started. This is the focus of the next section.

WHEN TO USE PRACTICE DEVELOPMENT AND HOW TO GET STARTED

Being involved in health care at any level and in any role means that almost any activity or intention to improve the patient's experience individually or collectively or improve the effectiveness of care provided by individuals and teams can lend itself to using practice development as an approach. Even though practice development is usually driven by practitioners and practice teams, external drivers, such as policies and/or guidelines that are expected to be implemented across organisations, can also be the impetus for practice development work.

Therefore, starting points can vary considerably. Story 3.1 illustrates how one individual who was addressing a challenge experienced in everyday practice was supported to begin to ask questions of herself. By recognising that the term 'patient care' was banded about without a common understanding about what this actually meant to everyone in the team led to the realisation that a common understanding and shared values were absent. To some, the label 'patient care' did not include documentation of care even though this is an expectation as an accountable practitioner. To others, 'patent care' did not include the provision of nutrition and hydration. This illustrates how easy it is to make assumptions that we have the same understanding of a commonly used term and the same set of values and beliefs. On exploration, people often do share the same values and beliefs but they just need time out to explore what the values and beliefs mean for everyday practice and to come to a shared understanding. Whilst it takes time to do this, more time is wasted when a common understanding is absent and consequentially patients and service users experience mixed messages, inconsistent standards from different providers and a lack of continuity.

Opportunities to embark on a practice development journey may arise from a spectrum of triggers that include your own individual or team role and the challenges you face on a daily basis. For example, if you are a specialist practitioner running clinics every day (and an 8 week lead time is required for cancellation) the type of questions that will challenge you are: How do you go about ensuring that my patients have access to the support they may require 24/7? How do you ensure that your patients have person-centred information that meets the government's information standards? How do you enable your team's expertise to benefit colleagues in general settings in a way that does not create dependency and rather nurtures learning and growth in others? How do you enable national guidelines to be implemented across your whole organisation so that care is experienced positively and consistently by all, not just a few? Such questions can be the starting points to individual and collective practice development journeys. Table 3.4 identifies the full spectrum of starting points that can trigger a practice development journey, classified under three headings:

- My practice, my team's practice
- My facilitation practice
- Workplace, local and national drivers

A multitude of possible starting points for a practice development journey have been identified, but as a beginner or a novice, you may want to select something that is small and well bounded to begin your first practice development project, guided by what you have learnt about what practice development is and the key elements of the practice development journey explored below.

THE KEY ELEMENTS OF THE PRACTICE DEVELOPMENT JOURNEY

In Chapter 1, seven elements of the practice development journey were identified. Each element will now be described and illustrated. Whilst the impression might be that these elements unfold in a linear process with one step following the other, this is usually not the case. First, the starting point can be any one of the elements, and second, some of the elements may occur in a different order based on learning and reflection that takes place throughout the project's journey.

Table 3.4   Starting points to a practice development journey.

Starting points in my practice and my team's practice

Developing my practice as a health care practitioner
1. What is my personal vision of care?
2. What are my values and beliefs?
3. Questions I am asking myself about my practice.
4. Challenges I am experiencing in my practice.
5. Issues arising from my self-evaluation.
6. Feedback I am receiving from my patients, or colleagues.

Developing our practice as a health care team
1. What is our purpose and vision of care?
2. What are our shared values and beliefs?
3. Questions we are asking ourselves about our practice and the service we provide.
4. Challenges we are experiencing as a team.
5. Issues arising from the team's own evaluation.
6. Feedback we are receiving from our patients, team or colleagues.

Starting points in my facilitation practice

How do I develop my practice as a facilitator of individuals:
- in the midst or moment of practice;
- as a critical companion;
- as a clinical supervisor;
- as a mentor or preceptor?

How do I develop my practice as a facilitator of teams/groups:
- as a team member/colleague;
- at patient handover;
- in formal meetings of teams/groups;
- in action learning;
- in active learning?

Starting points from workplace, local and national drivers

Drivers: workplace	*Drivers: local context*	*Drivers: national context*
Improving the patients experience	Involving and engaging the public organisational objectives	National strategy
Reducing infection rates		
Reducing readmissions	Local strategy	National objectives
Improving continuity of care	Local policies and initiatives	National policies, guidelines, priorities
Improving staff well-being	Using resources more effectively	
Developing innovations		
Evaluating initiatives and innovations		
Implementing local policy and national guidelines		
Working more effectively as a team		
Using the 'releasing time to care' freed up from participating in productive ward		
Improving the care of vulnerable people		

Element 1: knowing and demonstrating values and beliefs about person-centred care

Whatever the starting point in the journey, there will be a need to explore the values and beliefs and/or assumptions associated with the practice concepts and direction at some level or another. This is necessary if a common vision is to be developed and also as the basis for supporting and challenging each other in the implementation of agreed values. This is an aspect of embedding values and beliefs into everyday practice. It is inevitable in the world of health care, which is structured around people and relationships that practice development work will encompass, sooner or later, the values and beliefs around what being person-centred means. If a project is about explicitly improving the patient's experience and delivering person-centred care, then the focus of any values clarification would directly address the concept of person-centredness. Often, though, practice development projects may not start with such an explicit premise; for example, they may focus on developing more effective teams or implementing strategies to improve some aspect of care where the links to person-centredness are not the starting point. Whether as the basis of working in partnership with patients and service users or with team members in a person-centred way, what it means to be person-centred will inevitably be addressed, even if the values explored to start with provide a different way in. The key message is that one starts where the people are who you are working with, unless there are key issues with safety, human rights, dignity and compassion that require a direct and interventionist approach from which practice development can then build its approach.

Ten key values have been identified that underpin effective workplace cultures, and these are clustered into three interdependent groups: being person-centred; ways of working; and maintaining effectiveness (Manley et al., 2011b) (see Chapter 8). As we introduced in the beginning of this chapter, to work effectively as a health care provider requires an appreciation of not only the person in the patient but also the people within our teams if a culture is to be achieved that enables person-centredness. Whilst some teams have a clear purpose and direction, they may not function effectively because their ways of working are not effective and/or they do not know how to support each other in a person-centred way. In such instances, the focus may need to be on working with the values and beliefs that help the team identify how they want to work with each other.

Some of the ways that values and beliefs can be explored are through using tools such as picture cards and artefacts, values clarification, visioning or other creative approaches and expressions as you will see in a number of chapters in this book. In Story 3.1 (learning to recognise when a shared vision is absent), 'patient care' and what this meant was identified as a starting point for a practice development journey. The language used by practitioners in this setting was not couched in 'person-centred' terms, but through exploring the assumptions underpinning the language used, they found a way of establishing shared values and beliefs. Using tools to explore what 'patient care' means to different team members enables values to be surfaced, discussed and agreed around what the ultimate purpose of 'patient care' is; the values and beliefs held about how this purpose is achieved; and the enablers and inhibitors that impact on achieving the agreed purpose.

Element 2: developing a shared vision for person-centred care

Knowing one's values and beliefs enables a shared vision to be developed about the initiative or direction being focused on (see Chapter 2). Through using the CIP principles a shared vision can be developed about both the concept being focused on and the ways of working necessary to achieve the concept or direction in practice. In Story 3.2, the establishment of a creative space was achieved through focusing on values and beliefs using a collaborative creative expression to clarify the purpose of the creative space. This purpose was then shared in a way that would enable others interested in participating in the creative space to know what it entails. One of the challenges posed by the organisation when the creative space was established was how it would be evaluated. With practice development being a systematic activity this challenge was pertinent and led to the development of a simple evaluation approach that could be collectively addressed over the first year to provide insights into its outcomes, impact and participants' experiences, yet still maintaining confidentiality.

Element 3: getting started together – measuring and evaluating at each stage

The development of a creative space, in Story 3.2, was a new initiative for the organisation and one that may enable creativity and innovation to be nurtured – time will tell. However, much of practice development is about improving a situation or thinking and acting in different ways towards a more person-centred approach. Whilst having shared values and beliefs is a good starting point, the realities are that there is often a gulf between talking about them and experiencing them. The values and beliefs talked about are often referred to as 'espoused values'. In effective workplace cultures, the values and beliefs espoused are also experienced in practice by all stakeholders (Manley et al., 2011b). It is not until practitioners and other stakeholders get involved in measuring and evaluating together that the gulf between what is talked about and experienced becomes apparent (see Chapter 13, Randal's experience). Tools such as observations of care are particularly effective at helping practitioners come face to face with this gulf and the taken for granted aspects of their practice when looking at this care through a different lens – that of the observer. Collaborative measurement and evaluation, therefore, is a powerful engagement and motivational strategy for developing a shared direction, in addition to providing a baseline against which progress can be measured. Story 3.4 illustrates how asking questions about the patients' experiences of care acted as an incentive to use qualitative 360-degree feedback to find out how these experiences actually were perceived by patients and service users as well as other team members.

Story 3.4: Using qualitative 360-degree feedback to gain feedback on patients' experiences

Specialist practitioners participated in a self-assessment about the care they were providing as individuals and whether this care was person-centred, effective and evidence based. The specialists were also asked to identify the innovations they were involved in introducing and those they would like to take forward. In relation to person-centred care, many felt that they were providing this, but when asked how they knew that person-centred care was experienced by patients and service users they could only cite general patient experience surveys, the absence of complaints and the presence of compliments. None had actually asked their patients or service users for feedback in this respect. As a result a qualitative 360-degree feedback tool was developed and a hospital protocol established to enable specific feedback to be provided to the specialist practitioners by patients and service users, in addition to accessing feedback from other members of the health care team. Whilst having the feedback was a boost for the individual confidence of many of the specialist practitioners as it reinforced that they were doing a good job, it also enabled a number of actions to be identified that could further improve the patients' experiences by working together as a team. A further bonus was that staff began to give and receive feedback to and from each other, and therefore, also began to build greater team effectiveness.

Gathering feedback and making measurements of care at the beginning of a project collaboratively provides the basis of developing a practice development plan to address the insights resulting. Chapter 13 provides a thorough example of this in relation to the context and starting point described by Randal Parlour, one of the authors.

Element 4: creating a practice development plan

The CIP principles have guided every stage so far in the practice development journey and continue to be important in the remaining stages too. Developing a plan is a collaborative endeavour, something that needs to be co-constructed by key stakeholders so as to maintain continued engagement, shared responsibility as well as self-direction.

In a large organisational project that involved the development of a strategy and the measurement and evaluation of four parameters, described in Chapter 12 by Jill Down one of the authors, it was important to identify collaboratively the qualities of an effective action plan and what this would comprise. A concept analysis framework was used as a tool to develop a common vision and framework as well as capture the salient points of effective action planning, its enablers and consequences. The key success factor identified was that the plan is recognised as 'our' plan not just belonging to one or two people (O'Neal & Manley, 2007). The main attributes of an effective action plan are identified in Table 3.5. These were identified in workshops that tried to answer the questions, what is happening in good action planning? What are its characteristics/attributes?

Element 5: ongoing and integrated action, evaluation, learning and planning

Practice development is a continuous process and so action will continue to be ongoing in the form of spirals that take practice forward through integrating collaborative planning,

Table 3.5   The eight characteristics of an effective action plan (O'Neal & Manley, 2007).

1. *An issue/problem/change that can be addressed through action*
   (a) Clarity of the problem/issue/change exists.
2. *Collaboration and involvement of all stakeholders*
   (a) Team discussion across the health care team.
   (b) Involvement of all key stakeholders in change and development and implementation of the action plan.
   (c) Health care team committed to progressing action plan.
3. *Shared ownership*
   (a) Action plan is shared and owned by all key stakeholders.
4. *Specific, measurable, achievable, realistic, time-bounded, energising, recorded, shared goals*
   (a) Identified goals (shared).
5. *Identified individuals and responsibilities*
   (a) Identified lead/coordinator.
   (b) Identified individual for each intended action.
6. *Implementing action*
   (a) Putting the actions into practice.
   (b) Mechanisms for identifying and overcoming any barriers to action.
7. *Ongoing evaluation and reporting*
   (a) Reporting mechanisms for sharing progress.
8. *Documentation and audit trail*
   (a) Logical sequence of events from identification of the problem/issue to evaluation and ongoing action is evident.

implementation and evaluation, the use of multiple sources of evidence, collaborative reflection and learning.

Element 6: learning in the workplace

The workplace is the main resource for learning in practice development (Manley et al., 2009). Through reflection and critical dialogue on new and different strategies and approaches to developing practice, continued refinement occurs. Parallel to addressing the issues and challenges in practice towards the provision of person-centred care and cultures of effectiveness, where all can flourish, is the focus on facilitating learning in self and others. In a project with consultant and aspiring consultant practitioners (Manley & Titchen, 2012), ten principles were identified as the key mechanism through which these practitioners achieved increased effectiveness in others. The principles are identified in Table 3.6 and may be helpful to you when revisiting your own development plan following the self-assessment you undertook at the beginning of the chapter. You could even use the first principle as the basis for your first practice development journey in your workplace through identifying shared values and beliefs about what this would look like then developing and implementing a collaborative plan to enable this to happen.

If you are a novice facilitator, Chapter 6 provides a really good start to developing insights about what these principles mean for your own facilitation practice, as the ability to facilitate learning in and from practice is pivotal to enabling individuals and teams to move forward in the practice development journey.

Element 7: sharing and celebrating

The final stage in the practice development journey is sharing and celebrating, although this is something that should not be reserved just for the end of a journey but built in at every

Table 3.6 The ten principles for learning in the workplace that are influential when enabling self and facilitating others to become effective (Manley & Titchen, 2012).

Principle 1	Developing a learning and inquiry culture
Principle 2	Negotiating the learning objectives and action to be taken to achieve individual and collective goals
Principle 3	Optimising the use of appropriate resources
Principle 4	Helping participants to learn opportunistically in the group learning situation
Principle 5	Role-modelling and articulating own professional knowledge about being an active learner (involving mind, body, heart and soul), facilitator of active learning and practitioner researcher
Principle 6	Enabling the integration of knowledge and ways of knowing to develop professional artistry (see Chapter 14) and praxis (mindful doing with the moral intent of human flourishing) through using cognitive and creative approaches
Principle 7	Using a wide range of styles, processes and skills that match participants' level of knowledge and the context in which they are working
Principle 8	Enabling a working relationship/partnership built on mutual trust and high challenge and high support through paying attention to the whole person and processes as well as outcomes
Principle 9	Facilitating rigorous organisational, cultural and practice changes at individual and collective levels through practitioner research
Principle 10	Collaborating in project administration and management

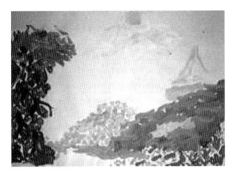

Fig. 3.1   'Land in sight' (Manley & Titchen, 2012).

stage so that it becomes the norm in your workplace. There are many ways that celebrations can occur and again this is something that provides a small and well-bounded opportunity for beginning or novice practice developers to engage colleagues in thinking about. Chapter 12 shows how celebrations can be built in.

Some teams start their meetings with individual and team celebrations as a way of recognising and enjoying the achievements of self and others. As you will see in this book, others use approaches such as *claims, concerns and issues* a stakeholder evaluation tool (Guba & Lincoln, 1989) to capture positive statements (claims) about progress en route through a journey of practice development with other stakeholders. And others will use poems and songs and other creative expressions. Figure 3.1 is one such expression from the consultant nurse project mentioned earlier. The consultant nurse called it 'land in sight'. For her, it conveys and celebrates the eventual coming together of the facilitation skills required by a consultant practitioner for enabling person-centred care.

Sharing successes, however small, is a way of life in practice development work, but sharing learning and exposing this learning and our new insights to collaborative critique and critical dialogue is a fundamental foundation. There are many ways that this learning can be shared.

CONCLUSION

This chapter aimed to take the novice practice developer on two journeys. The first was to help new practice developers develop an overview and practical insights necessary to grasp the essentials of practice development. This is achieved through exploring the evolution of practice development and the landscape in which the journey starts. The first concept analysis provides a good benchmark of the key practice development skills required against which one can assess oneself. Three methodological developments have led to clarity about the role of facilitation, using the CIP principles and methods within a critical creativity worldview in practice development work. Although these methodological developments, which may appear to be complex, have been presented at a superficial level for the purpose of highlighting the landmarks, other chapters in the book provide much deeper insights. This journey of understanding what practice development is has concluded with exploring practice development as a complex intervention in the context of challenges around demonstrating outcomes and impact that bring the reader bang up to date in our current understanding.

The second journey the reader has been taken on is that of a specific practice development project and the stages that one would expect to be embraced in this journey. Whilst presented as a series of seven steps, the reality might be quite different and hence the importance of being able to fall back on fundamental principles about what practice development is and is not when wrestling with the everyday challenges that will be experienced.

Whilst the importance of workplace learning, high challenge and high support as well as other practice development processes have been impressed on the reader, one key issue that has not been made explicit is the need to obtain your own support with your own journey. This question is, therefore, posed as the first of a number of reflective questions for you to consider to conclude this chapter and commence your own journey.

REFERENCES

Binnie, A. & Titchen, A. (1999) *Freedom to Practice: The Development of Patient-centred Nursing.* Butterworth-Heinemann, Oxford.

Commission on improving dignity in care for older people (2012) http://www.ageuk.org.uk/home-and-care/improving-dignity-in-care-consultation/ (Accessed 7 October 2012).

Dewing, J. (2004) Concerns relating to the application of frameworks to promote person-centredness in nursing with older people. *International Journal of Older People Nursing*, **13** (3a), 39–44.

Dewing, J. (2008) Becoming and being active learners and creating active learning workplaces: the value of active learning in practice development. In: *International Practice Development in Nursing and Healthcare* (eds K. Manley, B. McCormack & V. Wilson), pp. 273–294. Blackwell Publishing Ltd., Oxford.

Garbett, R. & McCormack, B. (2002) Focus. *A Concept Analysis of Practice Development, NT Research*, **7** (2), 87–100.

Guba, E.G. & Lincoln, Y.S. (1989) *Fourth Generation Evaluation.* Sage, Newbury Park, CA.

Kelman, H.C. (1961) Processes of opinion change. *Public Opinion Quarterly*, **25**, 57–78.

Kelman, H.C. & Hamilton, V.L. (1989) *Crimes of Obedience: Toward a Social Psychology of Authority and Responsibility.* Yale University Press, New Haven, CT.

Manley, K. (2000) Organisational culture and consultant nurse outcomes: part 2 consultant nurse outcomes. *Nursing Standard*, **14** (37), 34–39

Manley, K. (2004) Transformational culture: a culture of effectiveness. In: *Practice Development in Nursing* (eds B. McCormack, K. Manley & R. Garbett), pp. 51–82. Blackwell Publishing Ltd., Oxford.

Manley, K., Crisp, J. & Moss, C. (2011a) Advancing the practice development outcomes agenda within multiple contexts. *International Practice Development Journal*, **1** (1), 1–16.

Manley, K. & Hardy, S. (2012) Impact framework for practice development. Practice Development Master-class series 2012, Centre for Practice Development, Canterbury Christ Church University April. Unpublished.

Manley, K. & McCormack, B. (2004) Practice development purpose, methodology, facilitation and evaluation methodology. In: *Practice Development in Nursing* (eds B. McCormack, K. Manley & R. Garbett), pp. 33–50. Blackwell Publishing Ltd., Oxford.

Manley, K., McCormack, B. & Wilson, V. (2008) *International Practice Development in Nursing and Healthcare.* Blackwell Publishing Ltd., Oxford.

Manley, K., Sanders, K., Cardiff, S. & Webster, J. (2011b) Effective workplace culture: the attributes, enabling factors and consequences of a new concept. *International Practice Development Journal*, **1** (2), 1–29.

Manley, K. & Titchen, A. (2012) *Being and Becoming a Consultant Nurse: Towards Greater Effectiveness Through a Programme of Support.* RCN, London.

Manley, K., Titchen, A. & Hardy, S. (2009) Work based learning in the context of contemporary healthcare education and practice: a concept analysis. *Practice Development in Health Care*, **8** (2), 87–127.

McCormack, B. (2004) Person-centredness in gerontological nursing: an overview of the literature. *Journal of Clinical Nursing*, **13** (3A), 31–38.

McCormack, B., Dewar, B., Wright, J., Garbett, R., Harvey, G. & Ballantine, K. (2006) *A Realist Synthesis of Evidence Relating to Practice Development.* NHS Education for Scotland and NHS Quality Improvement Scotland, Scotland. Retrieved from: http://www.nes.scot.nhs.uk/ (Accessed 5 April 2011).

McCormack, B., Kitson, A., Harvey, G., Rycroft-Malone, J., Titchen, A. & Seers, K. (2002) Getting evidence into practice: the meaning of 'context'. *Journal of Advanced Nursing*, **38** (1), 94–104.

McCormack, B. & Titchen, A. (2006) Critical creativity: melding, exploding, blending. *Educational Action Research: An International Journal*, **14** (2), 239–266.

Medical Research Council (MRC) (2008) *Developing and Evaluating Complex Interventions: New Guidance*. MRC, London. www.mrc.ac.uk/complexinterventionsguidance (Accessed 8 May 2012).

Nolan, M.R., Davies, S., Brown, J., Keady, J. & Nolan, J. (2004) Beyond 'person-centred' care: a new vision for gerontological nursing. *International Journal of Older People Nursing in Association with Journal of Clinical Nursing*, **13** (3a), 45–53.

O'Neal, H. & Manley, K. (2007) Action planning: making change happen in clinical practice. *Nursing Standard*, **21** (35), 35–39.

Royal College of Nursing (RCN) (2011) Making a business case for ward sisters/team leaders to be supervisory. http://www.rcn.org.uk/__data/assets/pdf_file/0005/414536/004188.pdf (Accessed 7 May 2012).

Shaw, T., Dewing, J., Young, R., Devlin, M., Boomer, C. & Legius, M. (2008) Enabling practice development: delving into the concept of facilitation from a practitioner perspective. In: *International Practice Development in Nursing and Healthcare* (eds K. Manley, B. McCormack & V. Wilson), pp. 147–169. Wiley Blackwell, Oxford.

Titchen, A. (2000) *Professional Craft Knowledge in Patient-Centred Nursing and the Facilitation of its Development*. D. Phil. Linacre College Oxford. Ashdale Press Tackley, Oxfordshire.

Titchen, A. & Horsfall, D. (2011) Embodying creative imagination and expression in qualitative research. In: *Creative Spaces for Qualitative Researching: Living research* (eds J. Higgs, A. Titchen, D. Horsfall & D. Bridges), pp. 179–190. Sense Publishers, Rotterdam, The Netherlands.

Titchen, A. & McCormack, B. (2008) A methodological walk in the forest: critical creativity and human flourishing. In: *International Practice Development in Nursing and Healthcare* (eds K. Manley, B. McCormack & V. Wilson), pp. 59–83. Blackwell Publishing Ltd., Oxford.

Titchen, A. & McCormack, B. (2010) Dancing with stones: critical creativity as methodology for human flourishing. *Educational Action Research: An International Journal*, **18** (4), 531–554.

Wilson, V., Hardy, S. & Brown, B. (2008) An exploration of practice development evaluation: unearthing PRAXIS, Chap 7. In: *International Practice Development in Nursing and Healthcare* (eds K. Manley, B. McCormack & V. Wilson), pp. 126–146. Blackwell Publishing Ltd., Oxford.

4 Approaches to Practice Development

Theresa Shaw

Foundation of Nursing Studies, UK

INTRODUCTION AND OVERVIEW OF CHAPTER

This chapter builds on previous work presenting and contrasting methodological approaches of technical and emancipatory practice development (Manley & McCormack, 2004). Since this publication, there has been a great increase in both the use and reporting of practice development; alongside this, knowledge and understanding has also grown. After considering why practice development approaches are important, the chapter moves on to revisit some of the philosophical perspectives influencing practice development to date. Experience from practice and research are shared and some refined thinking presented regarding the process and outcomes of practice development in health care.

WHY CONSIDER HOW PRACTICE DEVELOPMENT IS APPROACHED

The demand for health care to be effective, efficient and focused on the specific needs of patients and their families has increased nationally and internationally. Within the UK health care context, there has been increased activity and investment to monitor and improve health care practice. Organisations including the Care Quality Commission, the NHS Institute for Innovation and Improvement and the National Institute for Health and Clinical Excellence all have specific and overlapping roles in supporting improvement, innovation and health care quality. Despite this investment and the espoused commitment to practice improvement and change, it is still the case that for many developments in practice, progress is slow and difficult to sustain (McKenna et al., 2004; Tolson et al., 2008; Shaw, 2011). The problem is compounded by a lack of good quality evaluation and research into both, the process and outcomes of practice development and change initiatives (Wilson et al., 2008). From listening to practitioners, it is evident that for some, activity to improve practice can be a positive experience that transforms ways of working and results in sustained improvement in patient care. For others, it can at times feel negative, be perceived as ongoing criticism of practice or just another unnecessary change. This de-energising and demotivating force has more recently been qualified further by Titchen et al. (2011) as a representation of the

Practice Development in Nursing and Healthcare, Second Edition. Edited by Brendan McCormack, Kim Manley and Angie Titchen.
© 2013 John Wiley & Sons, Ltd. Published 2013 by John Wiley & Sons, Ltd.

current nature of organisational and workplace change, which counters the opportunity for human flourishing and development.

More recently, the increased reporting and publicity accorded to poor practice suggests that to significantly improve practice, activities must address the fundamental issues of values, attitudes and culture (Patterson, 2011). This raises questions about the suitability of traditional approaches to change and improvement activities, which tend to focus on the task of change rather than the people involved. There is a growing sense that change and improvement could be more successful if initiated in the front line of care and led by the work of clinically based teams (Bevan, 2010). Furthermore, as Marshall (2011) emphasises, we need to deepen understanding of environmental elements that facilitate and/or block improvement, how they connect and how they can be changed. As Bevan (2010) suggests such learning and understanding can then be transferred across health care teams who continue to struggle to achieve best practice.

Reflecting on the experience of practice development and analysing the increased literature, the difficulties of practice change are perpetuated by the drivers of, and more significantly the approaches to, quality improvement activity (Shaw, 2009; Shaw, 2012). These include the following:

- The pressure exerted by service improvement and policy-driven targets.
- Too great an emphasis on quick fix approaches to change and development.
- The ongoing use of technical approaches to change and improvement.
- A perpetuation of the rational assumption that the presentation of evidence and knowledge leads people to embrace change.
- An unrealistic expectation placed on the individual leader or change agent to achieve change.

At times, there also remains an overarching unwillingness to acknowledge at both policy and organisational levels, the significance and impact of organisational and workplace context and/or culture within which change and development is proposed; so, even with a willingness to consider change, practitioners experience barriers that are difficult to overcome. As a result, of all these issues, many initiatives have a short-term or limited impact.

Just as the organisation of health care practice has evolved from a task-driven approach to a care improvement activity also needs to truly embrace change by moving towards activity that focuses on values and people (patients and staff) and a commitment to a longer term vision for culture change and human flourishing. However, as with the evolution of health care and nursing practice, the time line for realising such change should not be underestimated.

PRACTICE DEVELOPMENT: UNRAVELLING ITS THEORETICAL DEVELOPMENT

Practice development can now be described as a 'global movement' of quality improvement activity directed at enhancing patients experience of health care; developing practitioners; and enabling the transformation of workplace cultures that are committed to person-centredness, learning and effectiveness (McCormack, 2010, p. 189). However, unravelling the methodology, that is, the set or system of methods and principles used is central to understanding effectiveness and value.

Influence of and relationship with critical social theory

The early definition of practice development included several of the key tenets we recognise as practice development today, namely, that it is a facilitated and systematic process which, not only focuses on patient care and change but also emphasises person-centredness, enabling, transformation and emancipatory change (McCormack et al., 1999). McCormack et al. (1999) provided greater theoretical understanding by developing a conceptual framework for practice development underpinned by critical social theory (Habermas, 1972). Practice development was described as working across three interconnected interfaces, namely, organisational, strategic and client/patient, which together could create a patient-centred, learning and enabling culture through continuous reflexivity (McCormack et al., 1999).

Critical social theory is considered appropriate to practice development for a number of reasons. Firstly, there has been a growth of interlinked activities that encourage critical action-based working and thinking (McCormack et al., 1999), which includes the use of emancipatory action research (Binnie & Titchen, 1998), reflective practice (Schon, 1983; Johns, 2000) and action learning (McGill & Beaty, 1997). Secondly, critical theory is concerned with seeing the world critically (Habermas, 1972) and encouraging individuals and teams to examine situations and phenomena so that they can develop an understanding of themselves, the reality of the world they are working in and ways of moving forward to make changes (Carr & Kemmis, 1986). Fay (1987) argues through his complex framework of 8 theories and 20 sub-theories that critical social science is concerned with enabling processes towards enlightenment, empowerment and emancipation.

Although now more developed, all these theories/positions can be related to the earliest articulation of practice development, including: the value of inductive approaches to knowledge transfer and change, a commitment to working with people, and development in practice taking account of the complexity of contexts (Kitson et al., 1996).

Articulating a methodology

In order to provide greater clarity about the processes and outcomes of practice development, Manley and McCormack (2004) critically explored the methodology underpinning practice development approaches. Refined from previous work in the field (Kitson et al., 1996; McCormack et al., 1999), it appeared to be the first attempt to directly articulate a methodology for practice development and the theoretical assumptions that underpin it.

Manley and McCormack (2004) proposed that the way practice development is approached is influenced by different assumptions and values, and suggested that understanding these could help those engaged in practice development to act more effectively. Drawing on critical social theory and in particular the work of Habermas (1972) regarding different knowledge interests and Grundy's (1982) three modes of action research, they present two perspectives or 'worldviews' for practice development. These worldviews help to clarify the purpose of practice development, provide insights into methodologies that may be used, the style of facilitation and approaches to evaluation.

It is stressed that the intention is not to present a 'good versus bad' approach to practice development. Rather, these insights can help practitioners engaged in practice development activity to consider their approaches and the position of their organisation. However, Manley and McCormack (2004) do suggest that one approach may be more 'sophisticated' and have more far-reaching outcomes.

The first worldview, 'technical' practice development, is aligned to the perspective of technical knowledge interests (Habermas, 1972) and views the project leader or facilitator as directing an initiative to a pre-planned end point in order to achieve a known outcome or target; this way of working is often characterised by one-way relationships. Within this worldview, the notion of best practice is believed to be universally understood and accepted, and the outcome of the initiative is more important than the process. Ultimately, technical practice development represents a 'deductive' or top-down approach to change, driven by management and led by a single practice developer or project leader. Little consideration is given to the context or culture of the environment, and the evaluation of outcomes focus on measurement, such as waiting times, length of stay, morbidity and mortality (Manley & McCormack, 2004).

An excellent example of technical practice development in action and the impact such an approach can have is provided by Sanders' (2004) critical reflection on her experiences as the appointed project leader for a change in practice to support the care of vulnerable families by health visitors. A small group of senior colleagues developed a project plan by considering research evidence on the best practice, as the appointed project leader Sanders reviewed the evidence further and developed a frame for a new assessment tool. The project leader recognised that involving the practitioners would help foster ownership of the tool and therefore a project team was established to achieve this. The assessment tool and guidance was developed and a pilot was then undertaken. It was at this point that uncertainty, discontent and resistance began to emerge. The health visitors either found reasons for being unable to use the tool or expressed discomfort about its implementation. As is quite commonplace in health care today, organisationally, there was a tendency towards transactional leadership with the driving forces for change being top down. For example, following the identification of the practice problem, a solution was identified at a senior level. There was a belief that the change should happen, and there appeared to be evidence from research that this was the 'right' thing to do. The project leader was placed in the position of 'leading' what was perceived to be a clearly defined change with pre-determined outcome. Reflecting on the consequence of working within a technical worldview, Sanders (2004) concluded that it had led to a lack of shared purpose and vision (with regard to assessing vulnerability) within the team and, as a result, variability of implementation (Sanders, 2004).

This example shows that technical approaches to practice development may not be effective in improving or changing practice (Bates, 2000; Hooke et al., 2008). In practice, however, there are still many drivers for this approach, arising primarily from policy and health care targets, which demand rapid change, and the pursuit of guideline development, which continues to have 'questionable' outcomes for practice (Tolson et al., 2005). Research evaluating evidence-based practice programmes developed with the specific intention of getting evidence, guidelines and research into practice indicate that the appeal of linear, technical/rational approaches was their simplicity (Redfern et al., 2003). However, in reality, such approaches ignore several factors, in particular, the complex contexts in which care is provided and the complex nature of change (Kitson et al., 1996; McCormack et al., 1999; Redfern et al., 2003).

The second worldview Manley and McCormack (2004) presented was 'emancipatory' practice development aligned to emancipatory knowledge interests (Habermas, 1972), where acting collaboratively, collective decision-making and transformation are firm commitments. As a result, working *with* people is valued and the 'complexity' and 'messiness' of practice context and culture (Schon, 1987) is acknowledged. Whilst not disregarding research and evidence, understanding of best practice is formed from local knowledge, and ideas for change come from practice. Reflection and critique is central to achieving outcomes. The facilitator's role is equally valued within the team or group and is one of enabler so as to create a climate for enlightenment and empowerment (Fay, 1987). The process of change is regarded as equally important as the outcome and evaluation is an inclusive part of the process (Manley & McCormack, 2004).

Dewar et al.'s (2003a, 2003b) initiative to implement previously validated carer guidelines exemplifies practice development aligned to the emancipatory worldview. Having developed the guidelines with carers, the next stage was the implementation of the guidelines into a hospital setting using a framework of work-based learning to facilitate the process. Two clinical development nurses (CDN), who worked with older people in the hospital, were nominated because of their eligibility and willingness to participate. Each CDN worked with a team of practitioners to examine and develop practice in relation to the guidelines. Supported by an academic supervisor (external facilitator), the CDNs began by collecting data about current practice and shared this with all the staff. Ideas for change and development emerged. Action learning helped staff explore their work, their experience of involving carers and enabled the development of new understandings about the issues they were dealing with in practice. The staff eventually decided that they did not want to implement the guidelines; rather, they developed and shaped their own standards for practice as a result of working with the guidelines.

The particular strengths of this approach were the CDNs' commitment to working with the staff and their ability to observe and listen to their feelings, and those of the carers they worked with. As a result, they recognised that pursuing the original aims of the work would not lead to implementation of the guidelines or changes in practice. Instead, the staff were enabled (Harvey et al., 2002; Shaw et al., 2008) towards a practice change they felt was needed. In their report, the project team draw attention to the complexity of practice change, the value of creating ownership and the importance of facilitated support (Dewar et al., 2003a, 2003b).

Other accounts of practice development work show the consequences of taking either a technical or an emancipatory approach. Balfour and Clarke (2001) describe a year-long study in an ophthalmology unit, where the planned change of self-administration of medicines had failed following organisational change. The first attempt had been introduced to staff utilising an 'educational process' and was reliant on the leadership of the ward sister. When she left, practice had reverted to the previous way of working (Balfour & Clarke, 2001). In the second attempt, Balfour and Clarke (2001) focused more on understanding the 'context' and 'culture' of the care environment as well as introducing a 'supportive process' to achieve change (Manley & McCormack, 2004). They opted to use a participatory action research process and found it promoted greater 'involvement' and the use of reflective processes, which enabled 'deep professional change' based on the needs of patients rather than a 'superficial service change' (Balfour & Clarke, 2001), as often found when more technical approaches are used (Manley & McCormack, 2004).

Dewing and Wright (2003) describe how adoption of an emancipatory methodology enabled staff working with older people to begin a journey of empowerment, which focused on transforming the culture of care from one which was hierarchical and task-orientated to one that was more patient-centred and evidence-based. Pemberton and Reid (2005) also adopted an emancipatory approach to practice development by using the 'practice development diamond' developed by Binnie and Titchen (1998). To value and to be with patients was at the top of their agenda, and they worked systematically to support practitioners to learn from practice and from patients as a means of improving patient care over a 4-year period. The authors not only reported significant improvements but also offered a number of important 'lessons' learnt about practice development work of this kind. These included the importance of investing in the development of core skills such as communication and the need for 'substantial preparation and energy' (Pemberton & Reid, 2005) to achieve development, as well as ongoing support to sustain new ways of working. Working in cardiothoracic surgical care, Bouras and Barrett (2007, p. 162) found that an emphasis on emancipatory practice development provided a 'useful vehicle for enhancing patient-centred care', indicating that the approach helped practitioners challenge taken-for-granted practices and increased interdisciplinary team working. Henderson and McKillop (2008), working to develop services in cancer care, came to the conclusion that technical approaches were a feature of much of the service improvement activity that may not include commitment to cultural change. The differentiation between service improvement and practice development is significant for contemporary health care practice, in the light of the growing acknowledgement that the nature of workplace and organisational culture can be closely linked to the quality and standard of practice (Patterson, 2011).

   In summary, these differing examples of practice development in action show the contrasting ways of working to develop and improve practice. Under the worldviews of technical and emancipatory practice development, there are contrasting approaches to learning, namely, education/training versus reflective learning in practice, contrasting drivers, namely, top-down versus participative/bottom-up decision-making processes and contrasting styles of facilitation, namely, telling versus enablement. Taking account of the reality of practice, however, indicates a need for flexibility. Combined approaches that recognise the value of practice and practitioners, and that also utilise a rigorous, systematic approach, may be the best way forward. This could be achieved by drawing on the worldviews (Manley & McCormack, 2004) and the experience of Henderson and McKillop (2008), which suggest that the selection of an effective strategy begins with the consideration of (1) the purpose of any proposed practice development, (2) the underpinning evidence and (3) the context of the workplace in which it is intended. This could help ensure that the approach is appropriate and the outcomes of any development may be more sustainable. However, if agreed that the ultimate purpose of practice development is person-centred care and that it takes place in health care contexts that are complex, then approaches underpinned by or that make use of an emancipatory methodology may result in more significant, sustainable change together with transformation of attitudes and culture.

Using multiple methods in practice development through collaborative, inclusive approaches

Overtime, consensus has increased regarding the need for systematic, facilitated, collaborative and supportive approaches to improvement and change, and therefore, emancipatory practice development has attracted more interest. However, with much variation in the approaches adopted, the need for a systematic review specifically focused on identifying approaches to practice development and critically examining the underpinning evidence base was recognised (McCormack et al., 2006). Two phases of activity were undertaken. The first phase involved a review of published practice development literature and grey practice development literature used a methodology derived from realist evaluation (Pawson & Tilley, 1997). The second phase involved 47 telephone interviews with key informants from around the world (McCormack et al., 2006).

The key conclusion from the review was that 'no one methodological perspective' could support 'all practice development functions' (McCormack et al., 2006, p. 124). Rather, it was proposed that there should be evidence of 'participatory, inclusive and collaborative methodology' in all practice development work (McCormack et al., 2006). Furthermore, whilst the review found little to support a single methodology, interviewees described a plethora of methods and processes being used for practice development. These were themed into 18 essential processes or methods for practice development (see Box 1.1).

Although helpful, McCormack et al. (2006) pointed to the need for further research to test both relevance and impact. As part of an extensive review of literature, Shaw (2009) refined the list of methods into six values or areas of significance for practice development:

1. Person-centred care (1, 2, 3)[1]
2. Collaboration and partnership (1, 2, 3, 4, 5, 7, 8)
3. Enabling facilitation and support (10, 11, 15)
4. Commitment to active learning and development (9, 10, 11, 12, 13, 16, 17)
5. Transforming workplace culture (6, 18)
6. Evaluation (14, 17)

These values can be used to inform the decision to use practice development methodology and the subsequent choice of methods (as is demonstrated later in the chapter). These values might also be experienced through the values and beliefs of those taking part in practice development. Whilst each value or area can stand alone, there is an obvious interdependence indicating how far reaching an effective approach to practice development could be.

Expanding on the influences of critical social science and the evolution and relevance of critical creativity

In the last decade, practice developers have also begun to explore the role of artistry and creativity. Most notably, theoretical work led by McCormack and Titchen (2006) presents new thinking around the integration of critical theory and creative imagination, resulting in the articulation of critical creatively as a new theoretical perspective underpinning practice development. To further refine critical creativity, McCormack and Titchen (2006) interrogated the framework developed by critical theorist Brian Fay (1987) that enables the journey from enlightenment to emancipation, suggesting potential difficulties with its application to practice. Focusing on sub-theory 10, social transformation, they argue that there is an underestimation of the complexity of transformation. Rather, McCormack and Titchen (2006) argue that for practice be transformed, activity needs to focus and draw on a theory of 'creativity', which blends artistry, reflexivity and human flourishing. The refinement of this work is ongoing, and within a recent publication, Titchen et al. (2011) have expressed critical creativity as a worldview, the strengths of which extend beyond the confines of critical social science; they argue that when coupled with skilled facilitation, critical creativity results in human flourishing. This is significant for practice development because of the commitment there is for the development of people. Working in such a way as to enable people to flourish has tremendous implication for improving and maintaining the quality of health care delivery (Patterson, 2011).

---

[1] Methods selected from Box 1.1 are shown in brackets.

PRACTICE DEVELOPMENT AND SERVICE IMPROVEMENT: AN EXPLORATION OF CONTEMPORARY ACTIVITY TO IMPROVE PRACTICE AND INCREASE COMMITMENT TO PERSON CENTRE CARE

The remaining part of the chapter draws extensively from a study completed by Shaw (2009) that set out to understand the impact of practice development from the perspective of health care practitioners. The findings help to clarify some of the theoretical and methodological issues for practice development and demonstrate the contribution for person-centred health care.

The study, a qualitative descriptive exploration of the relationships between practice development approaches, practitioners' experience and practice outcomes, involved the participants (health care practitioners) of two named practice development projects (Boxes 4.1 and 4.2).

Box 4.1: Practice development project 1

Project 1: Introducing a ward-based exercise programme for older people across three in-patient care areas

This project focused on promoting exercise and aimed to make a contribution to healthy ageing by helping prevent falls, improve physical well-being, promote social interaction and promote positive mental health (Hayes, 2006).

Key characteristics:

- Small project team with experienced clinical leader
- Commitment to improving patient care
- Strong evidence base
- New role development and training
- Complex context

Box 4.2: Practice development project 2

Project 2: Improving mealtimes for older people in a ward for older people in an acute trust

The purpose of this project was to implement patient-focused mealtimes for older people within a hospital unit/ward. Whilst the team were directly focusing on nutritional care, they planned to tackle the issue by addressing the unit culture, and so it was anticipated to have a wider impact on patient care and other dimensions of older people's health (Dickinson et al., 2006).

Key characteristics:

- Ward-based team with two lead facilitators
- Involvement of all ward staff
- Wide evidence-based including patient experience
- Focus on learning in and through practice
- Complex context

Taking part in practice development: the experience of health care practitioners

From the data collected from the research participants, it was evident that participants experienced the highs, lows and complexity of taking part in practice development. With a commitment to improve the care of patients, they were involved in the type of practice development initiatives that can be said to be common to health care practice and clinical settings, and there were similarities across both experiences. All the practitioners experienced varying levels of frustration related to levels of involvement, resistance and organisational constraints. They also experienced a sense of satisfaction, as they could see changes happening and recognised that their efforts were making a difference to patient care.

Being involved in practice development was at times perceived to be extra work, either as a direct result of the implementation of a new practice/task or because of the additional activities required to support and sustain change. Some practitioners experienced the benefit of having a specific role to help move the practice development forward. Other benefits resulted from the creation of greater team working and collective responsibility.

In terms of the impact on practice, for all there was a strong sense that the practice development was reaching patients and having an impact on direct care. However, there was significant transition for one group of participants who appeared to become more aware of the people they were caring for and became more patient-centred in their attitudes. Other ways in which practice appeared to be influenced was through personal and professional development. It was interesting to note that one group experienced more professional development and the other more personal growth and development. A further way in which practice was influenced related to a change in attitudes and perceived progress in altering the workplace culture.

From early on in the projects, it was evident that one project took a more task- or outcome-focused approach (i.e. implementing the ward workout programme), and the other a more process-focused approach. As a result, differences in impact, that is, experience and outcomes, for practice emerged. Whilst both groups experienced the value of strong leadership, the emphasis on facilitation with one group of participants influenced the progress and involvement in the project overall. The challenge of transferring knowledge and skills from training was experienced by one group, whereas the other group seemed to benefit greatly from the opportunity to learn through practice. Both groups experienced the value of some form of stakeholder involvement, but significantly, through wide participation and collaboration, one group appeared to both sense and achieve greater ownership. Whilst both groups experienced the influence of context, one group felt they benefited significantly from organisational support. However, this group also experienced the tentative nature of context in a health care climate where organisational structures can quickly change. Values and decisions regarding evidence also influenced experience, the progress of the projects and sustainability of their practice development overall. Finally, both projects highlighted the benefit of having some form of external backing and support at a time when resources for practice development were limited.

It was apparent that both sets of project participants had experienced journeys in pursuit of improving patient care, but despite some common experiences, there were also some broad differences. Project 1, began with a strong impetus for change and development. There was a cohesive project team, a task (exercise programme) to implement and organisational support. The potential for achieving sustainable change seemed moderate to good, but throughout the project, participants' experiences remained a mix of positive and negative. By the end, it was evident that some impetus had been lost and with limited wider uptake of the exercise programme, participants were thinking about how to revitalise the initiative.

In Project 2, the impetus at the start of the project appeared more tentative with a more open focus on mealtimes and patient-centred care. The facilitators embarked on a whole care team approach that also involved a wide range of stakeholders. The initial experience was a mix of positive and negative, but towards the end of the project, this became more positive than negative. The impetus for change appeared stronger and ongoing, suggesting a greater likelihood of the new practice being sustained.

Through scrutiny, a number of micro level differences emerged, which when clustered together with the aforementioned broader differences, show fundamental and tangible differences in approaches used with resulting differences in terms of consequences or practice outcomes.

Unearthing the differing approaches to improving practice, the impact on and relevance for practice

Taking account of what is already known about practice development and reflecting on the two projects, it is suggested that there is a relationship between the practice development approaches observed in the two projects and the methodological perspectives relating to practice development described and explored by Manley and McCormack (2004), namely, technical (Project 1) and emancipatory (Project 2) practice development (Manley & McCormack, 2004).

Closer critical analysis of these real-world examples of activity to improve practice and patient care, provides greater insight regarding the similarities, differences and associated impact of the activities. The two projects represent characteristics of the two typologies or approaches for improving and developing practice, which resonate with current practice and have specific and significant consequences or outcomes for practitioners and practice (Shaw, 2009; 2012). The first, Project 1, whilst more aligned to technical practice development, would be better referred to as 'service improvement' (Typology 1, Box 4.3), a means of improving health care services that has a tendency to be both task focused and technical in its approach to achieving change or implementing a new service. There are connections here with the experiences of Henderson and McKillop (2008), who distinguished between practice development and service improvement as part of their work developing cancer services, and which arguably could have a much wider application to health care practice. Project 2 is more aligned to emancipatory practice development (Typology 2, Box 4.4), as defined by Garbett and McCormack (2002); Manley and McCormack (2004) and McCormack et al. (2006): a facilitated and collaborative process for enabling effectiveness in patient-centred care.

Box 4.3: Typology 1: service improvement

Service improvement

- Makes a contribution to improving practice and developing those involved.
- Methods and processes used may not enable collaboration, inclusion and participation.
- Potential for diminishing impact over time.

An activity contributes to the development and improvement of practice and practitioners, but the methods and processes may not enable the level of collaboration, inclusion and participation that could lead to culture change.

Box 4.4: Typology 2: practice development

Practice development

- Facilitated process, focused on enabling inclusion and participation of all stakeholders.
- Methods and processes used enable collaboration, inclusion and participation.
- Staff development and improvement in practice evident.
- Potential shift in values towards person-centredness.

A methodology underpinned by the key values of person-centredness, collaboration and partnership, enabling facilitation, active learning, culture transformation and evaluation for the development of health care practitioners and practice, for the ultimate purpose of achieving patient-centred care.

Service improvement and practice development: a critique

More specific features that discriminate between service improvement and practice development approaches using evidence from Projects 1 and 2 are demonstrated through adapting Stage 3 of Walker and Avant's (1995) concept analysis approach, presented in Tables 4.1

Table 4.1 Typology/Case 1 – technical/service improvement.

Antecedents	Critical attributes	Consequences (positive (+ ve) and negative (–ve))
What may need to be in place for the typology to take place	What key approaches, processes and strategies may be a feature in this typology	What are the likely key outcomes for practitioners and practice
		For practitioners
• Patient need identified from practice and policy	• Focus on new service provision	• Apprehension (–ve)
	• Project team responsible for implementing service improvement	• Frustration (–ve)
• Leadership (project leader)		• Achievement and pride (+ ve)
		• Professional development of project team members (+ ve)
• Cohesive project team with shared values relating to the project and to improving patient care	• Research evidence as the driver for change	• Staff interested in the new service but levels of participation variable (+ ve on a continuum/going in the right direction)
	• Systematic project plan developed and followed	
	• Project team members extend their knowledge, skills and roles, and develop new expertise to deliver the service improvement	• Lack of staff involvement and ownership (–ve)
• Research of the main evidence base and/or rationale for the service improvement		• New service perceived as extra work by staff (–ve)
• Organisational drive and management support	• Training provided for staff	• Differing agendas (in this case, lack of common vision and purpose) (–ve)
	• Specific team deliver the new service (in this case, the exercise programme)	For practice/service
• Team support process		• New service/development implemented by project team (+ ve)
• External support desirable	• Link nurses used as champions	• Care/practice improvements experienced by patients participating in new service/development (+ ve)
	• Support processes used by project team (in this case, team talked of action learning)	• Wider involvement variable (+ ve and –ve) (albeit moving in the right direction)

Table 4.2 Typology/Case 2 – practice development.

Antecedents	Critical attributes	Consequences (positive (+ve) and negative (–ve))
What may need to be in place for the typology to take place	*What key approaches, processes and strategies may be a feature in this typology*	*What are the likely key outcomes for practitioners and practice*

• Patient need from practice, service users and policy
• Leadership (ward team leaders)
• Whole team approach with willingness (in principle) to improve patient care
• Wide range of evidence[a] to underpin development
• Supportive ward manager and espoused organisational and management support (the degree to which this is lived or experienced may be ambivalent)
• Supervision and support seen as essential
• Internal facilitators available and predisposed to the following core values and beliefs:
  • Whole team approach
  • Inclusion and participation
  • Contribution of patient and staff experience
  • External support valued
	• Focus on becoming patient-centred
	• Collective responsibility for practice development
	• The patients' ongoing driver for development and change
	• Systematic plan focusing on processes and outcomes
	• Learning 'through' and 'in' practice
	• Facilitation approach enabling
	• Reflective practice used
	• Facilitators as role models
	• Inclusion and participation strongly evident
	• Full stakeholder involvement
	• Action learning principles used by facilitators to work with staff groups
		For practitioners
		• Frustrations (–ve) but decreasing (+ve)
		• Increase in person-centred attitudes toward patients and colleagues (+ve)
		• Personal growth (+ve)
		• Increased confidence (+ve)
		• Increased reflectivity (+ve)
		• Overcoming barriers to change (+ve)
		• Achievement and pride (+ve)
		• Sense of ownership (+ve)
		For practice
		• Care/practice improvements across practice, with evidence of care becoming more patient-centred (+ve)
		• Movement of workplace culture towards being patient-centred (+ve)
		• Perceived improvement in clinical effectiveness (+ve)
		• Team development: increased cohesion and understanding (+ve)
		• Participation and inclusion (became a lived value) (+ve)

[a]staff/clinical experiences, patients, policy, research.

and 4.2. Concept analysis provides the foundation for identifying and evaluating concepts and specific approaches. Stage 3 in Walker and Avant's (1995) approach offers a helpful tool to structure and critique information by focusing on the following:

1. The *antecedents* or conditions that precede the manifestation of a concept; in this case, what might need to be in place for the typology or case to take place?
2. The *critical attributes* or characteristics of the concept; in this case, what key approaches, processes and strategies may be a feature of the typology?
3. The *consequences* or outcomes relating to the concept; in this case, what are the likely key outcomes and consequences of the typology?

Adapted from Walker and Avant (1995)

Through critical discussion and with reference to Manley and McCormack (2004), and in particular, the systematic review of practice development (McCormack et al., 2006); six values were subsequently identified by Shaw (2009, 2012) (Box 4.5). The relative merits, influences and significance of both the typologies for quality improvement will now be expanded. New perspectives about the role and impact of service improvement are highlighted, along with new insights about practice development as a methodology and the identification of implications for future practice and health care quality improvement.

Box 4.5: Six values underpinning practice development

1. Person-centred care
2. Collaboration and partnership
3. Enabling facilitation and support
4. Commitment to active learning and development
5. Culture transformation
6. Evaluation

As previously stated, these values should inform the decision to use practice development methodology and the subsequent choice of methods. It is possible to determine the extent to which the work undertaken by Projects 1 and 2 represent service improvement (Typology 1; Table 4.1) as experienced in health care or practice development (Typology 2; Table 4.2); in turn, this may help those seeking to improve health care practice to consider how best to approach activity. Within the discussion, tentative phrases such as 'might' or 'may' are used rather than being definitive; these perspectives are open to further refinement and critique.

Person-centred care

In relation to the two typologies, there are several features that show the extent to which the activities are underpinned by the value of person-centred care. However, it is important to highlight that, in general, the projects (and therefore the typologies) referred to patient-centred care rather than person-centred care. The degree to which person-centred care and practice development are linked has been challenged by Dewing (2004) amongst others, because of the degree to which as a concept, it is universally understood. However, much of the literature does still refer to practice development alongside patient-centred care and practice including much of that contained within the systematic review (McCormack et al., 2006).

As Manley and McCormack (2004) suggest, improving patient care is a shared value, whether the focus is a technical one as in service improvement or (emancipatory) practice development. Both projects had identified an area for improving patient care based on a need that had been identified from practice. The additional influence and the value of policy in Typology 1 are also common in task-focused service improvement, where the impetus for change can come from policy directives and targets (Manley & McCormack, 2004). As Sanders (2004) experienced, the link with policy or targets can ensure support from the organisation as seen in Typology 1. However, the use of policy and targets can establish and perpetuate the use of strategies, where the dominate focus is the new service provision only (Sanders 2004), as was the case in Typology 1, with less if any regard for any wider issues related to patient care. A new service may subsequently be implemented with some benefits for patients, but as seen in Typology 1, the long-term sustainability may be variable (Sanders, 2004; Hooke et al., 2008).

In Typology 2, service users had influenced the identification of the need for change. Patient and service user involvement, as Dewar et al. (2003a, 2003b) found, can help root an initiative in practice and patient care and it is arguably an essential feature of practice development (McCormack et al., 2006). In Typology 2, the influence of the patient was seen as part of a strategy to focus on becoming patient-centred and this helped drive progress. As a consequence, the research findings indicated a movement towards more person-centred attitudes and behaviours, together with a movement towards a more person-centred workplace culture.

Collaboration and partnership

The value of collaboration and partnership, as indicated by McCormack et al. (2006), embraces the notion of practice development being an inclusive and ethical process, where person-centredness, shared vision, values and ownership are achieved through wide participation. An explicit example of partnership is stakeholder involvement and this featured in both typologies, perhaps indicating a wider recognition that cross-boundary working is more effective in complex health care systems (Henderson & McKillop, 2008). However, in relation to other aspects of participation and involvement, there were significant differences in the typologies.

Service improvement, as shown in Typology 1, is often enabled by a small project team who work well together and have a shared commitment to patient care. The project team act in a similar way to the single authority figure or project leader in technical practice development (Manley & McCormack, 2004), taking on the responsibility for the change. This was demonstrated in the findings relating to Typology 1, where the project team members extended their skills to be able to initiate the programme and support its delivery; intentionally or unintentionally, they became the main practitioners delivering the programme. Consequently, as Sanders (2004) experienced, the new service was not owned at the practice (in this case, ward) level and there was limited participation by the ward staff. This was frustrating for the team, who had been enthusiastic about the project: an indication of the kind of negative consequences that can occur as part of service improvement.

Typology 2, using a practice development approach, worked purposefully to involve the whole ward team. This was reflected in the methods they adopted, and whilst within the team, a very small number of people had specific roles and responsibilities, the use of action groups helped achieve collective responsibility for activity overall. Here, consequences that are more positive are seen, with participation and inclusion becoming 'a value' as well as 'an experience'. A further consequence of the 'whole team' participatory approach characterising Typology 2 was the evidence of wider improvements in patient care (Clarke et al., 2003; Moss et al., 2008).

Enabling facilitation and support

The value of, or commitment to, facilitation is primarily seen in Typology 2. Within the literature, there are many references to the presence and the importance of a skilled facilitator role (Dewing et al., 2004; Manley & McCormack, 2004; Webster & Dewing, 2007; Shaw et al., 2008). Facilitation that is holistic (Harvey et al., 2002) or enabling (Shaw et al., 2008) is a strong value and an intentional process in practice development, which is also demonstrated in Typology 2.

In Typology 2, as an enabling factor for practice development, facilitators need to be predisposed to a number of core values and beliefs specifically, participation and inclusion that also comprises patient and staff experiences (McCormack et al., 2006). It is also important to note that the core values held by the facilitators were not simply espoused, rather they were 'lived by' and experienced by others taking part. Linked to active learning, the facilitators of Typology 2 worked as role models and focused on learning in and through practice. Consequently, practitioners experienced personal growth, increased confidence and as previously demonstrated, attitudinal shifts towards person-centred care (Moss et al., 2008).

Other features in Typology 2 relate to facilitation and support, including a commitment to supervision, action learning and creating opportunities for support and challenge, which all appear consistent with the notion of enabling facilitation in practice development (Shaw et al., 2008). Some of these features are also experienced in service improvement (Typology 1), but are often limited, so that only a few key individuals benefit; for example, in Project 1 (Typology 1) it was only the project team that experienced the team support processes.

Leadership has a role in supporting and maintaining project progress in both typologies. Shaw (2005) suggests that there is evidence of a close relationship between the role of leadership and practice development facilitation. In Project 1 (Typology 1), the leader was noted to be essential to the success of the project. In contrast to what might be expected in technically focused service improvement, the leader was experienced (by other participants) to be visionary, influential and resourceful. These are all characteristics of transformational leaders (Manley, 2000) recognised as supportive of practice development (Binnie & Titchen, 1998), as well as qualities required for practice development (Garbett & McCormack, 2003). It could be argued that without strong and effective leadership, Project 1 may have floundered. Although not as strong a feature in the data of Project 2, leadership was present as a value that enabled practice development.

Commitment to active learning and development

A commitment to active learning and development embraces a range of methods (Dewing, 2008) for enabling purposeful learning through experience and practice. In the context of this value, Typology 1 is shown to be strongly consistent with service improvement in many ways because the processes and activities do not encourage active learning. Firstly, training was used as the key process for sharing information and gaining involvement in the new service. Whilst the Project 1 team members (Typology 1) benefited from professional development as a consequence of taking part in the initiative, but as described by Manley and McCormack (2004), in technical practice development, there was little explicit commitment to develop individuals outside of the project team. This remains true of many service improvement activities despite a growing appreciation that new skills and knowledge are unlikely to be transferred by teaching and training alone (Harvey et al., 2002; Rycroft-Malone et al., 2004; Karlsen, 2007). Secondly, the strategy of having link nurses, which is quite commonplace as part of service improvement, reduces the opportunity for others to learn, as the link person is seen as the expert advisor. In Project 1 (Typology 1), it was often the case that the link nurses delivered the exercise programme rather than promote its use by others in practice. Finally, active learning can be stifled where there is a focus on research evidence only and the technical rational belief that this should ensure practice change. It can be argued that all three aspects contributed to the consequences of apprehension and frustration, resulting in a lack of wider staff involvement experienced by the team in Project 1.

In Typology 2, commitment to active learning and development was demonstrated in a number of explicit ways, including the use of action learning principles, reflective practice, role-modelling and peer learning. Active learning was also evident in the way this typology used knowledge and evidence from patients and practice, and created opportunities for practitioners to generate ideas for ongoing development. It became clear that a commitment to active learning resulted in a number of positive outcomes consistent with practice development, including personal growth, increased confidence, greater reflectivity and, interlinked with all of these, a sense of achievement (McCormack et al., 2006; Dewing, 2008; Moss et al., 2008).

Transforming workplace culture

Practice development has the potential to transform workplace culture (Garbett & McCormack, 2002; Manley & McCormack, 2004; McCormack et al., 2006; Manley et al., 2011) and is often aspired to in reported practice development projects (Dewing & Wright, 2003). Service improvement, however, does not share this aspiration. Just as Henderson and McKillop (2008) suggest that service improvement may not have any commitment to culture change, so it is not surprising that there was no evidence of this seen in Typology 1. Rather, the focus in Typology 1 was the implementation of a new service, directly focused on an area of patient need. Whilst there was a sense of achievement and pride as a consequence of the benefits seen to care, there was also frustration as is often the case when the 'surface' rather than the 'culture' of practice is tackled. This relates to the limited involvement of the ward staff, which from the findings, the project team recognised had implications for the sustainability of the initiative. Sustainability is a key challenge for service improvement as found when using most technical strategies (Manley & McCormack, 2004).

Whilst in Typology 2, the aspiration of culture change is not explicit, participant data from the research indicated that it was an important outcome. The presence of several of the enabling factors, although not explicitly related to culture change, may have increased the opportunity in Typology 2 for culture transformation, for example, the whole team approach, the value placed on wide evidence (Manley & McCormack, 2004) and valuing the patient experience (Dewar et al., 2003a, 2003b; Tolson et al., 2006). Further opportunity for culture change may also have been facilitated by the use of strategies for inclusion, reflective practice and learning in and from practice. Overall, there was evidence of some shift in the workplace culture towards a greater focus on patient-centred care.

Evaluation

Evaluation that focuses on both the processes used and outcomes achieved is another key element of practice development (McCormack et al., 2006; Wilson et al., 2008). This contrasts with service improvement, which like technical practice development, tends to focus on audit and measurement of outcomes only (Manley & McCormack, 2004).

Surprisingly, within the research findings, and hence the two typologies, there was little referral to evaluation as a process. However, there was evidence in relation to both typologies that some evaluation of practice was undertaken; for example, practice outcomes are included in the reports produced by the project teams. Those outcomes referred to in the typologies arose mainly from research data gathered during focus groups with participants.

Process evaluation appears implicit in Typology 2 because of the commitment given to use methods such as reflective practice to gather evidence about the process, consistent with practice development. In Typology 1, the team support process was an opportunity to discuss and evaluate activity. What cannot be judged is the level to which this contributed to the project's evaluation.

Service improvement and practice development: in summary

Project 1 did appear to be more closely aligned to service improvement (Typology 1). It made a contribution to the improvement of practice and the development of those involved; however, the methods and processes used did not enable collaboration, inclusion and participation. As a result, the overall impact of the practice was diminished over time. Project 2 did have a range of features consistent with the values of practice development (Typology 2). The project was enabled by facilitators who valued inclusion and participation, as well as the experience and contribution of patients and staff. A range of methods that enable participation in learning through practice contributed to a number of outcomes that are consistent with practice development, including the development of staff, improvement in patient care and movement toward a more patient-centred culture (McCormack et al., 2006).

There are, however, questions that need to be answered in relation to the differences between service development and practice development. First, are there any scale, size or speciality issues that influence the selection of a service improvement or practice development approach? Second, at what point does service improvement become practice development? Both Projects 1 and 2 occurred in the same specialist area of older people care, and whilst Project 1 covered three wards and Project 2 just one ward, the selection of the approach related more to the underlying aims of each project. In Project 1, the aim was the implementation of evidence and a new service, whereas for Project 2, the aim was to increase commitment to person-centred care. Based on the research findings, Shaw (2009) suggests that the scale and size of the projects are not significant. With regard to the second question, Shaw (2009) argues that service improvement might become practice development when the processes and outcomes used in service improvement demonstrate integration with, and reflect the values of, practice development, as refined by Shaw (2009) from McCormack et al. (2006). Finally, as stated previously, the typologies do not represent complete types or cases because they were developed using only the findings data and as such may not contain all the features of practice development and service improvement. Whilst they offer insight for practice in their current form, further development using additional evidence from practice and the literature could increase their relevance and value.

Implications for practice

The articulation of these two typologies (through a research process) provides new insight into practice development as an emancipatory methodological approach for enabling improvement in person-centred health care practice and transformational, person-centred cultures. It also draws attention to the place and value of service improvement as an activity that contributes to the development and improvement of health care services.

Whilst McCormack et al. (2006) suggest that no one methodology best serves practice development, Shaw (2009, 2012) argues for some re-thinking. Whilst practice development has and will continue to be informed by a range of methods, the methodology has become much clearer, particularly when viewed from the perspective of building on the concept analysis of practice development (Garbett & McCormack, 2002) and the systematic review of practice development (McCormack et al., 2006). Yet it is also evident that some initiatives do not achieve the key outcome of increasing person-centred care, validated as part of practice development (McCormack et al., 2006) and seen in reported examples and research from practice (Dewar et al., 2003a, 2003b; Tolson et al., 2006; Moss et al., 2008). With this in mind, rather than being seen on a continuum with activities such as service improvement, practice development should stand independently as a methodology (underpinned by six key values) for enabling the development of health care practitioners and practice, through collaboration, inclusion and participation for the ultimate purpose of achieving patient-centred care as defined by Manley et al. (2008):

> *Practice development is a continuous process of developing person centred cultures. It is enabled by facilitators who authentically engage with individuals and teams to blend personal qualities and creative imagination with practice skills and practice wisdom. The learning that occurs brings about transformations of individual and team practices. This is sustained by embedding both processes and outcomes in corporate strategy. (Manley et al., 2008, p. 9)*

Secondly, it is perhaps time to move away from the notion and cease using the phrase 'technical' practice development, as this misrepresents both technical activities undertaken to improve health care service and practice development. Instead, those activities often called technical practice development are better represented by the term service improvement (Shaw, 2009, 2012), an activity that makes a valuable contribution to the development of quality health care services (Henderson & McKillop, 2008).

Making the distinction between service development and practice development is important in terms of understanding what enables improvement and change and how different ways of working may result in different outcomes. However, there is also a suggestion that by using the methods and processes of practice development methodology, service improvement could be strengthened by increasing participation in and hence achieving sustainability of health care service improvement initiatives. Indeed, Figure 4.1 shows how activity can progress from service improvement to practice development. In this sense, the approach to improving health care practice should not focus on an either-or approach, but consider purposefully, what would most effectively achieve the desired outcomes. So in essence, by engaging in systematic practice development, service improvement outcomes can also be achieved.

Transformational practice development

There is one further aspect of contemporary theoretical development to revisit, and that is the influence of critical creativity. With the development and refinement of this new theoretical perspective (McCormack & Titchen, 2006; Titchen & McCormack, 2010), the notion of practice development underpinned by emancipatory processes, as define within critical social theory, has been challenged. It is suggested that the needs of health care practice and people within it would be better fulfilled by transformational practice development:

> *… more a way of living, being, doing, inquiring and becoming in professional work (i.e. a practice ontology and epistemology) rather than a time-limited project or programme. It is not a set of tools (although it makes use of them); rather, it is through the use of self and one's knowing and being, in relationship with others, that brings about transformation. (Titchen & McCormack, 2010, p. 533)*

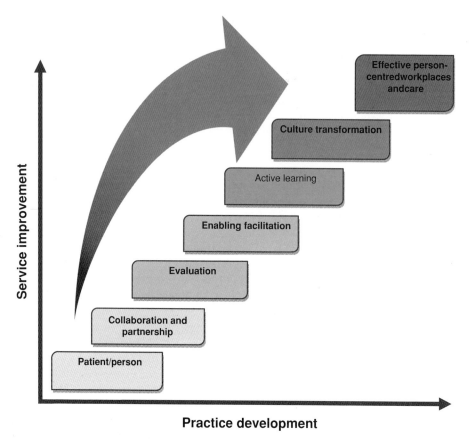

Fig. 4.1   From service improvement to practice development.

At the present time, when improvement activity in health care still continues to rely on traditional approaches to change, often in response to targets and policy, there would need to be a radical shift in values, attitudes and culture at all levels to move toward the use of transformative approaches. Indeed, for many, even mention of 'emancipation' can give rise to much cynicism. However, with an implicit focus on human flourishing (Titchen et al., 2011), transformational approaches would place emphasis on creating effective and person-centred cultures in health care where people (patients/families and staff) are the primary focus rather than tasks and services. In short, a shift towards acknowledging the need to invest in people really could make all the difference.

CONCLUSION

There have been tremendous advances in practice development from both theoretical and practice perspectives. Understanding of the influence of critical social theory has grown and new perspectives are emerging that could offer new challenge to how health care approaches the business of continuous improvement in health care practice. In addition, increasing knowledge and understanding about the 'practice' of practice development and the values and principles underpinning it have matched the methodological insights. For those working in the field of practice development and the enablement of others in the pursuit of high-quality patient-centred care, it is perhaps time to endorse the values and beliefs that underpin practice development and the achievement of effective person-centre practice. Furthermore, rather than dismissing some of the more technical and task-orientated service improvement activities as potentially ineffectual, the adoption of a more positive and supportive stance is required. The application of knowledge and skills from practice development can enable the ongoing development of health care services, alongside activity to transform workplace and organisational cultures towards a growing aspiration for person-centred health care.

REFLECTIVE QUESTIONS

1. To what extent do the typologies of service improvement and practice development represent the kind of approaches to improvement and change you experience in your workplace?
2. What could be the relative merits of practice development standing independently as a methodology (underpinned by the six key values) for enabling the development of health care practitioners and practice, through collaboration, inclusion and participation for the ultimate purpose of achieving patient-centred care (McCormack et al., 2006)?
3. Consider whether the phrase 'technical' practice development, misrepresents both the technical activities undertaken to improve health care service and practice development, and reflect on whether it should still be used?
4. Reflect on whether activities that to date have been referred to as technical practice development, are better represented by the phrase 'service improvement', a valuable activity that contributes to the development of quality health care services?
5. How can the range of methods within practice development methodology strengthen service improvement activity in relation to participation in, and sustainability of, quality health care service improvements?
6. What added value might be gained by further refining the (emancipatory) practice development towards transformational practice development through the application of critical creativity as articulated by Titchen et al. (2011)?

REFERENCES

Balfour, M. & Clarke, C. (2001) Searching for sustainable change. *Journal of Clinical Nursing*, **10** (1), 44–50.

Bates, G. (2000) The challenge of practice development unit accreditation within an elective orthopaedic ward. *Journal of Orthopaedic Nursing*, **4** (4), 170–174.

Bevan, H. (2010) How can we build skills to transform the healthcare system? *Journal of Research in Nursing*, **15** (2), 139–148.

Binnie, A. & Titchen, A. (1998) *Freedom to Practise: An Action Research Study of Practice Development in an Acute Medical Unit*. Royal College of Nursing, London.

Bouras, C. & Barrett, C. (2007) Strategies to enhance patient-centred care in a cardiothoracic surgical unit. *Practice Development in Health Care*, **6** (3), 150–164.

Carr, W. & Kemmis, S. (1986) *Becoming Critical: Education, Knowledge and Action Research*. Falmer Press, London.

Clarke, A., Hanson, E.J. & Ross, H. (2003) Seeing the person behind the patient: enhancing the care of older people using a biographical approach. *Journal of Clinical Nursing*, **12** (5), 697–706.

Dewar, B., Tocher, R. & Watson, W. (2003a) Enhancing partnerships with relatives in care setting for older people. *Foundation of Nursing Studies Dissemination Series*, **2** (2), 1–4.

Dewar, B., Tocher, R. & Watson, W. (2003b) Using work-based learning to enable practice development. *Foundation of Nursing Studies Dissemination Series*, **2** (3), 1–4.

Dewing, J. (2004) Concerns relating to the application of frameworks to promote person-centredness in nursing with older people. *International Journal of Older People Nursing*, **13** (3a), 39–44.

Dewing, J. (2008) Becoming and being active learners and creating active learning workplaces: the value of active learning in practice development. In: *International Practice Development in Nursing and Healthcare* (eds K. Manley, B. McCormack & V. Wilson), pp. 273–294. Blackwell Publishing Ltd., Oxford.

Dewing, J., Hancock, S., Brooks, J., Pedder, L., Adams, L., Riddaway, L., Ugloe, J. & O'Connor, P. (2004) An account of a 360 degree review as part of a practice development strategy. *Practice Development in Health Care*, **3** (4), 193–209.

Dewing, J. & Wright, J. (2003) A practice development project for nurses working with older people. *Practice Development in Health Care*, **2** (1), 13–28.

Dickinson, A.M., Welch, C. & Ager, L. (2006) Improving the health of older people: implementing patient-focused mealtime practice (eds T. Shaw & K. Sanders). *Foundation of Nursing Studies Dissemination Series*, **3** (10), 1–4.

Fay, B. (1987) *Critical Social Science*. Polity Press, Cambridge.

Garbett, R. & McCormack, B. (2002) A concept analysis of practice development. *Nursing Times Research*, **7**, (2), 87–100.

Garbett, R. & McCormack, B. (2003) The qualities and skills of practice developers. *Journal of Clinical Nursing*, **12** (3), 317–325.

Grundy, S. (1982) Three modes of action research. *Curriculum Perspectives*, **2** (3), 23–34.

Habermas, J. (1972) *Knowledge and Human Interests*. Heinemann, London.

Harvey, G., Loftus-Hills, A., Rycroft-Malone, J., Titchen, A., Kitson, A., McCormack, B. & Seers, K. (2002) Getting evidence into practice: the role and function of facilitation. *Journal of Advanced Nursing*, **37** (6), 577–588.

Hayes, N. (2006) 'Ward workout' – implementing nurse-led exercise programmes for in patients on rehabilitation wards for older people (eds T. Shaw & K. Sanders). *Foundation of Nursing Studies Dissemination Series*, **3** (9), 1–4.

Henderson, L. & McKillop, S. (2008) Using practice development approaches in the development of a managed clinical network. In: *International Practice Development in Nursing and Healthcare* (eds K. Manley, B. McCormack & V. Wilson), pp. 319–348. Blackwell Publishing Ltd., Oxford.

Hooke, N., Lewis, P., Kelly, M., Wilson, V. & Jones, S. (2008) Making something of it: one ward's application of evidence into practice. *Practice Development in Health Care*, **7** (2), 79–91.

Johns, C. (2000) *Becoming a Reflective Practitioner - a Reflective and Holistic Approach to Clinical Nursing, Practice Development, and Clinical Supervision*. Blackwell Publishing Ltd., Oxford.

Karlsen, R. (2007) Improving the nursing documentation: professional consciousness-raising in a Northern-Norwegian psychiatric hospital. *Journal of Psychiatric and Mental Health Nursing*, **14** (6), 573–577.

Kitson, A.L., Ahmed, L.D., Harvey, G., Seers, K. & Thompson, D.R. (1996) From research to practice: one organisational model for promoting research based practice. *Journal of Advanced Nursing*, **23** (3), 430–440.

Manley, K. (2000) Organisational culture and consultant nurse outcomes: part 1- organisational culture. *Nursing Standard*, **14** (36), 34–38.

Manley, K., Crisp, J. & Moss, C. (2011) Advancing the practice development outcomes agenda within multiple contexts. *International Practice Development Journal*, **1** (1) Article 4.

Manley, K. & McCormack, B. (2004) Practice development: purpose, methodology, facilitation and evaluation. In: *Practice Development in Nursing* (eds B. McCormack, K. Manley & R. Garbett), pp. 33–50. Blackwell Publishing Ltd., Oxford.

Manley, K., McCormack, B. & Wilson, V. (2008) *International Practice Development in Nursing and Healthcare*. Blackwell Publishing Ltd., Oxford.

Marshall, M. (2011) What has health service research done to improve patient care? *Journal of Research in Nursing*, **16** (2), 101–104.

McCormack, B. (2010) Clinical practice development. *Journal of Research in Nursing*, **15** (2), 189–192.

McCormack, B., Dewar, B., Wright, J., Garbett, R., Harvey, J. & Ballantine, K. (2006) *A Realist Synthesis of Evidence Relating to Practice Development: Final Report to the NHS Education for Scotland and NHS Quality Improvement Scotland*. NHS Quality Improvement Scotland, Edinburgh.

McCormack, B., Manley, K., Kitson, A., Titchen, A. & Harvey, G. (1999) Towards practice development – a vision in reality or reality without vision. *Journal of Nursing Management*, **7** (5), 255–264.

McCormack, B. & Titchen, A. (2006) Critical creativity: melding, exploding, blending. *Educational Action Research*, **14** (2), 239–266.

McGill, I. & Beaty, L. (1997) *Action Learning*. Kogan Page, London.

McKenna, H., Ashton, S. & Keeney, S. (2004) Barriers to evidence-based practice in primary care. *Journal of Advanced Nursing*, **45** (2), 178–189.

Moss, C., Walsh, K., Jordan, Z. & Macdonald, L. (2008) The impact of practice development in an emergency department: a pluralistic evaluation. *Practice Development in Health Care*, **7** (2), 93–107.

Patterson, M. (2011) *From Metrics to Meaning: Culture Change and Quality of Acute Hospital Care for Older People*. Report for the National Institute for Health Research Service Delivery and Organisation programme. HMSO, London.

Pawson, R. & Tilley, N. (1997) *Realistic Evaluation*. Sage, London.

Pemberton, J. & Reid, B. (2005) A systematic approach to the improvement of patient care. *Nursing Times*, **101** (24), 34–36.

Redfern, S., Christian, S. & Norman, I. (2003) Evaluating change in health care practice: lessons from three studies. *Journal of Evaluation in Clinical Practice*, **9** (2), 239–249.

Rycroft-Malone, J., Harvey, G., Seers, K., Kitson, A., McCormack, B. & Titchen, A. (2004) An exploration of the factors that influence the implementation of evidence into practice. *Journal of Advanced Nursing*, **13** (8), 913–924.

Sanders, K. (2004) Developing and implementing a family health assessment: from project worker to practice developer. In: *Practice Development in Nursing* (eds B. McCormack, K. Manley & R. Garbett), pp. 291–311. Blackwell Publishing Ltd., Oxford.

Schon, D. (1983) *The Reflective Practitioner*. Basic Books, New York.

Schon, D.A. (1987) *Educating the Reflective Practitioner*. Jossey-Bass, London.

Shaw, T. (2005) Leadership for practice development. In: *Effective Healthcare Leadership* (eds M. Jasper & M. Jumaa), pp. 207–221. Blackwell Publishing Ltd., Oxford.

Shaw, T. (2009) *A Qualitative Descriptive Exploration of the Experiences of Healthcare Practitioners Involved in Practice Development*. Unpublished Doctor of Nursing (NursD) thesis, University of Nottingham.

Shaw, T. (2011) Review: knowledge transfer and the integration of research, policy and practice for patient benefit. *Journal of Research in Nursing*, **16** (3), 271–273.

Shaw, T. (2012) Unravelling the consequence of practice development: an exploration of the experiences of healthcare practitioners. *International Practice Development Journal*, **2** (2), 1–25.

Shaw, T., Dewing, J., Young, R., Devlin, M., Boomer, C. & Legius, M. (2008) Enabling practice development: delving into the concept of facilitation from a practitioner perspective. In: *International Practice Development in Nursing and Healthcare* (eds K. Manley, B. McCormack & V. Wilson), pp. 147–169. Blackwell Publishing Ltd., Oxford.

Titchen, A. & McCormack, A. (2010) Dancing with stones: critical creativity as methodology for human flourishing. *Educational Action Research*, **18** (4), 531–554.

Titchen, A., McCormack, B., Wilson, V. & Solman, A. (2011) Human flourishing through body, creative imagination and reflection. *International Practice Development Journal*, **1** (1), 1–18. http://www.fons.org/library/journal/volume1-issue1/article1 (Accessed June 2011).

Tolson, D., Booth, J. & Lowndes, A. (2008) Achieving evidence-based nursing practice: impact of the Caledonian Development Model. *Journal of Nursing Management*, **16** (6), 682–691.

Tolson, D., McAloon, M. & Hotchkiss, R. (2005) Progressing evidence-based practice: an effective nursing model? *Journal of Advanced Nursing*, **50** (2), 124–133.

Tolson, D., Schofield, I., Booth, J., Kelly, T.B. & James, L. (2006) Constructing a new approach to developing evidence based practice with nurses and older people. *Worldviews on Evidence Based Nursing*, **3** (2), 62–72.

Walker, L.O. & Avant, K.C. (1995) *Strategies for Theory Construction in Nursing*, 3rd edn. Appleton and Lange, Norwalk CT.

Webster, J. & Dewing, J. (2007) Growing a development strategy for community hospitals. *Practice Development in Healthcare*. **6** (2), 97–106.

Wilson, V., Hardy, S. & Brown, R. (2008) An exploration of practice development evaluation: unearthing praxis. In: *International Practice Development in Nursing and Healthcare* (eds K. Manley, B. McCormack & V. Wilson), pp. 126–146. Blackwell Publishing Ltd., Oxford.

5 A Case Study of Practice Development 'The Practice Development Journey'

Brendan McCormack[1] and Jan Dewing[2]

[1]University of Ulster, Newtownabbey, UK
[2]East Sussex Healthcare NHS Trust & Canterbury Christ Church University, Canterbury, UK

INTRODUCTION

In the context of the practice development 'journey' metaphor that we have used to focus the chapters in this book, this chapter should be read as a holistic example of the whole journey. In this chapter, we present an overview of a national practice development programme – 'The Older Persons Services National Practice Development Programme'. This was a collaborative programme over 2 years between the University of Ulster and the Republic of Ireland Health Service Executive (HSE). It involved older people, families and multi-disciplinary staff (including, e.g., registered nurses, care support workers, catering, domestic, gardening, maintenance, administration, volunteer and medical staff). The programme was facilitated in eighteen residential sites where older people live across the four HSE Administrative Areas in the Republic of Ireland (ROI). The programme was led and facilitated by two nurse researchers from the University of Ulster and six nurses from the HSE Nursing and Midwifery Planning and Development Units (NMPDU)[1]. Funding for the 2-year period was obtained from the National Council for the Professional Development of Nursing and Midwifery[2] and the HSE.

Like many countries, the ROI has a mixed economy of residential care provision. Residential services are provided through a network of local community hospitals and publicly, voluntary and privately funded nursing homes. Across the sector, 'National Quality Standards for Residential Care Settings for Older People' (HIQA, 2010) have been introduced. These have person-centred practice as a central strategic direction for service delivery. The standards highlight the need for empowerment of older people in residential settings. Therefore, this person-centred practice development programme was consistent with the national priorities for the development of residential services and enabled the preparation for and enhanced implementation of the national quality standards.

---

[1] There are eight Nursing and Midwifery Planning and Development Units (NMPDU) in the Republic of Ireland. The NMPDU is an integral component of the Health Service Executive, coordinating continuing professional development, practice development, quality improvement and workforce developments in the Health Service Executive areas.

[2] The purpose of the Council is to promote and develop the professional roles of nurses and midwives in partnership with stakeholders in order to support the delivery of quality nursing and midwifery care to patients/clients in a changing healthcare environment.

Practice Development in Nursing and Healthcare, Second Edition. Edited by Brendan McCormack, Kim Manley and Angie Titchen.
© 2013 John Wiley & Sons, Ltd. Published 2013 by John Wiley & Sons, Ltd.

AIMS AND OBJECTIVES

The overall aims of the programme were to implement a framework for person-centred practice for older people across multiple settings in Ireland, through a collaborative facilitation model and to carry out an evaluation of the processes and outcomes.

For the purposes of this programme, the team defined person-centredness as:

an approach to practice established through the formation and fostering of therapeutic relationships between all care providers, older people and others significant to them in their lives. It is underpinned by values of respect for persons, individual right to self determination, mutual respect and understanding. It is enabled by cultures of empowerment that foster continuous approaches to practice development. (McCormack et al., 2009a)

Objectives

1. Coordinate a programme of work that can replicate effective PD processes in care of older people's settings.
2. Enable participants/local facilitators and their directors and managers to recognise the attributes of person-centred cultures for older people and key practice development and management interventions needed to achieve the culture (thus embedding person-centred care within organisations).
3. Develop person-centred cultures in participating practice settings.
4. Systematically measure or evaluate outcomes on practice and for older people.
5. Further test a model of person-centred practice in long-term care/rehabilitation settings and develop it as a multi-professional model.
6. Utilise a participant generated data set to inform the development and outcomes of person-centred practice (already designed and tested tools will be used to produce data set).
7. Enable local NMPDU facilitators to work with shared principles, models, methods and processes in practice development work across older people's services.

METHODOLOGY

The programme drew on numerous principles from different yet complementary theories and approaches: emancipatory practice development (e.g. Garbett & McCormack, 2004; Manley & McCormack, 2004; Titchen, 2004; Dewing, 2009; van de Zipj & Dewing, 2009), cooperative inquiry (Heron & Reason, 2001) and a specific person-centred nursing framework (McCormack & McCance, 2006). Additionally, through the programme another methodology, namely, 'active learning' (Dewing, 2008a, 2009; McCormack et al., 2009b) emerged, was systematically tested refined and expanded. Within the approach, and for the aims of this programme, particular emphasis was placed on evaluation and on learning.

Structure and processes

Eighteen residential units for older people participated in the programme. The programme commenced in September 2007. An awareness campaign was initially held in each participating site with an open invitation to attend extended to all staff, older people and their families. Although there were some similarities in what events took place, there were also local differences according to context and the creativity of staff for how they went about creating and building awareness about the programme. Following on from these sessions, practice development programme groups were established. The groups represented staff from different areas within the units and different grades, that is Clinical Nurse Mangers, Staff Nurses, Health Care Assistants, Housekeeping, Catering and Administration staff.

The participants from the groups at each site met with the internal facilitator from within their unit and the external facilitator from the NMPDU for a formal programme and skills development day every 6 weeks approximately. As the first year progressed a range of interim meetings and discussions groups were established within the workplace in between these days. In year 2, these sessions evolved into project working and action plan implementation groups. Overall, the programme days were well attended, and the rate of engagement with workplace activities designed to enable learning and model changes in practice remained high.

Programme activities

The programme had a number of visible activities that took place on a regular basis. These were as follows:

- Daylong workshops or programme days at each site (approximately 12 over 2 years)
- Two-hour interim sessions
- Project working groups or action implementation groups
- Managers Stakeholder Group
- National Reference Group meetings
- Meetings with NMPDU Directors
- Programme team development and planning days
- Site visits by the programme leads

Overarching these 'events' were programme activities that principally involved the following:

- Developing an understanding of what the work/practice development involves and the competence and confidence to role model the processes to be used.
- Becoming familiar with the Person-Centred Practice Framework and Practice Development Model as the frameworks used for the programme and for achieving the above.
- Developing an understanding of workplace culture and 'change' processes.
- Awareness raising activities for different staff groups, older people and families in the programme sites.
- Developing a shared vision using Values Clarification Exercises involving the residents/ patients families/carers and all staff within their workplace. Clarifying values and beliefs and agreeing common or shared values and beliefs is the first step in collaborative practice development work. Using values clarification exercises to give a sense of direction a common vision for the future. Developing and working with shared vision statements.
- Active Learning in the workplace. Examples included the following:
  - *Person-centred language*: At the beginning of year 1, participants were asked to reflect on how person-centred their everyday language was. This not only applied to the

language used when speaking to older people but also to each other and language used in documentation. Participants developed posters to generate group discussion amongst the programme groups. The posters were then displayed throughout the units, which again promoted discussion about person-centredness and workplace cultures.

- *Observations of practice*: Participants were all involved in carrying out several short observations of the care setting (how the environment worked) and of care practices ('see', 'hear' and 'imagine'). This helped the participants get a greater understanding of how person-centred the care was for the older person within their units. Seeing practice, raising consciousness about taken-for-granted practices and assumptions and reflecting on them are key components of the observation activities. Providing feedback to the staff in the form of a 'critical dialogue' was essential to challenging practice by highlighting the differences between values espoused and those observed in practice. These activities highlighted the need to see things from a different perspective and to facilitate therapeutic/relationship-based care that can be sustained and thus transform health care delivery. It enabled participants to reflect on how they practice and the things they take for granted. Participants also facilitated other team members to undertake these activities for themselves.
- *Environmental walkabouts*: Environmental walkabouts by the participants took place at all the sites. The purpose of these was for participants to look at how person-centred or not the environment was for older people. The basis for this was that unless we offer older people an environment that compensates for impairments and disabilities, as far as is possible, they are being made to be more disabled and dependent than is needed. The data collected were used to inform the development of action plans in year 2. Participants facilitated additional walkabouts with other staff. In some sites older people and family members were involved in this activity and in a few sites photography was used.

- *Structured reflection*: Participants were introduced to a model of reflection and the use of reflective questioning which they were encouraged to use at all programme events and every day. Participating in structured reflection showed some signs of assisting participants in both their personal and professional learning. At the end of year 1, a representative sample of written reflections were analysed. As a consequence more attention was given to this method in year 2.
- *Facilitation skills development*: Listening, the use of enabling questions, high challenge, high support, giving and receiving feedback are all components of facilitation that were explored and developed in the programme. Participants were introduced to these skills and were encouraged to develop their confidence further in using them in their every-day work and across their workplaces to help develop a more person-centred culture. Active learning methods were used to enable participants to enhance their skills in a focused way.
- Developing an understanding and gaining direction on how practice development processes would impact positively on the achievement of the National Standards for Residential Care developed by the Health Information and Quality Authority (HIQA). All the objectives and development processes were mapped to the HIQA Standards and these were used to explore the findings from the evaluation data and inform action plans developed.
- Developing greater appreciation of and skills in effective group and team working.
- Introduction to the evaluation methodology used for the programme and involvement in the collection of the evaluation data. A range of evaluation tools and processes were

used in this programme. Wherever possible, programme participants were involved in collecting and analysing these data and informing the identification of outcomes. This intention further contributed to changing the social power within their workplaces.

Programme evaluation

The processes and outcomes from the practice development programme were evaluated within a framework of cooperative inquiry (Heron & Reason, 2001), primarily drawing upon reflective dialogue data between lead facilitators, project participants and the project leaders; interview data with all participants and records of developments. In addition, a number of 'evaluative instruments' were used. These instruments have been developed as components of previous research and development in person-centred nursing and have established validity and reliability data. The project leaders, lead facilitators and project participants all acted as co-researchers in the collection and analysis of data. Thus, the framework has the added benefit of developing evidence gathering and research skills among participants.

Data were collected at three time points during the programme: approximately between December 2007 and March 2008 and again at two more time points (January–February 2009 and August–September 2009). The tools used were as follows:

1. *Person-centred nursing index* (PCNI; Slater & McCormack, 2007): This tool measures the processes and outcomes of person-centred nursing from both nursing and patient perspectives.
2. *Person-centred caring index* (PCCI; Slater & McCormack, 2007): This tool measures the processes and outcomes of person-centred caring from health care worker perspectives (including health care assistants and other care workers in the care setting who contribute to patient care). It was piloted in sites within the north-west region prior to national use.
3. *Cultural observation tool* (Workplace Culture Critical Analysis Tool (WCCAT); McCormack et al., 2009): This observation of practice tool explores the culture of a workplace at a number of levels in order to inform the degree to which changes in practice are achieving a change in culture.
4. *User narratives*: Utilising a framework developed by Hsu & McCormack (2011) for collecting and analysing older peoples' stories about the quality of care, these data would serve to bring richness and depth to the other data sets.

Data collected using the environment awareness and impact and the observation of practice tools were analysed at a local level only and the data used to inform the development of local action plans. Data collected using the PCNI, PCCI, cultural observation tool and user narratives were analysed at a local level to inform the development of action plans and collectively at a national level to inform the effectiveness of processes and outcome achievement across the programme as a whole. All the data were analysed using a participatory approach with programme participants, programme facilitators and programme leaders.

Ethical approval

Ethical approval was given by the appropriate body in all the regions involved in the programme. Approval included the use of process consent (Dewing, 2002, 2006, 2008b) that enabled the inclusion of older people with a dementia into the evaluation.

OUTCOMES

Learning and development outcomes arising from the facilitation activities

The overall aim of the programme days was to enable staff to have the confidence to become facilitators of practice development in their own workplaces. This was a complex and slowly unfolding process. In the first instance, staff who were attending the programme days needed to be able to self-facilitate in order to role model the new ways of being in their day-to-day work. Then they needed to find ways to influence their colleagues to adopt new ways of relating and being.

Each daylong workshop had a programme and facilitation guidance. For year 1, the external programme leads devised the workshop programme and produced the facilitation guidance. This had several benefits:

- It ensured educational quality in regard to the planning and organisation of learning for programme participants.
- It ensured national consistency in terms of how the days were delivered and the coordination of workplace learning activities.
- It enabled the NMPDU facilitators to focus of developing their skills in facilitating the workshops based on translating the pre-prepared facilitation guidance.
- The facilitators were able to share experiences within the team, as they had been working on the same programmes and drawing on the same guidance.
- It provided detailed written guidance and structure for new internal facilitators to work from and a theoretical background to enhance their knowledge.
- It contributed more readily towards evaluation of the programme.
- It enabled more diverse the testing of the methodology of Active Learning and some of the specific workplace learning activities.

The planning of the programme days/workshops evolved in year 2 – so that by the end of year 2, the NMPDU and internal facilitators were designing the programme day learning aims and some of the active learning activities.

The programme days were the most visible and regular feature of activity. However, they were not simply study days, instead they acted as a collective rehearsal ground for transferring learning into the workplace and introducing or enhancing a learning culture. This is known to be necessary for developing a person-centred culture. Indeed the learning activities were in fact the building blocks (Dewing, 2009) for the new ways of person-centred working. By enabling participants to experiment with these in a learning capacity, the participants and other staff were offered a safer way of exposing themselves and their work to critique. Getting these activities right – so that they help move the culture on but do not cause panic within individuals or for the team was vital.

The Active Learning methods were for many 'new' but were viewed as essential activities for developing and establishing new ways of working that are sustainable and evidence based. The concept of learning in this way was a journey for all members of the health care team, and it was a journey for many that took patience, made individual take risks by moving away from comfort zones but ultimately provided a learning style that approached the change process in a different way. This approach enabled different members of the team to learn and work together in a way that had not happened before.

Care environment outcomes

The 'care environment' is a key consideration in the development of a person-centred culture (McCormack & McCance, 2006, 2010). The PCNI and PCCI determine the impact of an intervention on creating a person-centred care environment. The intervention in this case was the programme of activities and set within the person-centred practice theoretical framework. A person-centred culture can be summarised as one that achieves a decrease in nursing stress, an increase in nursing satisfaction and organisational commitment, and a decrease in intention to leave the job in the following year. Using these criteria of change, the practice environment of each care setting was evaluated.

Nine factors measure aspects related to nurse stress levels (see Table 5.1, factors 1–9). Scoring ranged from 1 to 7 and a decrease in scoring indicates a decrease in stress levels. The overall stress levels were low among the sample of nurses' at all three time points. A heavy workload was deemed to be the main cause of stress among nurses on all three occasions and equally the scores decreased over the three time points but not at a statistically significant level. Conflict with other nurses was scored as causing the least amount of stress. Stress levels decreased at a statistical level on five of the nine constructs (inadequate preparation, lack of staff support, and uncertainty regarding treatment, lack of communication and support, and career development). All statistically significant changes reflected a positive change in the practice environment.

Nurses' level of satisfaction with their job was assessed using a 7-point scale that ranged from 'Very dissatisfied' to 'Very satisfied', with 'Neither satisfied nor dissatisfied' as the mid-point (a score of 4). Four constructs (18 statements) helped to measure specific areas of satisfaction (factors 10–13). Personal and professional satisfactions with the job were scored highest by the total sample. Both constructs increased by a small but statistically significant amount by the third time point.

There were four key indicators of positive change towards a more person-centred practice environment – adequate staffing and support, empowerment, professional staff relationships, and nurse management (factors 14–17). Scores above 4 or more indicate a positive growth in the practice environment. All four factors indicated a movement towards a more positive environment. The largest increase was recorded on the construct that was most negatively scored (adequate staffing and support). Further, this increase was at a statistically significant level. The professional relationship between staff also increased and at a statistically significant level, whilst the remaining two constructs also increased this was not at a statistically significant level.

Two factors were directly related to the turnover of staff: intention to leave and organisational commitment (factors 18 and 19). Slater et al. (2010) reported the two factors to have an inverse relationship. A positive change in each is represented by an increase in organisational commitment and a corresponding decrease in intent to turnover. The findings for the total sample reported here show similar findings, and a positive change across all three time points. Organisational commitment increased and intention to leave the job decreased with the changes at a statistically significant level. A summary of the total mean scores for each of the 19 constructs at each time point is presented in Table 5.1.

Overall, statically significant changes were observed on 12 of the 19 factors, all indicating the change to be in a positive direction. In the seven factors that changed but at a non-significant level, the modest change was in a positive direction with stress levels decreasing, job satisfaction levels increasing, and the practice environment being stronger and a better environment to work in. Whilst statistical analysis across the sites is limited to those sites

Table 5.1   Mean scores of each of the 19 constructs.

	Data collection points			
Factors	**Time 1**	**Time 2**	**Time 3**	**Significant change**
1. Workload	4.37	4.27	4.24	ns
2. Inadequate preparation	3.03	2.91	2.86	0.01; positive
3. Lack of staff support	3.43	3.37	3.25	0.05; positive
4. Conflict with other nurses	2.3	2.24	2.30	ns
5. Uncertainty regarding treatment	2.48	2.34	2.44	0.03; positive
6. Work–social life balance	2.72	2.63	2.62	ns
7. Working environment	2.63	2.61	2.57	ns
8. Lack of communication and support	3.11	2.94	2.96	0.08; positive
9. Career development	2.61	2.45	2.46	0.01; positive
10. Satisfaction with pay and prospects	4.25	4.68	4.37	0.00; positive
11. Satisfaction with training	3.83	3.75	3.82	ns
12. Personal satisfaction	4.92	5.1	5.17	0.00; positive
13. Professional satisfaction	4.91	5.04	5.06	0.02; positive
14. Adequate staffing and resources	3.02	3.3	3.45	0.00; positive
15. Doctor nurse relationship	4.45	4.58	4.69	0.02; positive
16. Nurse management	4.98	5.02	5.07	ns
17. Empowerment	4.72	4.76	4.78	ns
18. Organisational commitment	4.7	4.94	4.92	0.00; positive
19. Intention to leave	3.34	2.96	2.91	0.00; positive

ns, non-significant.

where data were collected on all three time points, examination of the impact of the intervention indicates variability in findings. The number of significant changes in factors across each of the sites ranged from a maximum of 12 and a minimum of none (see Table 5.2). The average number of construct changes was three. All sites reported at least one significant change. The largest impact was reported at site 10 with 12 constructs being changed. Examination of the impact of the programme on factors shows that significant changes were reported on each of the factors, but the biggest impact occurred on the factors 'satisfaction with pay and prospects', 'satisfaction with training' and 'intention to leave'.

Paying attention to the environment was an important part of the practice development programme. Whilst acknowledging that in most cases, the environment of the care settings in each of the participating units did not reflect contemporary evidence about residential care environments, an increased focus on developing the environment was seen to occur. Changes to the environment have included changes to the management of noise, better use of space, colour and light, and gardens, all with the impact of providing more comfortable spaces for living and reducing the institutional 'feel' of the care setting (e.g. seating arrangements):

The overall impression from the first observation carried out [4 months previous] was of a great improvement in the décor of the room. The room was bright, freshly painted and looked great. The tables and chairs and furniture in general in the room was very much improved. The small tables were much more conducive to a homely dining area. The tables were spaced out well with easy access for residents. In the room there were some pictures on the walls and some memorabilia displayed on shelves. (Observation note)

Calm music in residents' lounge. Very soothing, resident friendly, not loud. (Observation note)

Table 5.2 Statistically significant differences in factor scores in each of the sites (sites 7 and 17 did not provide data at all three time points and are not included in the analysis).

Constructs	Sites															
	1	2	3	4	5	6	8	9	10	11	12	13	14	15	16	18
Workload	Ns	ns	**	ns	ns	ns	ns	ns	**	ns	ns	ns	ns	ns	ns	ns
Inadequate preparation	Ns	ns	ns	ns	ns	ns	ns	ns	**	ns	ns	ns	ns	ns	ns	ns
Lack of staff support	Ns	ns	ns	ns	ns	ns	ns	ns	**	ns	ns	ns	ns	ns	*	ns
Conflict with other nurses	Ns	ns	ns	ns	ns	ns	ns	ns	ns	ns	ns	ns	ns	ns	ns	ns
Uncertainty regarding treatment	Ns	ns	ns	ns	ns	ns	ns	ns	ns	*	ns	ns	ns	ns	ns	*
Work–social life balance	Ns	*	ns	ns	ns	ns	ns	ns	*	*	ns	ns	ns	ns	ns	ns
Working environment	Ns	ns	ns	ns	ns	ns	ns	ns	ns	ns	ns	ns	ns	ns	ns	ns
Lack of communication and support	Ns	ns	ns	ns	ns	*	ns	ns	**	ns	ns	ns	ns	*	ns	ns
Career development	Ns	ns	ns	ns	ns	ns	**	ns	**	ns	ns	ns	ns	ns	ns	ns
Satisfaction with pay and prospects	Ns	ns	*	ns	**	*	**	ns		ns	ns	ns	ns	*	ns	ns
Satisfaction with training	Ns	ns	ns	**	ns	*	ns	ns	**	*	ns	ns	ns	ns	**	ns
Personal satisfaction	*	ns	ns	ns	ns	ns	ns	ns	**	ns	ns	ns	ns	ns	**	ns
Professional satisfaction	Ns	ns	ns	ns	ns	ns	ns	ns	**	ns	ns	ns	ns	ns	*	ns
Adequate staffing and resources	Ns	ns	ns	ns	ns	ns	**	ns	**	*	ns	ns	ns	ns	**	ns
Doctor nurse relationship	Ns	ns	ns	ns	ns	*	*	ns	*	ns	ns	ns	ns	ns	ns	*
Nurse management	Ns	ns	ns	*	ns	ns	ns	ns	ns	ns	ns	ns	ns	ns	ns	ns
Empowerment	Ns	ns	ns	ns	ns	ns	ns	*	ns	ns	ns	ns	ns	ns	ns	ns
Organisational commitment	Ns	ns	ns	ns	**	ns	ns	ns	ns	ns	ns	ns	ns	ns	ns	ns
Intention to leave	Ns	**	ns	ns	**	ns	ns	ns	**	ns	*	ns	ns	ns	ns	**

*, statistical significance at $p > 0.05$; **, significance at $p > 0.01$; ns, non-significant.

There are nice paintings and artwork on the walls . . . it is a warm day so the windows are open which leaves a pleasant breeze. There is toast being made for the residents, the smell is pleasant and fills the room. The residents seem happy to see each other and greet each other warmly as the two staff members do. There is a good 'banter' – a happy atmosphere. There are magazines on the coffee tables – some of them are out of date. There are bowls of fruit available. When each resident enters the room they are greeted warmly, often b other residents but the staff are friendly and cheerful too. (Observation note)

Chairs and space arranged in different settings throughout the room. Looks homely. Fish tank being cleaned, residents interacting with the man cleaning the tank. Photographs of the residents on the mantle. Decorations for St Patrick's Day up around the room . . . Nice radio (old style), pictures nice on the wall. (Observation note)

However, whilst it was evident that staff became much more aware of the need to create an aesthetically pleasing environment as a part of being person-centred and did much to address environmental issues, there was still much work to be done, as the following data extracts illustrate:

The visitors room feels sparse, chairs not comfortable. (Observation note)

The tables were very sparsely dressed with condiments and napkins and some cutlery on the table. Sugar was on the table, stored in a plastic Tupperware container. Lovely serviettes were placed on the table except for one table where 3 men sat and who had none (not sure why?). There were mugs but no drinking glasses or drinks on the table for residents. No refreshment/choice was offered to the residents during the meal except for tea at the end of the meal. (Observation note)

However, the issue of balancing a person-centred approach and meeting safety requirements is one that continues to complicate the extent to which a full person-centred approach can be maximised, and there is indeed an issue of managing risk, meeting regulatory requirements/demands and meeting individual needs in a person-centred way, as illustrated by this reflection from one of the internal facilitators:

> *During the observations there were a few issues with signage over resident's beds that privileged staff and not residents and were there as a risk management measure and were not very person-centred. While the signage was observed during the observations, it was in the feedback to the ward that it became apparent that this was for risk management. Another problem was that strip lighting was on and seemed very bright and harsh during an evening observation but it was only again during the feedback that staff stated that they wanted to have bedside lamps but in order to comply with HIQA hygiene standards and risk management of the hospital, they were unable to have them. The challenge of the relationship between risk and person-centredness became obvious when the action plans were being implemented, as participants had to address the risk in order to get approval for the action. (Internal facilitator reflection)*

Perceptions of caring outcomes

The PCNI and PCCI incorporate a sub-scale called 'the caring dimensions inventory (CDI)' (Watson et al., 1999, 2003a, 2003b). It evaluates nurses' and care workers' perceptions of caring over time. It comprises 35 operationalised statements designed to elicit the degree to which participants perceive these actions as representative of caring (see Table 5.3). The items included in the instrument have been categorised as 'technical care', 'intimacy', 'supporting', 'unnecessary practice' and 'inappropriate aspects of practice'. A description of each category is provided as follows:

1. *Technical care*: Items that indicate technical and professional aspects of practice (14 items).
2. *Intimacy*: Getting to know a patient and becoming involved with them (10 items).
3. *Supporting*: Items that indicate helping the patients with spiritual matters (2 items).
4. *Unnecessary practice*: Aspects of practice that are not inappropriate or unprofessional but would not normally be expected of care workers (4 items).
5. *Inappropriate aspects of practice*: Actions, which, in addition to being unnecessary, are not recommended aspects of practice (5 items).

The analysis of the CDI is completed using Mokken Scaling Procedure (Mokken, 1997). This helps to identify a hierarchy of statements that have all been rated positively. The hierarchy of responses to items in the Mokken scale indicates a cumulative scale, whereby the level of endorsement of any particular item in the scales indicates the level of endorsement of all the other items in the scale. For example, an individual who endorses 'Consulting with a doctor about a patient' in the CDI at time 1 should also endorse all the other items in the scale that are more strongly endorsed such as 'Being with a patient during a clinical procedure' and 'Providing privacy for a patient'.

Time 1

The majority (8) of the 17 items are related to 'technical' aspects of practice. 'Intimacy' aspects of care such as 'listening to a patient' or 'sitting with a patient' are included in the

Table 5.3 Thirty-five items of the CDI and category classification.

Statement	Statement classification
Being technically competent with a clinical procedure	Technical[a]
Observing the effects of a medication on a patient	Technical
Giving reassurance about a clinical procedure	Technical
Assisting a patient with an activity of daily living	Technical[a]
Making a nursing record about a patient	Technical[a]
Explaining a clinical procedure to a patient	Technical
Being neatly dressed when working with a patient	Technical[a]
Reporting a patient's condition to a senior nurse	Technical
Organising the work of others for a patient	Technical[a]
Consulting with the doctor about a patient	Technical
Instructing a patient about aspects of self-care	Technical
Keeping relatives informed about a patient	Technical
Measuring the vital signs of a patient	Technical
Putting the needs of a patient before her/his own	Technical[a]
Providing privacy for a patient	Intimacy
Involving a patient with his or her care	Intimacy
Being cheerful with a patient	Intimacy
Feeling sorry for a patient	Intimacy[a]
Getting to know the patient as a person	Intimacy
Sitting with a patient	Intimacy
Being with a patient during a clinical procedure	Intimacy
Being honest with a patient	Intimacy[a]
Exploring the patient's lifestyle	Intimacy[a]
Listening to a patient	Intimacy
Arranging for a patient to see his or her chaplain	Supporting
Attending to the spiritual needs of patients	Supporting
Praying for a patient	Unnecessary[a]
Staying at work after there shift has finished to complete a job	Unnecessary[a]
Keeping in contact with a patient after discharge	Unnecessary[a]
Appearing to be busy at all times	Unnecessary[a]
Coming to work if they are not feeling well	Inappropriate[a]
Assuring a terminally ill patient that he or she is not going to die	Inappropriate[a]
Dealing with everyone's problems at once	Inappropriate[a]
Making a patient do something, even if he or she does not want to	Inappropriate[a]
Sharing one's own personal problems with a patient	Inappropriate[a]

[a]statistical significance at $p > 0.05$.

ranking and comprise the three highest ranked items. A total of seven of a possible ten items were identified as caring. Two spiritual items form the highest rank ordering, indicating that 'supporting' aspects of practice were considered caring but below that of the 'technical' and 'intimacy' aspects of practice (Table 5.4).

Time 2

Nineteen items were identified at time 2 with 16 items shared with the findings reported at time 1. Nine items were categorised as reflecting 'intimacy' in the care relationship; nine referred to the 'technical' aspects of practice and one item was seen as being 'supporting'. Three new items emerged from the data at time 2. Watson et al. (1999) reported that this was not uncommon in a changing work environment when opinions and values fluctuate as new ideas of practice emerge. This fluctuation in supported by the changes in rank ordering of items at time 2 from time 1 (Table 5.4).

Table 5.4 The ranking of the caring dimensions index items at time 1 and time 2.

Rank	Statement	Mean	Mean time II	Mean time III	Statement classification
1	Providing privacy for a patient	6.67	6.64 (2)	6.65 (1)	Intimacy
2	Listening to a patient	6.63	6.65 (1)	6.57 (2)	Intimacy
3	Being with a patient during a clinical procedure	6.55	6.56 (3)	6.42 (4)	Intimacy
4	Reporting a patients condition to a doctor	6.55	6.47 (5)	6.39 (5)	Technical
5	Explaining a clinical procedure to a patient	6.54	6.34 (10)	6.30 (10)	Technical
6	Giving reassurance about clinical procedures	6.53	6.46 (6)	6.35 (6)	Technical
7	Observing the effects of medicine	6.50	6.42 (8)	6.33 (7)	Technical
8	Getting to know a patient as a person	6.50	6.37 (9)	–	Intimacy
9	Involving a patient with his/her care	6.46	6.48 (4)	6.55 (2)	Intimacy
10	Consulting with a doctor about a patient	6.45	6.43 (7)	6.33 (8)	Technical
11	Sitting with a patient	6.41	6.31 (12)	–	Intimacy
12	Instructing a patient about self-care	6.40	6.31 (11)	6.30 (10)	Technical
13	Being cheerful with a patient	6.35	6.23 (17)	–	Intimacy
14	Measuring the vital signs of a patient	6.34	6.27 (15)	6.24 (12)	Technical
15	Arranging for a patient to see a chaplain	6.32	6.27 (14)	6.31 (9)	Supporting
16	Keeping relatives informed about a patient	6.31	–	6.23 (13)	Technical
17	Attending to the spiritual needs of a patient	6.29	6.18 (18)	–	Supporting
18	Being neatly dressed	–	6.30 (13)	–	Technical
19	Being honest with a patient	–	6.26 (16)	–	Intimacy
20	Exploring the lifestyle of a patient	–	6.12 (19)	–	Intimacy

Time 3

The participants identified 13 items of the CDI as caring at time 3. Four of the items were related to aspects that were concerned with 'intimacy' in the caring relationship; eight items address 'technical' aspects of practice and one item was 'supporting'. The number of items identified was considerably lower than that of the previous two occasions indicating a much more focused perspective of the role of staff and the four top ranked items were all related to providing 'intimacy'. There was considerable and constant change in the ranking of item 9 'Involving a patient in his/her care' that moved from a ranking of 9th to 2nd (Table 5.4).

Resident outcomes

In total across the three time points, 180 periods of observation and 60 user narratives were collected. In the final analysis, four key categories were identified from across all data sets.

Choice

The theme of choice was a significant theme across the data sets and indeed it is something that featured in the work of the programme groups across the participating sites. The data demonstrate that over the period of the programme, residents were provided with a greater range and number of choices. Specific activities (such as resident and family groups) were initiated and established in the majority of settings as methods of enabling more choice for residents. However, the data also reflected a range of challenges and ongoing issues in the development of person-centred care environments that facilitate choice for older people:

> *Well it depends on my experience, it's a tough life being a patient . . . As regards my control, they'd say they are scared in case I'd go to the toilet on my own in case I'd have a fall and that*

way. Two years ago I had a fall and they are still referring to that as if it was recent . . . I am able to get up and go to bed when I want. I have people coming in and I suppose I can go out – I don't know if I want to . . . (Resident story)

Whilst there was increasing evidence of choice being facilitated, for example, greater choice of mealtimes, more choice of recreational activities, individualised waking and retiring times, there continued to be a sense of this being inconsistent and individual nurse/care worker dependent:

It would be good if people could remember or know when films like the westerns are on because all of the men like them. They were films you would have gone to see in the picture houses – John Wayne is great. You can talk for hours about them. A keg of Guinness would be good too – I do not like the cans. He [pointing to another resident] has one when a friend or sister comes into visit. (Resident story)

The involvement of families in the life-world of the residential setting and of residents was a challenge and one that was considered to be critical to the ongoing development of practice in residential settings. At some stage in the majority of the stories, residents recounted family-orientated experiences – experiences that they valued, missed, still wanted or felt sad about. In all cases, these family-related experiences provided a significant source of reminiscence for residents:

I became a widow 44 years ago. My husband was only 39. He had cancer and we didn't know at the time and we were not expecting him to die. I got a phone call at 2 o'clock in the morning and was told he was dead, I was all alone when I got the phone call. I worked in [shop name] in the boot section – we made loads of money. I had no kids so I had a lonely life, but I had my sister's kids. I spoilt them really. I was good to them and now they are good to me. I go to my sister's every Sunday for dinner and my nephew/nieces call nearly every day to me. They ask do I want anything and they'll always bring it to me (Resident story)

The explicit encouragement of families to visit was one that was identified as necessary in all settings as it was felt that there was often a lack of visiting from families:

My kids used to visit me a lot when I was in hospital first, but now I don't see them very often. I suppose they are busy with their own lives. My wife visits every day for an hour or so and takes me for a walk in my wheelchair. I used to go out once a week with the wheelchair people but they find me too heavy to manage so that outing has stopped (Resident story)

In addition, the need for the environment to support family engagement with the care setting was also necessary and the observations of practice highlighted efforts that teams had made to make the environment more 'homely' for both residents and visitors, but the environment continues to be a challenge that needs ongoing attention:

Feels relaxed today in the sitting room. Three men snoozing in chairs – look comfortable. There is a student nurse playing cards with two residents, laughter and positive interaction. Residents greeted me when I came into the sitting room and welcomed me . . . Chairs and space arranged in different settings throughout the room. Looks homely . . . (Observation note)

Throughout all the data sets, the issue of meaningful activity and prevention of boredom was a recurring issue. The observation data in particular highlighted the lack of meaningful activity for residents, particularly those who had high levels of physical need or who had a dementia. Developing meaningful activities and alleviating boredom were key components of most action plans in all sites. The data reflect a significant shift in the range of activities available to residents and this was noted in the observation data in particular:

> *I asked M [resident name] if she ever goes out of the unit or visits other areas and she stated 'no'. 'I like my own space here, I never was one for socialising or mixing. I have been to their [family members] homes a couple of times but the children running around and the noise, I prefer them to come here . . . I don't do any of those activities like painting or bingo. I don't enjoy that kind of thing . . . I just like the peace and quiet and staying in my room. I have always been that type, just a quiet person' (Resident story)*

> *. . . I would like to be able to go out in the sun. (Resident story)*

Overall, the data demonstrated that a range of processes were put in place to facilitate residents' choices including the use of biography and reminiscence. There was a general sense from the data of staff trying hard to pay attention to choices and to respecting individual preferences.

Belonging and connectedness

Belonging and connectedness reflects an observation of the data as reflecting the way in which the practice development programme enabled movement towards a greater sense of belonging and connectedness among residents and staff in the residential settings. The practice developments and culture changes initiated and implemented over the 2-year programme were seen to instil a greater sense of belonging and connectedness in most of the participating sites. At an individual level, the data reflected a greater sense of 'knowing the person':

> *J says that she enjoys getting her hair done. She was a brunette when she was young. He does not colour her hair as 'the grey ones are as easy to carry as the white'! She enjoys living in this house – there are 'special doors' (she looks down at her co-tag). J says that she likes the garden and the birds that come in to the feeder – 'I like to walk around the garden'. She says that she would like an open fire and someone to talk to when she is back in her room . . . (Interview with resident)*

This progress was evident in the range of activities planned in action plans and in the focus on knowing the person that featured in the observations. In addition, the narrative data demonstrated a sense of belonging by residents and more engaged relationships with care workers and teams.

Alleviating loneliness due to boredom and isolation is a key theme in the data. The data reflect an increased focus on alleviating loneliness and reducing isolation:

> *Across all three sites, programme facilitators at unit level worked with residents and staff on the development of individualised activity plans. These plans were based on activities/programmes the resident wanted to partake in. For some residents, trips to the local pub, local cinema, the resident's home place, local matches has now become the norm. Other activities have been introduced within the units based on the specific identified need of individual residents. (Midlands area evaluation data)*

It was generally reflected by participants in the analysis of the data, that the care environments were largely 'monotonous' and that there was a need to pay more attention to activities that act as diversions from day-to-day worries that residents may have and that lead to a greater sense of belonging and engagement. Paying attention to the life-world of the residents was increasingly recognised as important by participants, as illustrated by this poem, written with a resident:

Meanwhile in St Josephs Unit
In the unit of St Joseph's you won't hear too much noise
Some of us are silent an odd one sits and sighs
But look behind the faces and put away the chart
I'm sure my pulse is normal but try to read my heart.

In my years before St Josephs' I had some golden hours
and I walked with my true love among the leafy bowers
and if my eyes look vacant and sometimes I don't hear
I may be gone to shelter from the rain that fills my tears.

There was a time believe me when friends were near and dear
And I drank the cup of kindness and laughed without a fear
So when you think I'm hungry and I push away the food
I am struggling with my demons and don't mean to be rude.

And, staff, I do take notice when you greet me with a smile
And I really mean to thank you when you go the extra mile
But sometimes I am angry though I know it doesn't help
And when you lose your patience I can only blame myself.

In the unit of St Joseph's there are some who dare to hope
And some whose hopes are fading feel like giving up the ghost
But life is very precious though the deal you got is raw
There's no room or self pity with your back against the wall.

So please listen to my story and try to make the time
You might just learn a lesson and be a bit more wise
I will try hard to respond and not be such a pain
With a little understanding we both can stand to gain.

In the unit of St Joseph's life may seem very bleak
But life is still worth living for the sad and for the weak
And one thing is for certain as you go about your chore
The day is so much brighter when you look into my soul.

A significant finding in the baseline data was the lack of connection between the older person and various dimensions of their life. In the final data set, participants recognised a number of themes that reflected the attention to re-connecting and maintaining relationships – with family, past life, past role and to the outside (similar to social outlets theme) as illustrated through the following data extracts:

When I was seventeen I was told I was going on holiday and that is when I came to here where the nuns were, to the big grey building. I worked for the nuns looking after the flowers and the vegetables. I like my music, I like to listen to it and play the mouth organ. I am very happy here and everyone is very good to me. I go to Knock and to Lourdes (Religious Shrines) every third year. I have my own television and I watch lots of films. I watch it when everyone is in bed. I put the sound down low and watch the picture. I like all sorts of films . . . (he proudly showed off his collection). Every evening I listen to my music while having a cup of tea. Most days I don't think about my past experiences, however, some days it just comes in to you. But I am very happy here [Narrator's note: he also showed off his picture album which had photographs of all his birthdays since he came to (hospital name) and there was also photographs of day trips out they have had. He could name everyone and told us those who had died and those still alive]. (Resident story)

However, this is an area of practice that needs much more consideration and continuous planning based on an assessment of individual resident's needs, wants and desires with respect of their social connections – a key aspect of being person-centred. Engaging in these activities helps to maintain a sense of inclusion in the community and a greater sense of belonging that enables the older person to grow and change as well as experience change in their daily life.

Hope and hopelessness

The category of 'hope and hopelessness' reflected the contradiction that was evident in the data, that is a greater sense of hope being instilled into residential care settings, seeing them as a place of growth and development, whilst at the same time a prevailing sense of hopelessness existing.

The theme of 'hope' was reflected in the variety of activities that had been developed to enable older people in residential care settings to have a more meaningful life, irrespective of disability (physical and/or cognitive). However, overall there continued to be a prevailing sense of hopelessness, predominantly reflected in the themes of loss, hopelessness, acceptance and voicelessness.

The theme of 'loss' is unsurprising as it is recognised that loss is a common experience for older people. The areas of loss identified in the data are also not surprising – loss of health, independence, identity, self, life, freedom:

I like reading and doing crosswords. I tend to spend a lot of time in my room but I get involved in activities when they are available. I enjoy listening to classical music . . . in the afternoon I go for a nap just before tea time I don't sleep very much so I tend to read quite late into the night. My sleep is always broken waking during night to go to toilet. This is very tiring and I feel 'sick of it all'. I feel obsessed. I feel I am troublesome because of going to the toilet. The incontinence has become a phobia. I am absolutely shagged and my bones are like biscuits and I feel very apprehensive about the future . . . I feel inept in my life, I have been a perfectionist. Little things make me intolerant. I constantly compare how I would do it myself. I feel I need to relax more . . . I miss my old home and I am still unable to let go . . . (Resident's story)

Participants in the programme recognised the difficulties inherent in addressing these issues as they are often at the core of older persons' life experiences. However, activities that enabled greater participation in the daily life of wards/units, activities to enable social connection and activities that enabled connection with past lives were implemented and were successful in addressing issues of loss for many residents.

The implementation of these activities has an added benefit of dealing with issues of hopelessness. The first and second round of observations of practice identified how 'hopeless' some residential care settings are, often reflected by a lack of meaningful activity, a lack of meaningful social engagement and a lack of attention to maximising the older person's ability to do things for themselves (no matter how small). Whilst much effort by programme participants went into addressing these issues, hopelessness continued to be seen in resident's narratives through their worries, sadness and depression and a feeling of being ignored. Older people seemed to accept their lot and make the most of their loss of independence and were content with where they were at. Their voicelessness was underpinned by fear – fear of the future, fear of dying, fear of function and fears of not being included or fitting in:

> *Time is long, boredom sometimes. I'd love to get home but there would be no one there. Just to get out would be great – great to get away from it. I will go out in the weather when the weather is good. I go down in the lift but my husband used to come down four times a week before he died. He is a terrible loss. The girls are working and live off away from here. I'd like to get out while I'm able . . . No, I don't feel I have a say in how things are done here – No say, no, just get on with it . . . (Resident story)*

Paying attention to narratives and stories enabled the sense of older people being voiceless to be addressed. Some facilitators viewed the sense of hopelessness as a bleak view of residential care and despite the range of activities put in place to address these issues, recognised that instilling a sense of hope needs to be a key strategic issue for the ongoing development of residential services for older people.

Meaningful relationships

The final category 'meaningful relationships' links with and in many ways consolidates the previous three categories (choice, belonging and connectedness, and hope and hopelessness) as the focus of the category is that of the place of older people having the opportunity for meaningful relationships. Key themes underpinning this category include – communication, teamwork, routinised care and intentionality.

In the practice development programme, a key focus of development activities was that of 'language'. The baseline observation data demonstrated the contradiction that existed between the person-centred values espoused and the language used in everyday 'talk'. The use of words such as 'feeding', 'nappies', 'the heavies' are all illustrative of a non-person-centred approach to practice. Throughout the programme this language was challenged and staff were facilitated using high challenge/high support strategies to change this language to more person-centred talk, such as 'helping residents to eat and drink', 'having a meal', 'incontinence aids/pads' and so on. The data demonstrate that significant changes did occur in the way language was used by staff:

> *The care worker is helping a resident out of bed. She is working in a calm way and giving the resident lots of encouragement. The language she is using is very person-centred and is focused on the resident's needs – very respectful. (Observation note)*

The use of more person-centred language was seen to enable active listening and engagement with residents on a more equal footing:

> *Staff chatting to residents as they wheel them in the wheelchairs. All seems very friendly. Nurses communicating well with each other and with support staff. Handover appeared professional. Residents referred to by name, communication appeared very person-centred and respectful.*

Meaningful conversations, e.g. 'Mary would you like to attend the exercise class?' Staff called each other by their first names and were respectful. (Observation notes)

The person-centred practice framework used in the programme places equal emphasis on the development of meaningful relationships among team members as it does between team members and residents. Indeed it is argued that the development of person-centred relationships with residents is predicated on those same relationships existing among staff. The data demonstrate that the 2-year programme resulted in more evidence of teamwork and this was also supported by the PCNI/PCCI data.

However, issues of a dominant focus on tasks with a routinised approach to care, challenges of planning time in a person-centred way, lack of autonomy over decision-making and staff attitudes and behaviours all impacted on the extent to which the positive benefits of teamwork were realised:

9 am in the morning and the staff are very busy. There is one nurse and two carers working in the 4th cubicle. One carer takes out the 'morning trolley' and checks that the trolley is set up. Another attendant wheels a patient into the shower and the nurse pulls the curtain and then and then asks the attendant to aid her with the resident . . . there is a resident sitting on her bed and she is saying her prayers, I can see the rosary beads in her hand. The care attendant asks her if she is ready for a shower and she replies 'yes' but does not want her hair washed as she is going out in the afternoon and her family is taking her to her own hairdresser to get a colour in her hair. The resident is sitting on the shower chair, she is wearing her nightdress and has slippers on her feet, she is holding a towel, wash-bag and clean clothes. She is now wheeled out and another resident is at the hand basin cleaning her dentures . . . (Observation notes)

In some respects, managers and leaders were less concerned with 'authority and rules' than they were with the development of a service that focused on the needs of individuals:

Some evidence that some staff find it difficult to work with other staff. But staff on duty today are very happy and enjoying work. Some hierarchy but no overt distinction. Staff seem to be clear about what they are doing, asking for help from colleagues easily but discretely. The leadership evident today is transformational – it feels like an organised team. Staff look relaxed and are interacting with residents at a slow pace . . . good evidence of resident involvement in [named] assessments and personal profiles. (Observation notes)

The extent to which practices existed that compromised residents privacy, dignity and personhood was influenced by the active participation of managers and leaders in the programme and the reinforcement of agreed ways of working by senior staff. The data further illustrate and emphasise the importance of a continuous developmental approach to team development and team effectiveness as well as commitment from managers and leaders for this work.

Where there was intentional practice, that is, intent to engage in a meaningful way with residents then positive practices existed and meaningful relationships were developed and maintained:

Conversation taking place in CNM II's office – gentle voice and door is open. Can hear resident calling out for someone to help with their napkin. Very prompt response from two members of staff . . . Tone of voice appropriate during interaction . . . encouragement of staff with residents to eat meals. Interaction between support staff and resident re-dinner/dessert, 'what type of jelly is it?' Answered – diabetic jelly. Resident said they would prefer something else. Reply was – 'let me see what I have, maybe tart?' 'That would be lovely'... relationship with the relatives at mealtimes was good and they were included in the meal. Nice friendly banter between staff member and relative. Visitors appear to feel comfortable and at ease. The Chef visited the ward and spoke with the staff in a quiet voice. Nice to see care assistant and staff nurse engage with one another and check that everybody had their meals – good practice. (Observation notes)

In summary, when undertaking the analysis of the data sets, programme participants felt that there was significantly more evidence of positive relationships with residents, between staff members and with visitors/relatives than in previous data collections. The narrative data also suggest that most residents are content with the extent of the relationship they have with staff. However, there is still much work to do in this aspect of residential care. It remains the case that the extent of the existence of these positive interactions is largely dependent on individual staff member practices and further developments are needed to embed such practices in the system generally and realise it as 'standard practice'.

SUMMARY

Given the complexity of person-centred practice, it is important that any evaluation of it takes account of each of its different attributes and the inter-relationship between them. In this practice development programme, we worked with several models: practice development model (Garbett & McCormack, 2004) and the person-centred practice theoretical framework of McCormack & McCance (2006). Additionally, emerging from this programme is a new model of learning in practice development: *Active Learning* (Dewing, 2008a, 2009; McCormack et al., 2009). In addition, we actively experimented with scale of the programme and the programme leads being outside the local delivery of the practice development interventions and data gathering.

The person-centred practice theoretical framework is predicated on the conceptual stance that suggests – that in order for a person-centred culture to exist a number of pre-requisites need to be in place/attended to in a systematic way. A care setting that focuses on these pre-requisites will have the foundation attributes of a team in place who can pay attention to the care environment, its management, leadership and learning. The combination of pre-requisites and the positive attributes of the care environment, then enable effective care processes to be realised and sustained in practice. The evaluation of this practice development programme, whilst not explicitly structured on the concepts that make up the theoretical framework, does go some way to articulate the attributes of person-centred practice in residential care settings for older people, from the perspectives of staff, residents and their families.

The data from the programme days, site-specific reports, observations of practice and resident stories affirm the reality of the shift in focus towards a more person-centred culture. The data from the programme days demonstrate that over the period of 11 facilitated programme days and related development activities in practice, the priorities for care changed among staff teams. Activities such as observations of practice, reflection on the language used among teams and with residents/families and 'cats, skirts, lipsticks and handbags' increased staff awareness about a more holistic approach to care that went beyond the doing of tasks:

... For me person-centred care has been in the main about the staff. About developing them to deliver care to our patients that is of the best quality possible. It's about them learning about

their own values and beliefs in order to be able to realise that the patients as people also have a set of values and beliefs that need to be met. My role of facilitator has been in facilitating the growth of the staff at the hospital and supporting them to provide person-centred care. I am very glad I had the opportunity to participate in this programme albeit that on occasion it broke my heart. All I have learned and the networking I have been able to avail of have been of tremendous benefit to me and will continue to be used to benefit the patients lives at this hospital . . . (Internal facilitator reflection)

This reflection and the programme days evaluation clearly demonstrates that making these changes is not easy. This evidence is consistent with the international practice development evidence that demonstrates that changing cultures of practice from a routinised to a person-centred approach is challenging at individual, team and organisational levels (McCormack et al., 2007). Because the essence of emancipatory and transformational development is that of changing 'self', that is adjusting my perspective(s) of situations, then to do this requires considerable commitment and dedication of staff to engage the analysis of 'self'. For the most part, we exist on a day-to-day basis within largely routinised ways of engaging and behaving – the 'crisis' (Fay, 1987) that occurs when the comfort of such routines is challenged requires skilled facilitation. The crises that occur and the facilitation interventions necessary are not a one off event but reoccur to form a pattern until the individual can transcend it. The facilitation interventions to work with these crises are evident in this practice development programme. The evidence from the programme illustrates just how challenging it is for facilitators to engage staff who are feeling threatened by the approach being used, and to 'hold' staff as they make their own journeys in coming to terms with the realities of practice and maintaining momentum so that real changes can occur within a set time frame:

When I began the programme 2 years ago I had totally underestimated the commitment required to be part of the programme. I've always welcomed new challenges and looked forward to this one. I found the weekend in <name of town> to commence the programme was absolutely vital to give me a great foundation towards facilitation and practice development. Having a mentor in [NMPDU Facilitator] and [external facilitators] always available was crucial to my 'survival'. There were times when I felt like I was the only person in our unit that was interested in PCC. Without this sounding negative, if I knew at the start of the programme all the challenges I would meet, I'd have found it difficult to enlist . . . (Internal facilitator reflection)

REFERENCES

Dewing, J. (2002) From ritual to relationship: a person centred approach to consent in qualitative research with older people who have a dementia. *Dementia: The International Journal of Social Research & Practice,* **1**, 156–171.

Dewing, J. (2006) Wandering into the future: reconceptualising wandering? *International Journal of Older People Nursing,* **1** (4), 239–249.

Dewing, J. (2008a) Becoming and being active learners and creating active learning workplaces: the value of active learning. Chapter 15. In: *International Practice Development in Nursing and Healthcare* (eds B. McCormack, K. Manley & V. Wilson), pp. 273–294. Blackwell Publishing Ltd., Oxford.

Dewing, J. (2008b) Process consent and research with older persons living with dementia. *Association of Research Ethics Journal,* **4** (2), 59–64.

Dewing, J. (2009) Moments of movement: active learning and practice development. *Nurse Education in Practice,* **10** (1), 22–26.

Fay, B. (1987) *Critical Social Science.* Cornell University Press, New York.

Garbett, R. & McCormack, B. (2004) A concept analysis of practice development. In: *Practice Development in Nursing* (eds B. McCormack, K. Manley & R. Garbett), p. 29. Blackwell Publishing Ltd., Oxford.

Health Improvement and Quality Agency (HIQA) (2010) National Quality Standards for Residential Care Settings for Older People in Ireland. http://www.hiqa.ie/publications.asp (Accessed 21 July 2010).

Heron, J. & Reason, P. (2001) The Practice of co-operative inquiry: research with rather than on people. In: *Handbook of Action Research: Participative Inquiry and Practice* (eds P. Reason & H. Bradbury), pp. 179–188. Sage Publications, London.

Hsu, M.Y. & McCormack, B. (2011) Understanding the experiences of older people in hospital through narrative interviewing. *Journal of Clinical Nursing*, **21** (5–6), 841–849.

Manley, K. & McCormack, B. (2004) Practice development: purpose, methodology, facilitation and evaluation. In: *Practice Development in Nursing* (eds B. McCormack, K. Manley & R. Garbett), pp. 33–50. Blackwell Publishing Ltd., Oxford.

McCormack, B., Dewing, J., Breslin, L., Coyne-Nevin, A., Kennedy, K., Manning, M., Peelo-Kilroe, L. & Tobin, C. (2009a) Practice development: realising active learning for sustainable change. *Contemporary Nurse*, **32** (1–2), 92–104.

McCormack, B., Dewing, J., Breslin, L., Coyne-Nevin, A., Kennedy, K., Manning, M., Peelo-Kilroe, L. & Tobin, C. (2009b) The Implementation of a Model of Person-Centred Practice in Older Person Settings. Final Report, Office of the Nursing Services Director, Health Services Executive, Dublin, Ireland.

McCormack, B., Henderson, E., Wilson, V. & Wright, J. (2009) The workplace culture critical analysis tool. *Practice Development in Healthcare*, **8** (1), 28–43.

McCormack, B. & McCance, T. (2006) Development of a framework for person-centred nursing. *Journal of Advanced Nursing*, **56** (5), 1–8.

McCormack, B. & McCance, T. (2010) *Person-centred Nursing: Theory, Models and Methods*. Blackwell Publishing Ltd., Oxford.

McCormack, B., Wright, J., Dewer, B., Harvey, G. & Ballintine, K. (2007) A realist synthesis of evidence relating to practice development: findings from the literature review. *Practice Development in Health Care*, **6** (1), 25–55.

Mokken, R.J. (1997) *Handbook of Modern Item Response Theory*. Springer, New York.

Slater, P. & McCormack, B. (2007) An exploration of the factor structure of the Nursing Work Index. *Worldviews on Evidence-Based Nursing*, **4** (1), 30–39.

Slater, P., O'Halloran, P., Connolly, D. & McCormack, B. (2010) Testing of the factor structure of the nursing work index-revised. *Worldviews on Evidence Based Nursing*, **7**(3): early view; 123–134.

Titchen, A. (2004) Helping relationships for practice development: critical companionship. In: *Practice Development in Nursing* (eds B. McCormack, K. Manley & R. Garbett), pp. 148–174. Blackwell Publishing Ltd., Oxford.

van de Zipj, T. & Dewing, J. (2009) Learning to become a facilitator in the school context. *Practice Development in Health Care Journal*, **4**, 200–215.

Watson, R., Deary, I.J. & Lea, A. (1999) A longitudinal study into the perceptions of caring among student nurses using multivariate analysis of the caring dimensions inventory. *Journal of Advanced Nursing*, **30**, 1080–1089.

Watson, R., Deary, I.J. Lea Hoogbruin, A., Vermeijden, W., Rumeu, C., Beunza, M., Barbarin, B., MacDonald, J. & McCready, T. (2003a) Perceptions of nursing: a study involving nurses, nursing students, patients and non-nursing students. *International Journal of Nursing Studies*, **43**, 133–144.

Watson, R., Lea Hoogbruin, A., Rumeu, C., Beunza, M., Barbarin, B., MacDonald, J. & McCready, T. (2003b) Differences and similarities in the perception of caring between Spanish and UK nurses. *Journal of Clinical Nursing*, **12**, 85–92.

6 Getting Going with Facilitation Skills in Practice Development

Angie Titchen[1], Jan Dewing[2] and Kim Manley[3]

[1]Fontys University of Applied Sciences, Eindhoven, The Netherlands
[2]East Sussex Healthcare NHS Trust & Canterbury Christ Church University, Canterbury, UK
[3]Canterbury Christ Church University, Canterbury, UK

This chapter is written as a novelette. It follows a group of health care workers from different organisations. They are attending an introductory practice development learning programme organised by their organisations. The novelette is, of course, fiction. We have peppered it with influences from published research and reflections by others (e.g. Eldridge, 2011; Hunnisett, 2011; Jackson & Webster, 2011; Snoeren & Frost, 2011), and our own practice development research and experience (e.g. Manley, 2001; Titchen, 2004; Dewing, 2009). The characters and workplaces are imaginary, although they may share a resemblance to people and workplaces we have worked with on our own journeys. Writing fiction has enabled us to show the interior (what people are seeing, feeling, thinking and imagining), as well as the exterior (the visible actions and activities and the contexts people work in). The meaning of the novelette title, 'Making a path by walking it' and its contents are introduced through an imaginary 'arts review'.

INTRODUCTION

Facilitators are a vital connection in achieving a vision of a person-centred culture in our health care workplaces. They help stakeholders, including practitioners, to integrate, in continuous spirals, planning–action–evaluation–learning through the key elements or steps of the practice development journey as set out in Chapter 1 (Figure 1.3). Moving through the spirals requires practitioners to be reflective and evaluative of their own values, beliefs, feelings, motivations and actions, if the vision of a person-centred culture is to be fully achieved. Facilitators must grow a comprehensive skill set to help all of these activities to happen. Growing the skills does not happen overnight or by chance, so new facilitators need to get started somewhere at some point on the practice development journey.

First a bit of background . . .

We believe that to be effective with practice development, practitioners need help to reflect on, and come to understand, themselves and what is happening, before they can change anything significantly. This is where facilitation comes in. Facilitators help practitioners to come to such understanding by supporting them whilst they take things apart and put them

Practice Development in Nursing and Healthcare, Second Edition. Edited by Brendan McCormack, Kim Manley and Angie Titchen.
© 2013 John Wiley & Sons, Ltd. Published 2013 by John Wiley & Sons, Ltd.

back together in new ways that make things have more meaning and work better. Facilitators help others to use these new understandings to inform their action plans to change themselves, their practices and eventually their workplaces. They also help practitioners to understand why new ways of doing things that appear to work, do work, so that they can build on it. As practitioners progress along the practice development journey, facilitators help them to learn new skills, for example, how to gather and learn from patients' and colleagues' experiences, and use the new understanding to address any unsatisfactory aspects, for example, patients feeling disempowered by being excluded from decision-making about their care or feeling that their personal identity has been taken away.

The reality is that in many workplaces, there are not enough practitioners who have well-developed facilitation skills. So, the purpose of the chapter is to offer novice facilitators (whether a new graduate or someone who has worked longer but has no practice development experience) an opportunity to understand and try out the fundamental skills of a facilitator in their own workplace. It is important to note that novice facilitators are unlikely to be taking the overall lead on a practice development journey within an organisation, unit or workplace, but that they can contribute by helping their colleagues to reflect during their everyday work, as well as during specific activities associated with the elements of the journey. As introduced in Chapter 3, it is important to recognise that this contribution is not only about *what* facilitators do, for example, leading a values clarification exercise, but also about the *how* or the *way* they do it. Even if your organisation has not taken a strategic approach to practice development with someone who has experience of working at different levels in the organisation taking the overall lead (see Chapter 12), you can help bring about change in your workplace as shown by the characters in the following novelette.

We also want to make it clear that it would be inappropriate for novice facilitators to be facilitating, on their own, practice development learning programmes for large groups of people as depicted here. Working with large groups of people with different learning needs requires expertise in a range of skills. We encourage the practice developers beginning facilitation to find someone in their workplace or external to it who can act as a role-model for them and offer support or negotiate more formal supervision, mentoring or critical companionship (Titchen, 2003; 2004).

Becoming a work-based facilitator requires would-be facilitators to develop their self-knowledge and awareness of the impact that they have on others and a set of fundamental skills that are used consistently in both practice development activities and everyday work. These key skills are:

1. Active listening
2. Giving and receiving constructive feedback
3. Asking enabling questions
4. Doing all these things in ways that offer high challenge and high support

The skills are used within an approach called active learning (Dewing, 2009), an umbrella approach that brings together ideas about different learning styles and strategies and the integration of head, heart, body and, for some, the soul in their learning. We have found over many years that novice practice development facilitators struggle to use these key facilitation skills for promoting active learning.

Review

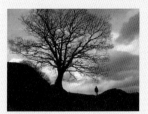 No doubt the authors of the recently published novelette, 'Making a path by walking it', used this intriguing title to entice newcomers to take a look at work-based facilitation within a practice development context. The title seems to imply that becoming such a facilitator is a unique journey for each person and that it requires some courage and risk-taking to step into what sounds like uncharted territory. However, it soon becomes clear that there is an overall map, but because would-be facilitators are unique and have different starting points, they will need to create their own paths towards becoming skilled facilitators of learning. The novelette acts as reference points for the beginning steps. Two experienced facilitators, Abbie and Mike role-model and verbalise their practical 'know-how' as the story unfolds.

Just as it is when working with patients and families as a practitioner, it is essential for facilitators to get to know the people they work alongside. It is the first step to creating the conditions for people to learn, grow and flourish through the changes to come. In the opening of the novelette, 'Getting to know you', Abbie and Mike show how this can be done with groups of practitioners. Then the novelette focus is on the importance of active listening and being yourself. This is central to getting to know where people are starting from in their practice development journey because they will be making their own paths too and you have to know how to help them walk it as unique individuals. Given that giving and receiving feedback is vital to learning and developing practice, the next part of the story is about how to do that in constructive, helpful ways that challenge and support practitioners at the same time. At the heart of skilled facilitation also is the ability to ask enabling questions: questions that help people to go further and deeper in their thinking and understandings. Novice facilitators find it one of the hardest things to do, so watch out for this. You can see, at the end, how the characters in this story got on 6 months after attending a programme facilitated by Abbie and Mike.

MAKING A PATH BY WALKING IT

1: Getting to know you

The practice development journey begins by establishing the conditions to enable person-centred relationships to grow:

- *Listening and hearing, so as to learn about others*
- *Sharing appropriately things about yourself*
- *Being authentic*
- *Being caring*

There is an expectant hum in the room. The faces of those already there variously reflect excitement, uncertainty and curiosity. A table stands in the middle of the room and on it are picture cards, all laid out like treasures waiting to be discovered or left for another occasion. Abbie and Mike, the practice development programme co-facilitators, greet participants at the door and, smiling, invite more people individually to come into the room. On their way to a seat, the participants are invited to choose any picture card that attracts them for an introductions activity and to finally take a seat in the circle. Snippets of conversation can be overheard, as participants begin to talk to those sitting next to them.

Abbie is a very experienced facilitator, who works between a practice development centre based in a university and one of the health care trusts involved in this programme. Mike is an experienced facilitator who has been working with Abbie in the trust. This is the first practice development programme he has facilitated and Abbie is his critical companion during the programme, helping him to learn from this co-facilitation opportunity. Mike remembers his first day as a participant. He can even see where he sat in this very room and thinks to himself, how much can happen in a year. He knows he needs to focus and remember to act like a facilitator. He also feels this might be wrong – as he is meant to BE a facilitator. However, today, right now, he does feel he needs to put on a show. Nerves, he guesses.

The last participant arrives. Making eye contact with Mike to cue him in to the start and with other people, Abbie says enthusiastically, 'Welcome to this introductory practice development programme!' Abbie and Mike, apparently confidently, introduce themselves and share something of their values and experience of practice development. They acknowledge that there are different approaches to practice development, but that, in this programme, they will be exploring an approach that resonates with their own values and principles about person-centredness, collaboration, inclusion and participation, high challenge/high support and human flourishing. Mike is unaware that Grace, a participant, wishes she could have his self-presentation skills. They briefly outline the purpose and aims of the programme this week and the shorter follow-up sessions that will take place every 6 weeks over the next 9 months. Then, picking up their own picture cards, they invite each person to say something about themselves and why they have joined the programme, using the card(s) they have chosen, if they want to.

Silence . . . then,

'OK, let's go for it! My name is Charlie, short for Charlotte. When I was a kid, I wanted to be a boy and told everyone that my name was Charlie. Now I like being a girl, but the name has stuck!'

A little giggly laughter, probably of acknowledgement and some release of tension, goes round the circle.

Charlie continues, 'I qualified as a nurse 2 years ago. I have chosen this card of two very pretty sheep (holds up card), all curls, looking very cute and appealing! But what the picture doesn't show is the pile of . . . that they are standing in! The card represents the team that I joined 6 months ago, in the care of older people unit I work in, where the appearance of harmony and working together is promoted to the outside world and everyone bleats to the same tune, when in fact, the very opposite is true. There's a lot of conflict between team members and the leader, but it never comes out into the open. It just gets talked about behind closed doors, but not between the people who have the issue and so it just festers. The hospital is a mess too. What really gets me is that all that stuff about providing the patients with choice and high-quality care is fake at the top. It's all about saving money and balancing the books. Anyway, 6 months into the job, I am beginning to realise that it is wearing me down and I find I am beginning to behave in the same way as some of the others in my team.

Before it's too late, I want to challenge and change the way we work, so that we give care that is centred around the patients and their families and not us. This is why I'm here. I want to learn how to do practice development. That's me!'

'That's great, Charlie. Thank you for this insightful introduction and for being so open and honest', said Abbie. 'Who would like to go next?'

Some more silence follows.

'Shall I go?' Abbie locates the slightly unsure voice and nods encouragingly.

'My name is Jalal, which means glory! I have been working for 5 years as a nurse and I have been a team leader for the last 3 in an acute medical ward in a large hospital. This card shows me, sitting on my surfboard (I love surfing and even won a competition last year!) and I am looking out to sea. Really, I feel "all at sea". Normally, I can read the weather, the tides and the waves and I know what to do. That is how I was at work until a few months ago. I am good at my job and used to be so sure about how to care for patients. We registered nurses do a lot of the "high-tech" work that used to be done by junior doctors and I love it. But recently, my father was very ill and was admitted to hospital. When I visited him on the ward, I was shocked to hear from him and my mother that although the nurses were great on the tasks, they were very impersonal and distant. My mother felt that they lacked compassion. She thought they seemed 'too busy' to give personal care. Now I know the way things are going in the health service today, means that a lot of bedside care is given by health care assistants, which is what happens in our ward, but the reality was that my father wasn't even getting that. My mother and family were taking care of him, helping him to wash and eat. My father is fine now, but that was a real wake-up call and I started to look more carefully at what was happening on our ward, and I talked to some patients and their relatives. I was shocked to find out that some of them were experiencing something similar to my father and, even worse, when some family members started to give personal care, they said that some of the nurses and the health care assistants were very shirty and disapproving. So like Charlie, I guess, I want things to change. And being a team leader, I feel very responsible, and that I should be very clear about how to do it, but the reality is I don't. So I am all at sea.'

And so, encouraged by Mike and Abbie's explicit and warm valuing of what each person has said, the participants, one by one, introduce themselves. There is Grace, a physiotherapist, who is there because she wants to work with the occupational therapists and nurses around discharge planning; she had made an attempt and felt she had failed miserably. Before this programme, Grace had said to herself, 'This is what we should be doing; we should be including patients and families in their own discharge planning'. And Lauren, an occupational therapist, and Marek, a health care assistant, respectively, work in an organisation that has recently built practice development into their corporate strategy and they had been invited by their unit leader to join a practice development coordination group for the unit. They had been asked to come along to the programme to learn how to do practice development and particularly, how to do audits.

All this while, Abbie and Mike give the impression that they have plenty of time for these introductions. Even though the introductions are going over the planned time, they both listen attentively to what each person says and respond authentically. Later on, in their debrief, Abbie tells Mike that she thinks it was wonderful that the introductions had been so vibrant; although, she had felt like a swan gliding on the surface of the water at that point, but all the time paddling furiously underneath it to work out how they would make up the time.

'It's so important to listen to people describing their starting point on their practice development journeys, so that we can help each person move forward during the programme.

We just couldn't skimp on that. I was amazed how open people were and feel we very quickly created a space where people felt safe enough to reveal something of themselves and their situations. We need to learn from what we did well there so that we can recapture this again'.

Mike replied, 'I feel that their responses showed how powerful active listening is in terms of helping people to open up. I liked it when you pointed this out to them later. I could see that making group processes explicit helps the participants learn'.

Abbie added, 'Thank you ... now we can weave their ideas into some of the examples we use, as we facilitate learning activities. Our active listening today was role-modelling a facilitation skill for them.'...

Had we been there in the room, observing, we would have seen Abbie moving on to talk about practice development as a journey. Whether setting out to improve one's own practice or that of a team, it's all about working towards becoming more effective within an organisation. The journey, whatever the context, has key elements that help everyone who has a stake in achieving the vision that they have helped to create and agree with. We would have seen Abbie point to a poster of Figure 1.3 on the wall and heard her explain that the elements are not a series of steps that people take, one after the other. Rather, the elements recur in a backwards and forwards, round and round spiral. A practice developer is someone who helps stakeholders, that is, everyone who has some kind of an interest in the change. So, this includes helping those receiving care as well as those giving it, to journey towards the vision. The practice developer is a facilitator helping people to develop a shared sense of where they want to go, in other words, the agreed vision or the destination of the journey. Then, building on the agreed vision and the evaluation, practice development facilitators help others to make plans for learning and action and carry them out. When people are implementing the action plans, they generally need challenge and support through the following:

- Constantly checking in to assess where they are on the journey (continuous evaluations to follow the impact of the learning and action as changes are made).
- Constantly refining what they are doing and identifying new learning to be done (continuous evaluations inform decisions, whether the actions are working or whether new action and/or learning plans need to be made).

Abbie notices, at this point, that many participants are looking blankly at the poster and others look frankly worried.

'Now, Mike and I know that this bigger picture of the journey shown in the poster is daunting, especially when beginning in practice development. But don't worry, no one is expecting you to go off and lead a big project. Practice development is complex because it involves many different people across an organisation, so taking an overall lead on it is too much for a beginner. But we need all of us to be doing things that will make a positive difference. So within practice development, everyone is considered to be a leader of something. Mike and I, and all of you, will be leading and facilitating different aspects of practice development across our care settings. To begin with, we would invite you all to start developing or more likely redevelop your relationships with stakeholders in your area. Focus on what you can do and on what you can influence. So, for example, Charlie here might decide that she wants to work with her fellow team members, leader and patients (the stakeholders) to develop a vision (that they all can own) for the way they want to work with patients and with each other.' Charlie stands up making a defiant pose and says, 'Bring it on' and there is more laughter around the room. Abbie pauses momentarily, so Charlie can have the group's attention, and then continues. 'This would involve using practice development tools and processes to help people to become aware of and talk about their values about care. And Jalal over here, might want to start by getting some different types of conversations going in his team, for instance, about doing technical care in a person-centred way and seeing personal care as providing moments of opportunities for person-centredness to emerge that makes a difference to patients and families. That could very well then lead on to discussions about developing a person-centred culture as a team vision.' Jalal is nodding. 'Sounds like something I can do.'

Seeing everyone relax a bit and with some encouragement from Abbie, who physically turned to Mike and gestured an invitation for him to join in, Mike continues, 'We will also be helping you to contribute to the bigger picture of practice development across your organisation. For example, if your organisation is working towards improving the patients' experience, or encouraging innovation strategically like Lauren and Marek's organisation is, there is likely to be a governance group that this strategic work is accountable to and also opportunities for experimentation through participating in creative spaces to test your ideas out'.

Lizzie speaks up, 'What I hear you saying, Mike, is that whatever our experience, that we can make a contribution to a practice development journey – whether the journey takes place just within a team, a ward, a unit or the whole organisation . . . . Have I got that right?'

'Spot on, you have been listening carefully!', Mike replies.

Pointing at the poster of the practice development journey on the wall, Dillon, a nurse working in community nursing, asks, 'Are you saying that practice development is not only about helping people to do all the things in the picture like demonstrating their beliefs and values or whatever, that it is also about helping people to learn and perhaps change the way they approach their work and relationships and even their values?' Most of the participants move slightly to get a view or a better view of the poster.

'Yes, and in relation to working with values, this is one of the most important things we do as practice developers.' Mike suddenly becomes self-conscious and feels he is at the front leading on this, has a bit of an emotional wobble (which he later regrets) and feels the need for support. 'Abbie, do you want to say anything here?', he says at the same time as hoping that Abbie picks up his uncertainty.

'Yes, I think this would be a good time to have a look at the practice development framework (see Figure 1.1) handout that we sent you in advance. It is the one with circles within circles, with 'person-centred culture' in the middle and 'values and vision' on the outside'. People find the handout and Dillon remembers wondering what the arrows with 'facilitated active learning' and 'authentic engagement' written in them meant. Abbie goes on. 'This model – which is an adaptation of Rob Garbett and Brendan McCormack's (2002) work – shows what you do as a facilitator to help people to change themselves and their settings, which we term workplaces. By facilitating active learning and being authentic, in other words, being yourself, you help people to change themselves and their workplaces, so that a person-centred culture is created.'

Abbie continues, 'When people are helped to become aware of and/or think about their own values or beliefs and what they mean for person-centred practice, they may consider re-examining how they go about their work. So, the practice developer might help them to become aware that they demonstrate a staff-centred rather than patient- or person-centred approach to care. Or the practice developer may help people become aware of a gulf between what they say and do. For example, a staff member may say in public that they value patient-centred care, but they don't show this in practice.'

Charlie thinks to herself, 'Oh no, this is what is beginning to happen to me!' And says out loud, in a bit of an exaggerated way, 'Thank goodness, I managed to get myself on this programme'. She tunes back into what Abbie is saying and asks, 'I read something somewhere about how we have to think about our language, as this is often an indictor of our underlying values and beliefs. What do you think?'

'Mike, would you like to respond to this comment and question by Charlie?' asks Abbie.

Mike, although paying attention to the conversation, as well as what was going on around the group, picks up another level, 'The practice developer might gently challenge, for example, labelling language that staff use to describe others like, "that difficult woman or family", "the trouble-maker on Ward 5", "the stroke" or "that man who keeps complaining". Helping people to come to hear and recognise that this is what they are saying and to realise that this has a potentially negative impact, needs skilled work and preparation. Really listening to people and valuing them as a person without necessarily sharing their values needs some navigation. But if you don't listen to people, you won't be able to work effectively with their values.' Mike decides to use a question, to take the attention off him, to engage participants in thinking about this a bit more for themselves.

'Have you experienced this kind of thing happening?'

'Yes,' responded Grace, 'that is exactly what happened to me when I tried to get the occupational therapist and the nurses working with me to explore how we talked about discharge planning. They shut me out, saying it wasn't that important.' Mike asks others to have a talk about other experiences with people around them for a few moments and see what comes up. After a few minutes, Abbie and Mike ask for any key points people want to share. Then Abbie explains that the programme will help them to step onto a path that will develop their own practice development skills through helping others with these sorts of things . . .

As we leave the group discussing the core skills of a practice development facilitator, it is possible to hear Lauren and Marek tell Grace how the language at the first practice development coordination group meeting they went to was very impersonal and technical, all about how best to do audits, 'When we mentioned talking with patients about their experiences, they just carried on as if we hadn't spoken.' And then almost unable to resist, Charlie chips in, 'While I have been listening to you three talk, it struck me that in my workplace people don't listen to me or my colleagues either. They come in with their own agendas and don't even ask us what we think. I think that practice development should focus on listening. And that is something that is within my reach. I can improve the way I listen and help people to say what they really want to say, because it isn't always easy to put things into words.'

With Charlie's words ringing in our ears, here is a summary of all the core skills practice development facilitators need to develop and enhance:

- Noticing.
- Active listening.
- Asking a wide range of effective questions that enable critical reflection in self and others.
- Receiving feedback from others and asking others for feedback.
- Offering constructive and supportive feedback.
- Working in ways that demonstrates a combination of high challenge and high support to self and others.

2: Active listening

The facilitator's practice development journey continues by listening and hearing to find out where:

- *team members are starting from, in terms of their own values, skills, practice and learning;*
- *patients and families are, in terms of their values and experience of care;*
- *the workplace is, in terms of structure, culture and how these influence the care experience and service delivery.*

After a morning break, Abbie suggests that it would be good to develop some terms for engagement or ground rules, 'whatever you want to call them', for the way they are going to work together on the programme. Abbie explains what the activity is about and how participants can contribute. Within small groups, they could start sharing ideas and come up with shared terms or rules, and then each small group could share their ideas with the whole group. When all the ideas were heard, they could work together to reach an agreement on the ideas and the wording of the terms or rules. Abbie adds, 'This activity gives you an opportunity to practise active listening skills even though you are all being asked to say what ground rules or terms of engagement you want to have. How do feel about working this way?', she asks. People say they can see the value of this activity and agree on using the name, 'ground rules'. They want to start off in small groups to give them confidence.

After the allocated amount of time and judging that the small groups were making progress, Abbie says, 'How did that go?' There is general laughter and some people say how difficult it was to concentrate on what the other person was saying because there was so much going on for them in their heads after the programme introduction or they were focusing on what they wanted to say more than listening to others. Abbie and Mike nod their head empathetically and Abbie says, 'Yes, that is often the case when we become more conscious of what we are doing. That is why it is important for us to agree on some ground rules for the way we engage with each other on this programme, like really listening to each other and hearing what is said. We would suggest that all teams and groups involved in practice development need to have their own ground rules or terms for engagement'.

Abbie and Mike had agreed that Mike would lead on this activity, so he comes in now and suggests that the small groups can share their ideas for ground rules with each other. 'How does that sound?'

Dillon says, 'But what about if we find we value different things, like someone might prefer a more top-down performance management style of working with people and not the collaboration that you have talked about and shown us in the way you have facilitated us in this activity? As a person-centred facilitator, what would I do?'

'That is a really good point, Dillon.' Mike recognises the contribution Dillon has made, assessing that Dillon is really thinking through the implications of listening to and working with people who have different values to his own.

He continues, 'The skill in facilitating this activity is about really listening to people's values, that is, what is important for people, and looking for commonalities in people's values. These points of connection become the group's ground rules; they guide how people work together as well as the directions they want to go in. And because you revisit them regularly, they can be changed and added to as people's values evolve. So, as we work together now to agree our own ground rules, we might want to hold Dillon's point in our minds as we develop them.'

Mike continues facilitating the activity. By the end of a short period of discussion, the group has a set of ground rules for learning and working together on the programme written up on a flipchart. Mike checks that everyone agrees with them and is committed to trying to work with them, although some of them might be challenging. They agree. All participants sign up to the ground rules in various colourful and creative ways and a spontaneous round of applause takes place in the group.

Mike concludes, 'Thank you for engaging in this activity. This is a good first list of ground rules. They match the working relationships I would expect to see in a person-centred culture. Just thinking about Dillon's earlier challenge, if your team had agreed to develop a person-centred culture, what would you do if someone in the team proposed a ground rule that might not be very conducive to such a culture, such as, "It is inappropriate for patients and their families to be asked to provide evidence about practice in our team". Such a ground rule goes against the values of collaboration, inclusion and participation. What might you do?'

Amy, a nurse manager, speaks up, 'You would have to tell them that it doesn't match, so they can't do it. After all, they have agreed to the culture.' Grace responds, 'But isn't that a bit directive? I've done something similar with the nurses and occupational therapists and it didn't work, they just got resistant.'

Mike asks Amy what she thinks might happen if she did that, what might be the consequences. Amy thinks for a while and says that definitely, it would not work if someone said that to her! Smiles break out around group members and they wait for her to continue. Then she thinks Grace is right, it would not work – 'But to be honest it wouldn't be what I'd want to do anyway.' Mike, nods, and asks her what else she could do. Silence prevails. 'Does anyone else have any ideas?' Silence, which Mike feels a bit more uncomfortable about. Then Grace asks Mike what he would do. Quickly, Mike decides if he's going to give the question back but thinks that the group needs help, so he will answer the question. Later, when he reflects with Abbie he recognises that he could have asked the participants to chat about the options for a couple of minutes before he gave an answer.

'OK, as you've asked me directly, I would ask people how they felt about this mismatch. In much the same way, I gently challenged Amy just now. In the discussion, I would be careful not to impose my own values, but I would point out the possible consequences of having such a ground rule. Then the seeds are sown. Even if they decide to stick with the rule for now because they don't feel able to work with patients, it is likely that they will move to this later. As they, in effect, exclude patients and families, they will begin to feel the implications for themselves and their vision. Then, it is likely that they will decide to include patients and families.'

Emma, an experienced palliative care nurse, has been listening carefully, 'But isn't that just skilful manipulation! If you are a facilitator committed to the values of person-centredness and so on, even if you listen to and work with other different values that stakeholders hold, aren't you in danger of engaging in a skilful manipulation of others?'

'Another really good question!' Mike continues, 'This is something we constantly have to examine within ourselves to check that we are not doing this and where we need to own up when we do. Skilled facilitators make their values explicit to themselves and to those they are working with. For example, Abbie and I did this intentionally in our introduction to you – do you remember? We do this so others can judge our actions in the context of our espoused values. If facilitators are more concerned with achieving what they think is best in a particular way and will countenance no other and they succeed, then that is skilful manipulation. On the other hand, they are authentic person-centred facilitators if they make explicit and put into practice their own personal values or those agreed in the vision, but also help people to go in their own directions based on thinking through actions and consequences based on shared values.'

Abbie adds, 'Emma, what does your challenge, and what Mike said in response, tell you about power?'

'Now you are asking me a very difficult question – my mind has gone blank . . . I hate being put on the spot.' Abbie and Mike look relaxed and wait.

'Well, I think you are showing that you are aware of power in the relationship with stakeholders. Normally, a teacher or leader holds the power. But from what you and Abbie have said, a person-centred facilitator works in partnership with stakeholders, rather than telling them what to do.'

'That's brilliant, Emma', says Abbie. 'We try to create the conditions so that stakeholders can share power with us in the relationship. And that power circulates according to where people or a group are at and who has the capability and competence for the particular thing at hand.'

'What if a group of stakeholders agree to a set of ground rules for working together and then people don't stick to them?' asks Lauren. A buzz breaks out around the group as various participants start making remarks to each other.

'OK, let's keep focused and remember, one of our ground rules stated here is not talking over others in the group.' The noise reduces.

'What could you do, Lauren?' asks Mike.

Emma thinks to herself, 'I am beginning to get this now, these practice developers don't just tell you something or give you advice, they make you work it out for yourself' . . . She watches to see what happens next.

'Well,' Lauren says, 'building on what you just said to Amy, I suppose when you think someone is not keeping to the ground rules, you could ask the person or group whether they think they are working within the ground rules they have agreed to. Then they can own up themselves that they are breaking the rules.'

'Yes you could do that, Lauren, and then . . . anyone else?'

Charlie quickly retorts 'You can lighten the situation by reminding everyone that it is a common human condition that we all have values that we espouse and that we don't live them perfectly all of the time.'

Abbie summarises saying, 'Challenging in a supportive way is fundamental to facilitating practice development. And it requires a lot of practice to do it so that people feel genuinely supported at the same time as their thinking or behaviour are being challenged. All we can do is strive to live up to our values and, of course, we can help each other to do that as we create our practice development path by walking the talk.'

Afterwards, they went on to evaluate the activity. Members in the group said that Mike had given them space to disagree, discuss and come to common agreements. He did not impose his own values on them. He also created the conditions so that Emma felt she could challenge him. They felt pleased with themselves that they had helped each other to express their values by asking questions and listening to what they were saying. This is close to focused attention. Focused attention means being truly present for and really hearing another person, even if this is only for a moment. It is often visible through stillness of the relaxed body and the flow of kindness and energy through eye contact. Focused attention is often experienced as the listener/facilitator acknowledges a common humanity with, and genuinely wants to help, the other. It is at the heart of being person-centred and getting to know and engage with the whole person including their hopes, dreams and values.

* * *

Later, back in her workplace, Grace was having a conversation with a patient called Freda about how she thought her rehabilitation was progressing. It was a typical conversation, but it came to Grace that she was not really listening to Freda, who was rather dejectedly sitting in front of her. Time to take a risk, thought Grace, why not use some of her developing facilitation skills with this patient, like active listening and giving focused attention?

'Can we start again, Freda? I feel we're not helping you in the way you want, for which I'm very sorry. I do really want to help you'. Seeing Freda nod, Grace took a deep breath and said, 'Tell me how you see your future . . . '

Freda started talking, slowly and hesitantly at first, and then started to say what really mattered to her and something she was hoping to achieve before it was too late. Grace listened until Freda stopped. She was processing a mound of things Freda had said.

'I bet you wish you hadn't asked me now – but I do feel better for saying all of that.'

Grace and Freda had a laugh about this.

Grace went on to say, 'I'm really so pleased I've listened to what matters to you. I feel this gives us a meaningful goal that we can help you work towards. Let me have a talk with the team, that is, if I have your consent to share what you've told me?'

'Yes of course', replied Freda.

'OK, I will come back tomorrow and maybe we can look at your goal and see how we work towards it – together.'

As Grace walked away she also knew she felt better about herself for that moment.

3: Feedback opportunities

Giving and receiving feedback to individuals, groups and teams along the practice development journey is vital for integrated evaluation–learning–planning–acting spirals. Using the high-challenge/high-support principle, we can work with critique rather than criticism. It is definitely not about blaming or being judgemental. The intention is to help the other person(s) to learn so that they can be more effective in their engagement with practice development. So, feedback needs to be clear and useful. It is given in an intentionally supportive and kind way and it requires honest and open communication. The process is often led by a practice development facilitator. Practice development facilitators can offer feedback both formally, for example, in clinical supervision or team and stakeholder meetings, and informally, for instance, in all sorts of day-to-day conversations.

The practice development programme seemed a long way away when, about 2 weeks later, the opportunity to give feedback in her workplace to her colleagues hit Charlie firmly between the eyes. As she gathered herself, she mused that this was what Abbie probably meant by an opportunity to influence. Miriam Turnball was walking around the unit again. This was likely to be a flashpoint for some of the team members who had difficulties with patients with dementia being out of their rooms. Charlie saw one of her colleagues approach

Ms Turnball and say in a parental tone 'Come on, back to your room, you naughty girl.' It grated with Charlie. She strode across to Miriam and the nurse.

'Miriam Turnball, how nice to see you' she said in an animated voice.

Miriam turned to see who was addressing her, 'Oh, you know me then?'

'Well, enough to know you're looking for something.'

'I think I was but she won't let me move. Look at what she's doing to me' and she indicated to the other team member . . . 'It's like a prison in here.'

Charlie put her hand out for Miriam to hold if she wanted to. 'That's awful. I'm very sorry to hear you say that. How can I, and my colleague here, help you?'

Having rescued the intervention and put the brakes on it becoming an increasingly negative experience for Miriam, Charlie engaged Miriam until she looked more relaxed and was beginning to smile. After a few more minutes, Miriam said she needed to go back to her house as it was getting chilly out here on the street and slowly walked back. Charlie looked at her colleague, 'OK, Maria, let's talk about this please to see what we can both learn.'

Maria rolled her eyes towards the ceiling and said nothing.

In a quiet spot, Charlie asked Maria to summarise what had just happened. As Maria reluctantly talked, Charlie listened carefully without interrupting.

'Thanks for sharing this as you saw it, Maria. I heard you address Miriam as "a naughty girl". How do you think that might affect her dignity?'

Maria looked stumped for a moment. Collecting herself, she shrugged her shoulders, 'Is it that important? She has dementia, what does it matter?'

'Maria, come on now, I have heard you say many times you believe in person-centredness. And that it happens here. So, I'm asking you now how addressing an older adult as "a naughty girl" relates to being person-centred?'

Charlie kept telling herself to stay focused on the language, as this was something Maria could address. The other aspects like challenging Maria about her 'professional knows best' attitude would need to wait. Charlie was also mindful of keeping the conversation to about 10 minutes at the most. After a short exchange between them, Maria said that she hadn't meant to say those things, that it just happens without her thinking about it and that everyone did it. Charlie then negotiated with Maria that Maria would pay more attention to how she addressed patients and that she would listen out to see how other team members did this too. Charlie said that she and Maria needed to follow up in about 2 weeks' time to see how she was progressing. Both Charlie and Maria then continued with their work, both sighing deeply, but for different reasons.

Charlie reflected on her way home from work that she would have to think more about how to balance her high challenge with high support when challenging one of her colleagues. Did she come over as too dictatorial? And she did not find out from Maria how she felt about the challenge and the actions Maria would take. She would see how effective she had been if and when they meet in 2 weeks' time.

* * *

It started like most workdays. Jalal had walked around to see his assigned patients and spoken to all the patients regardless of their recorded responsiveness level. The morning progressed pretty well. The daily ward round was taking place as usual and, as happens, a conversation began about treatment options for a particular patient who was not responding to treatment and brain death was being considered. Jalal listened to the different team members making their points. This was his opportunity to say what he had been wanting to say for a long while . . .

'How do we know what the patient might want for himself in this situation?' That was it, he had said it now. He assumed he had said it out loud as there was the silence he had expected. A senior team member spoke with curt authority, 'We will decide what is in this patient's best interests, thank you.'

'I agree with you that the patient's best interests are key here.' Jalal remembered the technique of finding a shared interest with stakeholders, 'I believe these extend beyond the immediate medical needs, so we may need to look more broadly in this case.' Another pause.

'I think you will find that the patient's clinical needs are being well taken care of.'

'Again, I agree, I am not questioning the clinical care, but asking about what is in this person's best interests and how we decide a direction that reflects the patient's best interests when they can't tell us. What do others think?'

Jalal, determined to have one more try, went on, 'I feel, since we have all signed up to shared values about patient care in which we state we will work with what is in the person's best interests, I guess this is a real test for us as a team, especially when there is no living will and the patient can't tell us what they would want for themselves.' He continued, 'I would like to discuss this with the patient's immediate family and find out what they believe their relative would have wanted. Maybe we could invite the patient's next of kin and another close family member to participate in a Best Interests meeting or small case conference on the ward?'

Although there was some reluctance from members of the ward round, quite a few people agreed, so it was decided to wait another day before revisiting the way forward, and that a case conference was a good idea. Jalal felt buoyant, he had practised his challenging questions by working with common ground, but more importantly, he had acted for the first time on the gap he had frequently experienced between the shared values and beliefs talked about by the team and actual actions in everyday work. Jalal reflected, 'Now that I have given the team this feedback in what was clearly a constructive way, at least for those who agreed with the case conference idea, I really have to follow through this commitment I have made. I will find out when the patient's next of kin is coming in so that I can talk with them.'

However, Jalal felt worried about the defensiveness and visible reluctance of some members of the ward round and thought that he should be thinking about what else was needed. He reflected that this test case could be used to raise consciousness about the importance of a person-centred team culture. In such a team culture, there would be agreement about and commitment to the values underpinning their work in the best interests of patients, and feedback would be given constructively and received non-defensively.

* * *

Lauren thought carefully about the group meeting she was going into. Such groups had been set up around the unit by the Practice Development Coordination group. She was as determined as she could be that it was not going the way of all the other recent meetings that were used as one big moaning session by the team. She felt she needed to give some constructive feedback to the team and owned that she was part of the problem.

Lauren picked up courage and said she would like to say something. Clearing her throat and determined to be authentic, she said, 'I would like to make an observation. When we get together in these meetings, we seem to just have a moaning session, nothing constructive happens and we don't take any actions forward. We don't have any shared purpose for these meetings or any ground rules for how we work together.'

A stunned silence resulted . . . Lauren, remembering the importance of silence when offering high challenge, stopped herself from further outpourings that might prevent others from thinking about the challenge she had just made. Then after what seemed an eternity, a couple of people spoke. 'I agree, I was thinking about not coming to this meeting. I am so busy, I have so much to do and it seems such a waste of time.' 'But it does give us a chance to let off steam – I feel so 'done to' in this hospital, there's no support and everyone takes us for granted.'

Lauren, relieved that her intervention had stopped people in their tracks and caused them to think, continued . . . 'I think we should use some of those practice development principles that Marek and I learned about at the practice development programme and which we have recently shared with you. We could use them to really think about what we want from this meeting and how we can support each other and what we want to achieve.'

One member of the group concurred, 'I heard about how one team went through this process of using postcards to identify how they wanted to work with each other. It really worked – they developed some ground rules in about 15 minutes flat and then moved on to developing a framework and objectives collaboratively. Now they are working really effectively together, no one misses a meeting because they are so productive. I think it could work for us, but who would facilitate this?'

Silence. Lauren was thinking . . . 'Maybe I could do this . . . . No . . . . I feel so strongly myself about how we should be working together, I might not be able to both identify my values and facilitate the group. Maybe Mike would facilitate this for me and then I can be a participant too and get more experience of observing Mike in action, so I can learn more too? . . . '

Lauren spoke, 'I could ask Mike; he is one of the facilitators who leads the practice development programme. I could see if he is free to come to our next meeting and help us with this.' To Lauren's surprise, everyone agreed that this would be a good idea and would provide a fresh start. Leaving the meeting Lauren reflected on her experience of using honest feedback to challenge ineffective team meetings, trying to be authentic, as well as using silence. She is certainly going to do more of this.

4: Enabling questions

Through working with enabling questions facilitators can enhance their effectiveness in helping practitioners to both reflect more deeply and put learning into action in the workplace. For new facilitators asking enabling questions takes practice as it is an acquired skill.

Emma is lying in bed after a busy day. She had decided to keep a notebook after the first week of the programme to write down her reflections and action plans for becoming a facilitator in her unit. She props herself up in bed and writes:

Asking questions?????

Today I thought about what questions I've asked at work and how good they are. Quick conclusion is, I'm a bit rubbish at asking questions . . . That's my surface stuff out, so now the real stuff.

I can recognise when and where a question needs to be asked. I can even ask one or two questions. In a few situations, I feel I have a small stock of enabling questions I can draw on. Probably, I do this best in the care planning meetings – actually, if I can do it there in front of the whole team, why can't I do it in other situations?

If I reframe that question:

What is it I do there that I can do elsewhere? That makes it more positive . . .

It's a sit down discussion that seems more planned and the team seems to have more time. I'm not good at thinking up questions quickly or when I'm put on the spot.

Patience . . . I need to build on my strength some more.

I'm still left wondering. How do I know what an enabling question is?

When Abbie and Mike asked questions, they seemed to be so good at getting to the heart of the matter quickly; they really help people find new directions and insights for themselves. Maybe I am using questions that are more about things I am curious about myself, rather than questions that would help the person to move on and think about the situation themselves. I always seem to relate to the person's situation and I think if I could find out if their situation was like mine then I could give them some really good advice . . . Oh, I forget that we are not meant to give advice . . . and I suppose that is why we aren't meant to ask questions to satisfy our own interests.

Abbie and Mike always seemed to sense what people are feeling, to pick up the paradoxes between what people say and do. They are also good at recognising and drawing on peoples' past experiences – I have noticed this always makes people feel good, as they realise that they do have the answers themselves.

So, what sort of questions would be enabling and help people to move forward themselves? Maybe it's things like really carefully listening to the story and then asking, 'What do you want to achieve?' Or, 'What worked for you in the past?' 'What options are open to you?' These seem to be all 'what questions', although, I've noticed that asking, 'How do you feel about this?' always seems to enable a cathartic release of emotion. And every time, when asked at the end (that's evaluation!!!), the person always says how relieved they feel to have shared their situation. This must be a good enabling question to start with as it clears away the emotion, so that they can move on to other things, such as helping people identify what question they are asking themselves.

Some people don't seem to know what questions they are asking, they have such messy situations that they don't know where to start. So, I suppose helping people to identify all the questions they are asking themselves may also be enabling because then they can choose to tackle one at the time, depending on what they see to be most important in the moment. I think I am getting this and I must start practising and evaluating so that I can learn! And when I ask for feedback on my facilitation questions, I must make sure I receive it non-defensively!!

* * *

A few months have now passed and we pick up with Charlie again. We find her reflecting on something that has happened at work.

Charlie chews her pencil for a minute or so and then starts writing:

'Rather than telling people what is going on and what to do, I need to ask open questions to help the people to find their own answers. Sometimes I might give advice, but not before I have helped people, through my questions, to work things out for themselves. Then, when they have gone as far as they can go with the help of the questions, I might offer some suggestions.'

Charlie closes her eyes and can recall Abbie inviting them to share what enabling questions meant to them. She remembers Abbie saying, 'As you have already grasped, enabling questions will help you to become more independent and effective learners in your workplace. As you say, this is because they help you to go further in the way you think or feel. Then you can use new understandings to develop your workplace or your work more effectively. You've really got it that enabling questions will help you to learn things for yourself rather than remaining dependent on others to tell you what to do or for advice. And that using enabling questions in your daily interactions with team members and patients as well as in active learning sessions will help contribute to creating a person-centred learning culture in the home.'

Charlie looked through her notes:

Enabling questions encourage reflection and can lead to action.
They are open questions in that they do not make any assumptions.

Compare, for example, the open, enabling question, 'How do you feel about what happened?' with the closed question, 'Did that make you feel angry?'

She remembers Dillon saying something about a closed question making the assumption that you felt angry and that you were made to feel in a certain way – as if you had no choices or control. She had noted that closed questions do not help the person to become reflective. Further scribbles showed that a leading question also tends to invite a yes or no answer, but it goes further in closing off opportunities for reflection. For example, 'What you did in that situation was inappropriate, wasn't it?' or 'You should have given that person feedback about their behaviour, shouldn't you?' Such judgemental, leading questions run the risk of defensive responses. They may also prevent the person from exploring the situation, reflecting upon and evaluating their own behaviour and developing action points about how they could behave more effectively in similar situations in the future.

Charlie goes back to writing:

'When I am more aware about asking enabling questions, I can see that I tend to ask leading questions as my first attempt to help others to learn. These leading questions point others in a direction the questioner believes is the best one. I know the trick is to try and avoid them, as well as closed questions and direct advice giving. But just a minute, I do remember Mike saying something positive about leading questions! He said, 'When a person has explored, reflected and evaluated for themselves and is still stuck, leading questions can then be used positively as an alternative to merely giving advice like, "What you must do first is give that person feedback about their behaviour before going to tell someone else" or "What I have found is that you need to ask patients or residents what they think?"

In coming up with helpful leading questions, you still use your experience to think up the questions, but you are opening up the opportunity for the person to think for themselves and draw their own conclusions. So, you might ask, "In these circumstances, would it be helpful to give that person feedback about their behaviour?" or "Have you thought about asking patients what they think? Is that a possibility?"

But what I remember most is that both Abbie and Mike stressed the importance of us building up a bank of enabling questions for ourselves. So here goes!

How do you feel . . . ?
It sounds as though you are feeling . . . ?
Perhaps it would be more helpful to turn that comment into a question?
What question does that raise for you?
What question was the most helpful?
What do you think is really going on here?
What sense are you making of . . . ?
What does . . . mean for you?
How would you know if . . . ?

What are we trying to do here?
What could you do . . . ?
What does that really mean?
Are you saying 'they' when you mean 'you'?

What do you think would happen if . . . ?
Do you think that . . . ?
How can you . . . ?

Can we stop for a moment and check on how we are doing?
How helpful was that comment?

Energy levels seem low – shall we take a break?
Perhaps we should check our agreed ground rules?

How can we help you (or someone else) move forward on this issue?
How can we make this relationship more effective?
How can I help you?'

Charlie notes, 'This seems to be a definite learning experience for me, which is very similar to that of other beginning facilitators from what I can gather. The high challenge/high support I get from my practice development peers helps me to identify what I need to learn.'

* * *

Going back to the final day of the practice development programme, we can see Abbie and Mike summing up the programme so far . . .

'And just to really emphasise', says Abbie, 'practice development is not only about using tools and processes like Values Clarification and Claims, Concerns and Issues to help stakeholders go round the integrated spiral (pointing again at the practice development journey poster on the wall), it is what you do and who you are in your everyday work as a nurse, pharmacist, therapist, health care assistant, and so on. As you become more experienced in these fundamental facilitation skills, you may be interested in experimenting with some ideas from facilitation theories developed in education and health care fields that we will introduce to you and give you some practice in over the next 9 months. We've been talking for a while, are there any comments or questions so far?'

Then the group shared the key facilitation principles that they had been exploring together:

- Facilitators get to know the person(s) they are helping and their contexts and situations through multiple methods, including active listening. They do this through engaging with the whole person with the whole of themselves.
- Active listening requires the facilitator to acknowledge but set aside their own thoughts on what they are hearing, so that they can offer focused attention and really hear what the other is saying. Focused attention is often experienced by the other as supportive.
- Active listening enables the facilitator to think through the relevant enabling questions that get to the heart of the matter and challenge the person's thinking.
- High challenge is balanced by high support to energise and motivate learning. It is enacted through the core facilitation skills.
- Giving feedback requires facilitators to develop high-level observation skills.
- Facilitators ask for feedback about their developing skills and then model receiving it non-defensively.
- Being able to ask appropriate enabling questions in a smooth, seemingly effortless way takes a while to develop and become part of who the facilitator is. When it does, facilitators find that they are asking such questions easily in their everyday work (and often in their personal lives).
- As facilitators have more experience of practice development, they are able to ask questions that get more quickly to the heart of the matter. The capacity to see what is significant develops from being able to see similar patterns emerging in individuals and situations. Facilitators always check out assumptions that they might be making based on their experience through asking enabling questions.
- Facilitators help people to learn in and from practice in the workplace (i.e. work-based and workplace learning) using active learning approaches (Dewing, 2009; Middleton, 2012). They help people to develop and implement their own learning at work action plans. If they occasionally adopt a teaching role, they build in active learning opportunities and use their facilitation skills as appropriate.
- Facilitators intentionally role-model facilitation skills and explain the methods and processes they are using to enable others to have insight into this for themselves. They encourage people to observe them and ask them questions about what they have observed like, 'What was in your head when you asked that question?', 'What options were open to you?', 'Why did you choose that option?' and 'What were you noticing when [name] responded . . . ?'

5: Postscript – 6 months later

Charlie

After 6 months, Charlie put herself forward to facilitate several practice development projects for the next 6–9 months, including leading a group to introduce and then evaluate intentional rounds on the unit. After she received consistent positive feedback about her ability to challenge and support, she undertook preparation to become a clinical supervisor in the trust.

Jalal

Jalal, with support from Mike, facilitated the development of a team vision using a values clarification and visioning method. Everyone signed up to the shared vision. Then the team went through a period of instability, including changes in nursing and medical management. The vision that he thought was shared did not seem to be taken seriously by the new members. The team reverted to a model whereby 'the professionals know best', rather than working in true partnership with patients and families. Jalal decided he needed to find another team to work with who really want to develop and work towards a shared vision.

Grace

Found herself becoming increasingly interested in patient experience and in how patients' stories could be used to develop the service and improve discharge planning. She found someone in the trust who encouraged her to set up a patient story project and also helped her get through the ethical approval. Grace is now coaching her physiotherapy team members to learn how to collect and analyse patient stories. The project has been put forward for a trust award.

Recently, the occupational therapist and some of the nurses with whom she tried to improve discharge planning (before she went on the practice development programme) have asked to join the project. Their involvement in actively listening to patients' stories has stopped their use of labelling language. They now see how disrespectful such language is and can be heard challenging others when they hear it.

Amy

In her role as unit nurse manager, Amy set up a practice development coordination group in the unit. They met a few times and developed a vision that they could all agree to, but since then, a funding crisis has developed in the trust. Amy feels pulled apart in all directions with demands from every level of the organisation. The work of the group has sunk low in her priorities and she has let it lapse. Although she has a vague sense that practice development could be a sound strategy for addressing cost-effectiveness and thus making savings in the unit, the initial investment in getting it going is too much for her right now. She has decided to withdraw from the practice development programme.

Lauren and Marek

Lauren and Marek succeeded in enabling the teams they worked with to become really effective. They became known for providing each other with peer support and review, as well as for taking forward an important hospital agenda. This agenda is about showing how improvements in care are experienced by patients, service users and staff. Lauren has decided that she will do a master's degree in practice development at the university where Abbie works and then move into a practice development role. She plans to use all the practice development skills she will learn in this way to develop organisation-wide care for patients and to help others in the development of their skills.

> **Emma**
>
> Emma was asked to start facilitating some of the palliative care multi-disciplinary care planning meetings. Her ability to ask good questions that made the palliative care team think more carefully about their discussion and decision-making was noticed and appreciated. Triggered by Jalal's disappointing experience of consciousness-raising of the team he worked with in the acute care setting, Emma learned how to become more involved in Mental Capacity work and especially with Best Interests meetings. She and Jalal are now collaborating in this work. Emma is also working with a mentor to become an After Action Review facilitator for the palliative care unit she was working in.

REFERENCES

Dewing, J. (2009) Moments of movement: active learning and practice development. *Nurse Education in Practice*, **10** (1), 22–26.

Eldridge, P. (2011) Reflections on a journey to knowing self. *International Practice Development Journal*, **1** (1), 5. http://www.fons.org/library/journal.aspx (Accessed 17 May 2012).

Garbett, R. & McCormack, B. (2002) A concept analysis of practice development. *NT Research*, **7** (2), 87–100.

Hunnisett, H. (2011) From fixer to facilitator: going round in circles promotes change! *International Practice Development Journal*, **1** (2), 9. http://www.fons.org/library/journal.aspx (Accessed 17 May 2012).

Jackson, C. & Webster, A. (2011) Swimming against the tide – developing a flourishing partnership for organisational transformation. *International Practice Development Journal*, **1** (2), 7. http://www.fons.org/library/journal.aspx (Accessed 17 May 2012).

Manley, K. (2001) *Consultant Nurse: Concept, Processes, Outcome*. Unpublished PhD thesis, RCN Institute/Manchester University.

Middleton, R. (2012) Active learning and leadership in an undergraduate curriculum: How effective is it for student learning and transition to practice? *Nurse Education in Practice*. [Epub ahead of print].

Snoeren, M. & Frost, D. (2011) Realising participation within an action research project on two care innovation units providing care for older people. *International Practice Development Journal*, **1** (2), 3. http://www.fons.org/library/journal.aspx (Accessed 17 May 2012).

Titchen, A. (2003) Critical companionship: part 1. *Nursing Standard*, **18** (9), 33–40.

Titchen, A. (2004) Helping relationships for practice development: critical companionship. In: *Practice Development in Nursing* (eds B. McCormack, K. Manley & R. Garbett), pp. 148–174. Blackwell Publishing Ltd., Oxford.

7 How You Might Use PARIHS to Deliver Safe and Effective Care

Jo Rycroft-Malone

Bangor University, Bangor, UK

INTRODUCTION

Whilst evidence-based practice has become a policy imperative and, in parallel, the research base for practice has grown massively, you may know from your own experience that the use of best evidence in practice remains patchy. In most developed countries around the world, there has been considerable investment in an infrastructure to support the development of knowledge products such as guidelines, standards and protocols; however, the literature is full of examples of patients receiving treatments and interventions that are known to be less effective or even harmful to patients. A few years ago, researchers identified that patients do not always get the most up-to-date care, even though there are many guidelines and protocols available to use (e.g. Grol, 2001; McGlynn et al., 2003). You may find the same in your workplace today. Patient safety is an international concern with preventable adverse events having significant human and medical costs for those who are harmed and their families and friends who care for them (Bucknall, 2011). It is very likely that your organisation puts a lot of emphasis on patient safety too. Additionally, we have seen health care costs increase, changes in professional and non-professional roles and accountability related to widespread workforce shortages, and limitations placed on the accessibility and availability of resources. A further development has been the increased access to information via multimedia, which has promoted greater involvement of service users in their treatment and management (Bucknall & Rycroft-Malone, 2010). All these factors focus attention on the need for health services to develop approaches to care delivery and practice that are safe and effective.

However, practitioners and the health system struggle to incorporate new knowledge into practice for achieving better outcomes for patients. Whilst practitioners genuinely wish to do the right thing for patients, robust research is just one of several components to inform health professionals in their everyday practice, and many factors influence this process. This chapter begins with highlighting some of those challenges, demands and complexities in achieving safe and effective care. The Promoting Action on Research Implementation in Health Services (PARIHS) framework is then introduced as a way you might incorporate and consider these challenges in your practice development activity.

Practice Development in Nursing and Healthcare, Second Edition. Edited by Brendan McCormack, Kim Manley and Angie Titchen.
© 2013 John Wiley & Sons, Ltd. Published 2013 by John Wiley & Sons, Ltd.

THE CHALLENGE AND COMPLEXITIES OF ACHIEVING SAFE AND EFFECTIVE CARE

Unlike the rapid spread associated with some forms of technology, which may simply require the intuitive use of a gadget and a little persuasion to purchase it, many health care changes are complex interventions requiring significant skills and knowledge to make clinical decisions prior to integration into practice. Not surprisingly then, implementation of evidence into practice is mostly a protracted process, consisting of multiple steps, with varying degrees of complexity depending on the context (Bucknall & Rycroft-Malone, 2010). However, for many years, the use of evidence in practice was seen as a linear and technical process, which focused at the level of an individual's ability to critically appraise research articles and put the findings from these into practice (Rycroft-Malone, 2008). You may have been on the receiving end of training in the critical appraisal of research; on reflection, did this approach encourage you to think differently about research, or more importantly, how you might use research within your practice? Findings from systematic reviews that examined individual nurse characteristics and how they influence research utilisation, found that apart from attitude to research, there was little to suggest that any potential individual determinants influence research use (Estabrooks et al., 2003; Squires et al., 2011). Arguably, this is because the individual practitioner cannot be isolated from all the other bureaucratic, political, organisational and social factors that affect care and the practice environment. Evidence use is beginning to be recognised more widely as a highly contingent process, which varies across settings and time. There has been an increasing awareness that there are a number of factors that might make a context more conducive to change and evidence use.

Views have been shifting over time about what constitutes evidence for evidence-based practice, and this has seen an acknowledgement that evidence is an inclusive concept (e.g. Lomas et al., 2005; Rycroft-Malone et al., 2004b; Scott-Findlay & Pollock, 2004). Authors recognise the appropriateness of the randomised controlled trial for evidence of effectiveness, but that other forms of evidence also inform clinical decision-making and the delivery of health care. Findings from research also support an expanded view of evidence indicating that evidence is socially and historically constructed, which means that different people will view 'the' evidence differently (Dopson et al., 2002; Dopson & Fitzgerald, 2005). The view about what evidence is has been expanding to recognise that clinical experience, patient views and experiences, and local information are part of the evidence base for practice (Rycroft-Malone et al., 2004b; Lomas et al., 2005). These issues are significant when thinking about achieving safe and effective care. For example, guidelines are viewed as an important clinical tool in promoting evidence-informed practice and their development has been prolific; however, research is not a product that can be taken off the shelf and readily applied in its current state. Guidelines and protocols are *one* of the catalysts to the process of situated decision-making and service delivery. This means that if you take an evidence synthesis such as a clinical guideline, it cannot automatically be assumed that the recommendations will mean the same thing to individuals and groups – some work needs to be undertaken to make them clinically relevant. Have a think about the sort of information that you use in your daily practice, what kind of evidence comes to mind? Then think about the organisation in which you work, is it clear to you what kind of evidence is most valued in your workplace?

The challenges that arise from the processes involved in promoting safe and effective care can be categorised into five areas (Greenhalgh et al., 2004). Challenges associated with: (1) the evidence or information to be implemented; (2) the individual clinicians who need to learn about the new evidence; (3) the structure and function of health care organisations; (4) the communication and facilitation of the evidence; and lastly, (5) the circumstances of the patient who will be the receiver of the new evidence. This categorisation is helpful in starting to think about what aspects need to be paid attention to during practice development processes, particularly in relation to developing a shared vision, describing and measuring where we are starting from, developing a plan, and in the ongoing evaluation and learning from and for action. Of course, fundamental to all these aspects are the prevailing values and beliefs of individuals and the organisation. The values and beliefs of individual patients, professionals, health care and education organisations, as well as local and national policy makers, including budget holders, will be critical in the relative success of achieving safe and effective care, and are therefore fundamental aspects to pay attention to in the practice development journey.

The previous text begins to highlight the multi-faceted nature of improving care through the use of evidence. The PARIHS framework presented in the following sections represents this complexity, and provides a map of the factors that need to be paid attention to during development and implementation activity. Additionally, how others have used PARIHS in implementation activity is described, in this way PARIHS can become a practical tool for you to use on your practice development journey.

PROMOTING ACTION ON RESEARCH IMPLEMENTATION IN HEALTH SERVICE (PARIHS) FRAMEWORK

The PARIHS framework was developed in an attempt to reflect the interdependence and interplay of the many factors that appear to play a role in the successful implementation of evidence in practice. Originally conceived through collaboration of Kitson et al. (1998), the framework has been evolving and developing for over a decade (Harvey et al., 2002; McCormack et al., 2002; Rycroft-Malone et al., 2002, 2004a, 2004b; Rycroft-Malone, 2004; Kitson et al., 2008).

Table 7.1 provides an overview of the various stages of development of PARIHS and associated publications.

The PARIHS framework is premised on the notion that the implementation of evidence-based practice depends on the ability to achieve significant and planned behaviour change involving individuals, teams and organisations. It serves as both a practical and conceptual heuristic to guide and evaluate research implementation and the practice development journey. As PARIHS is currently presented, it is a conceptual, rather than a process-orientated framework, although the inclusion of 'facilitation' as one of its core concepts indicates that process is a necessary ingredient. PARIHS maps out the elements that need attention before, during and after practice development efforts.

The title of the framework privileges the implementation of *research* evidence in health services, however, as mentioned earlier and the following sections show, evidence is conceived more broadly than just research, that is, it is acknowledged that decision-making and service delivery are also informed by other types of evidence. Despite a broad view of what constitutes evidence, an implicit assumption of the framework is that the implementation of good quality, relevant research in combination with clinical and patient experience, and local information is more likely to result in improved outcomes for patients and health services (Rycroft-Malone et al., 2002).

Table 7.1   Stages of development of PARIHS.

Phase	Activities and related publications
Development	• Retrospective and theoretical analysis of four case studies. • Development and publication of original framework. • Kitson et al. (1998).
Concept analysis	• Undertaken on the three core concepts of PARIHS: *Evidence, Context* and *Facilitation* using Morse's (1996) concept analysis approach. • This resulted in changes to the way that facilitation was conceptualised, and some changes to the content of context. • Harvey et al. (2002), McCormack et al. (2002), Rycroft-Malone et al. (2002) and Rycroft-Malone et al. (2004b).
Empirical enquiry	• Case studies of evidence into practice projects to check out the content validity of PARIHS. • This resulted in the addition of local information to the concept of evidence, and some additions to context, including fit with strategic priorities and resources. It also strengthened the rationale for the need of facilitation and/or a facilitative process. • Rycroft-Malone et al. (2004a).
Empirical testing	• Evaluating the impact of different types of facilitation (enabling and technical) on the implementation of recommendations for continence care: a process and outcome evaluation. • Funded by European Union Framework 7, involving centres in the United Kingdom and Northern Ireland, Ireland, Sweden and the Netherlands (2009–2013). • Seers et al. (2012)
Development of tools (by PARIHS group and others)	• Development of diagnostic and evaluative tools for use in research and practice. • Development of facilitation toolkits. Some initial items for tools can be found in Kitson et al. (2008). • Context Assessment Index – McCormack et al. (2009). • Alberta Context Tool – Estabrooks et al. (2009). • A guide for applying a revised version of the PARIHS framework for implementation – Stetler et al. (2011).

Successful implementation – SI = f(E,C,F)

Successful implementation (SI) is represented as a function (f) of (i.e. dependent upon) the nature and type of *evidence* (E), the qualities of the *context* (C) in which the evidence is being introduced, and a process of *facilitation*. This relationship is represented as: SI = f(E,C,F). If you look at Figure 7.1, you will see that the three elements (1) evidence, (2) context and (3) facilitation are each positioned on a 'high' to 'low' continuum. Within the practice development journey the aim is to move towards the high end of the continuum to optimise the chances of success.

The proposition is that the most successful implementation occurs when evidence is scientifically robust and matches professional consensus, patients' experiences and preferences and informed by local information/data ('high' evidence); the context receptive to change with sympathetic cultures, appropriate leadership and robust monitoring and feedback systems ('high' context); and, when there is appropriate facilitation of change with input from

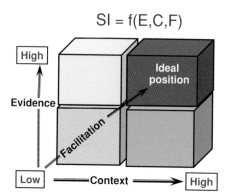

Fig. 7.1   Evidence, context, facilitation continua.

skilled external and/or internal facilitators ('high' facilitation). This ideal position is illustrated in Figure 7.1. On first glance at Figure 7.1, and considering the main elements of evidence and context, where would you place your organisation/service on the figure? We will explore ideas about how to move to the ideal position later in the chapter.

With a commitment to the development and refinement of the framework over time, its content has evolved. The most up-to-date content can be found in Rycroft-Malone et al. (2004b), which is summarised in Table 7.2 and described in more detail in the following sections. As the contents are described, you might want to think about how they relate to you as a practitioner, practice developer and the organisation/service in which you are working.

Evidence

Evidence is conceived in a broad sense within the framework including propositional and non-propositional knowledge from four different types of evidence: (1) research, (2) clinical experience, (3) patients and carers' experience and (4) local context information (see Rycroft-Malone et al., 2004b for detailed discussion). For evidence to be located towards the 'high' end of the continuum, certain criteria have to be met.

Research evidence within PARIHS is only one part of decision-making, and indeed, there are many issues where there is either a lack of research or the quality of it is poor. It is not advisable to be acting on evidence and changing practices based on poor quality research. For research evidence to be situated at 'high' on the continuum, whether it be qualitative and quantitative research, it should be well conceived and conducted, that is robust and judged to be credible. To enable you to judge the quality of the research, you should undertake some form of quality assessment (some suggestions about this are made in later sections). Additionally, you will remember, evidence is socially and historically constructed and individuals and professionals will likely think differently about the same piece of research evidence. Therefore, to increase the likelihood of implementation, a local process of tailoring and consensus building needs to take place. For example, in your workplace, you might be interested in implementing some recommendations from a national guideline, it would be important to incorporate a phase of working with colleagues (practitioners and manager) and service users and/or carers to agree on how those recommendations might be interpreted within the local context, and what needs to be done to prepare the ground for their use.

Table 7.2   PARIHS framework elements and sub-elements.

Elements		Sub-elements	
Evidence		**Low**	**High**
	Research	• Poorly conceived, designed and/or executed research • Seen as the only type of evidence • Not valued as evidence • Seen as certain	• Well conceived, designed and executed research, appropriate to the research question • Seen as one part of a decision • Valued as evidence • Lack of certainty acknowledged • Social construction acknowledged • Judged as relevant • Importance weighted • Conclusions drawn
	Clinical experience	• Anecdote, with no critical reflection and judgement • Lack of consensus within similar groups • Not valued as evidence • Seen as the only type of evidence	• Clinical experience and expertise reflected upon, tested by individuals and groups • Consensus within similar groups • Valued as evidence • Seen as one part of the decision • Judged as relevant • Importance weighted • Conclusions drawn
	Patient experience	• Not valued as evidence • Patients not involved • Seen as the only type of evidence	• Valued as evidence • Multiple biographies used • Partnerships with health care professionals • Seen as one part of a decision • Judged as relevant • Importance weighted • Conclusions drawn
	Local data/ information	• Not valued as evidence • Lack of systematic methods for collection and analysis • Not reflected upon • No conclusions drawn	• Valued as evidence • Collected and analysed systematically and rigorously • Evaluated and reflected upon • Conclusions drawn
Context		**Low**	**High**

	Culture	• Unclear values and beliefs
		• Low regard for individuals
		• Task-driven organisation
		• Lack of consistency
		• Resources not allocated
		• Not integrated with strategic goals
			• Able to define culture(s) in terms of prevailing values/beliefs
			• Values individual staff and clients
			• Promotes leaning organisation
			• Consistency of individuals role/experience to value the following:
			  • Relationship with others
			  • Teamwork
			  • Power and authority
			  • Rewards/recognition
			• Resources – human, financial, equipment – allocated
			• Initiative fits with strategic goals and is a key practice/patient issue

(continued)

Table 7.2   (Continued)

		Leadership	Low inappropriate facilitation	High appropriate facilitation
		Leadership	• Traditional, command and control leadership • Lack of role clarity • Lack of teamwork • Poor organisational structures • Autocratic decision-making processes • Didactic approaches to learning/teaching/managing	• Transformational leadership • Role clarity • Effective teamwork • Effective organisational structures • Democratic inclusive decision-making processes • Enabling/empowering approach to teaching/learning/managing

		Evaluation	• Absence of any form of feedback
			• Narrow use of performance information sources
			• Evaluations rely on single rather than multiple methods
				• Feedback on:
				  • Individual
				  • Team
				  • System
				  • Performance
				• Use of multiple sources of information on performance
				• Use of multiple methods:
				  • clinical
				  • performance
				  • economic
				  • experience
				  • evaluations

Facilitation			**Low inappropriate facilitation**	**High appropriate facilitation**
	Purpose		**Task**	**Holistic**
		Role	Doing for others: • Episodic contact • Practical/technical help • Didactic, traditional approach to teaching • External agents • Low intensity – extensive coverage	Enabling others: • Sustained partnership • Developmental • Adult learning approach to teaching • Internal/external agents • High intensity – limited coverage
		Skills and attributes	Task/doing for others • Project management skills • Technical skills • Marketing skills • Subject/technical/clinical credibility	Holistic/enabling others • Co-counselling • Critical reflection • Giving meaning • Flexibility of role • Realness/authenticity

Evidence from clinical experience tempers research evidence, for example, you may not believe findings from research because they do not fit with your clinical experience. Therefore, clinical experience is another strand of evidence. Clinical common sense needs to be evaluated to the same extent that you would evaluate research evidence. Additionally, within the practice development journey, you are encouraged to draw on your experience of local leadership and management, and your experience as a facilitator. Therefore your experience of these issues, as well as of clinical practice, needs to be made explicit and verified through critical reflection, critique and debate with a wider community of practice to be considered at the high end of the continuum. How might you go about this process within your workplace, who would you include and how would you identify them?

Evidence from patients is situated towards high when patients (and/or significant others) are part of the decision-making process during individual interactions and when patient narratives/stories are seen and used as a valid source of evidence. Much has been discussed about patient and public involvement, and there are many useful resources available (e.g. http://www.invo.org.uk/). You might want to consider and find out what sort of patient and public involvement take place where you work. It might also be useful to think about how carers are involved in care processes.

Local information/data such as audit, performance, quality improvement and evaluation information could be considered as part of the evidence base for practice if it has been systematically collected, evaluated and reflected upon. If you work in an organisation where this happens, your local information/data element would be considered 'high' on the PARIHS continua.

PARIHS' conceptualisation of evidence indicates the need for an interaction between the scientific and experiential through the blending of various types of information; this requires an interactive, participatory process guided by skilled facilitation. This evaluation of the evidence base takes place across the practice development journey, from describing where we are starting from, to evaluating any impact of action.

Context

Context refers to the environment or setting in which the proposed change is to be implemented (see McCormack et al., 2002 for detailed discussion). The quality and nature of the contexts in which we work can have a more or less facilitative influence on our ability to change and develop practices. Therefore, within the practice development journey, developing a comprehensive understanding of the practice context is critical to knowing what action needs to be undertaken. Within PARIHS, the contextual factors that promote successful implementation fall under three broad sub-elements: (1) culture, (2) leadership and (3) evaluation, which operate in a dynamic way.

Culture: Within PARIHS, it is proposed that organisations that have cultures that could be described as 'learning organisations' are those that are more conducive to change ('high'). Within the context of practice development as promoted in this book, this would include person-centredness. Such cultures contain features such as decentralised decision-making, a focus on relationships between managers and workers, and management styles that are facilitative.

Leadership: Leaders have a key role to play in creating such cultures. In PARIHS, leadership summarises the nature of human relationships in the practice context. In this sense, leadership has the potential to bring about clear roles, effective teamwork and effective organisational structures. Transformational leaders, as opposed to those that command and control, have the ability to create receptive contexts and challenge individuals and teams in an enabling way ('high'). It is transformational leadership that is promoted in emancipatory or transformational practice development.

Evaluation: Contexts with evaluative mechanisms that collect multiple sources of evidence of performance that feed back at individual, team and system levels comprise the third element of a 'high' context. This is because such contexts not only accept and value different sources of feedback information, but also create the conditions for practitioners to apply them into practice as a matter of course. As you can see from the practice development journey picture presented in Chapter 1 (Figure 1.3), evaluation and feedback are key elements of practice development.

The context of practice is complex and dynamic, but it needs to be understood as part of practice development activity. An evaluation or measurement of where a context is 'starting from' is critical in the planning of subsequent actions and interventions. It would also be important to capture how contexts might develop as part of engaging in practice development activity, hence, the integrated evaluation–learning–planning–acting–evaluation cycles of the practice development journey. Take a few minutes to reflect on the type of organisation/service you work in and consider the elements of culture, leadership and evaluation on a low–high continuum – where would you place it?

Facilitation

Facilitation refers to the process of enabling or making easier the implementation of evidence into practice (see Harvey et al., 2002 for detailed discussion). Facilitation is achieved by an individual carrying out a specific role; a facilitator, with the appropriate skills and knowledge to help individuals, teams and organisations use evidence in practice. Facilitators have a key role to play in developing contexts that are conducive to evidence use – part of this process is also about working with practitioners to help them make sense of evidence (in its broadest sense). The purpose, role, skills and attributes of facilitators are absolutely critical to the practice development journey.

How the facilitator role is carried out will depend on the underlying purpose, stakeholders, nature of evidence and context being worked with and in. Within PARIHS, the purpose of facilitation can vary from being task orientated, which requires technical and practical support (e.g. administrating, taking on specific tasks), to enabling, which requires more of a developmental, process-orientated approach. It is argued that the skills and attributes required to fulfil the role are likely to depend on the situation, individuals and contexts involved. Therefore, skilled facilitators are those that can adjust their role and style to the different elements of a practice development project, the features of the context and the needs of those they are working with.

Facilitation is being tested as part of an international multi-site pragmatic process and outcome trial. Within this study, two different facilitation interventions are being evaluated based on aspects of technical and enabling approaches to facilitation for the implementation of continence recommendations for people living in long-term care settings (Seers et al., 2012). This study should provide evidence about some of the critical active ingredients of facilitation that is likely to lead to the refinement of the facilitation element within the PARIHS framework.

USING PARIHS TO GUIDE PRACTICE DEVELOPMENT PROCESSES, ACTION AND EVALUATION

The PARIHS framework has good face and content validity, which probably accounts for its growing use in practice development, implementation, evaluation and research. Because

PARIHS is a framework that represents the elements that play a potential role in the successful implementation of evidence into practice, the intention is that it could be used by anyone either attempting to improve safe and effective care and/or trying to better understand the processes and influences involved in such activity. Those who are actively attempting to implement evidence into practice, could use the elements and sub-elements as a guide to what should be paid attention to, including the development of interventions/actions, and evaluation approaches/tools. Therefore, PARIHS could be usefully applied as a framework or guide for planning, action, learning and evaluation, and aligns to all elements in the practice development journey.

Planning

The practice development journey begins with making sense of the situation. This diagnosis phase includes understanding the evidence base for practice, the characteristics and quality of the context and then deciding on appropriate strategies and processes for action. There are many ways to approach this phase; the PARIHS framework provides some structure to think about the questions that you could ask to provide helpful information for planning.

Tools

A number of questions have been developed that could be used in this diagnostic – or where are we starting from – phase of a practice development journey. These questions identify what it is about evidence and context that need attention so that appropriate (i.e. 'bespoke') facilitation interventions can be planned and implemented (see Table 7.3) to reach the ideal position (Figure 7.1). They are best asked of stakeholders working within the practice context who will be part of the practice development journey, and of those in facilitation roles. These questions could also be asked during evaluation, to help you determine what sort of effect your facilitation approaches have had.

There are three other tools that you could use in the planning stages. McCormack et al. (2009) have developed a context assessment index (CAI), which links to PARIHS through examination of the three sub-elements in context: (1) culture, (2) leadership and (3) evaluation. A five-stage instrument development and testing approach was used to develop a psychometrically acceptable 37-item, 5-factor instrument. The purpose of this tool is to assist facilitators and practitioners with assessing and understanding the context in which they work and the effect this has on practice development. McCormack and colleagues encourage others to use and further test the instrument in other settings and with different clinical topics. Importantly, the use and interpretation of this tool might require the support of colleagues in other parts of the organisation and/or your partner higher education institution.

Stetler et al. (2011) have also developed a guide for applying a revised version of the PARIHS framework in implementation. The purpose of the guide and set of reference tools is to help others apply the framework in evidence-based practice implementation projects by focusing on each element (evidence, context and facilitation) and to interpret them at each stage of implementation (including evaluation).

Helfrich et al. (2009) have developed an organisational readiness tool based on the core elements of the PARIHS framework. The Organizational Readiness to Change Assessment (ORCA) instrument is currently being validated, and to date has been tested with data from three quality improvement projects conducted in the Veterans Health Administration.

Table 7.3 Diagnosis and evaluation questions.

Evidence	Characteristics of evidence in the PARIHS framework (see Table 7.2)	Evidence: diagnostic/evaluative questions
Research	Well-conceived, designed and executed research appropriate to the research question	Is the research evidence of sufficiently high quality? Use appropriate critical appraisal tools – there are many to choose from, but the Critical Appraisal Skills Programme is a good place to start (http://www.casp-uk.net/)
	Seen as one part of a decision	Will research be used as part of the decision-making process?
	Lack of certainty acknowledged	Do we value the research evidence?
	Social construction acknowledged	Does the research evidence fit with our understanding of the issue?
	Judged as relevant	Is the research evidence useful in thinking about the issue?
	Importance weighted	Is there consensus amongst colleagues about the usefulness of this research to this issue?
	Conclusions drawn	Are we clear about key messages from the research?
Clinical experience	Clinical experience and expertise reflected upon, tested by individuals and groups	Have we reflected on our own clinical experience in relation to this issue?
	Consensus within groups	Have we have shared and critically reviewed our clinical experience in relation to this issue in our workplace?
	Valued as evidence	Have we have shared and critically reviewed our clinical experience with knowledgeable colleagues outside of this (clinical) workplace?
	Seen as one part of the decision	Will we use clinical experience as one part of the evidence base for action?
	Judged as relevant	Is there a consensus of experience about this issue amongst colleagues?
	Importance weighted	Do we believe that experience is useful in thinking about the issue?
	Conclusions drawn	Are we clear about what the key messages for the planned intervention are?
Patient experience	Valued as evidence	Do we routinely (and systematically) collect users'/patients' experiences about this particular issue?
	Multiple biographies used	Will we use service users'/patients' and/or carers' experiences as part of the evidence base?
	Partnerships with health care professionals	Is our approach to care delivery one that embraces a partnership with patients/service users and/or their relatives?

Table 7.3 (*Continued*)

Evidence	Characteristics of evidence in the PARIHS framework (see Table 7.2)	Evidence: diagnostic/evaluative questions
	Seen as one part of a decision	Do we value patient experiences as part of the evidence base for action? And is there a consensus amongst colleagues about the usefulness of patient experiences to this issue?
	Importance weighed	Do we believe that patient experiences are useful in thinking about the issue?
	Conclusions drawn	Are we clear about what the key messages for the planned intervention are
Information/data from local context	Valued as evidence	Is data/information routinely (and systematically) collected about this issue in this organisation?
	Collected and analysed systematically and rigorously	Will data/information from the local context be used as one part of the evidence base for action?
	Evaluated and reflected upon	Do we value data/information from the local context? Is the date/information from the local context useful in thinking about the issue?
	Conclusions drawn	Are we clear about the key messages for action?

As described earlier, within the practice development journey, there is a need to draw on different types of evidence, make a judgement about these and then make a judgement about the best way to approach action. Asking these questions to yourself and the stakeholders you are working with will help make sense of the evidence base for action. Fundamentally, this will require a collaborative process to develop a consensus about how available research fits with prevailing clinical experience, patients' experience and preference (e.g. their story about the issue), and other existing local information/data. See Chapter 9 for the articulation of these processes.

Action

As described earlier, facilitation is currently being evaluated in a large international study. Additionally, Brown applied PARIHS in her doctoral study in which pain management services were being developed (Brown & McCormack, 2005). In a review of the literature about the factors that have an influence on getting evidence into practice in post operative pain assessment and management, PARIHS was used an organising framework to guide an analysis of the evidence. Using the main elements and sub-elements of the framework, an exploration of the factors that might influence the successful development of an evidence-based pain management service were elicited under the broad headings evidence, context (including culture, leadership and evaluation) and facilitation. These findings were then used as a guide to develop appropriate change strategies through action research, including facilitation.

Evaluation and research

The questions in Table 7.3 could be used to evaluate implementation efforts *post hoc*; what worked, what did not work and why. Most commonly, PARIHS has been used with research and implementation activity as a conceptual and theoretical framework, that is as an organising framework to underpin and/or guide implementation research. For example, Ellis et al. (2005) used PARIHS as a conceptual framework to evaluate a training programme delivered in Western Australia. In this study, the aims were to explore the relative and combined importance of context and facilitation in the implementation of a protocol and to establish individual and organisational change based on the principles of evidence-based practice. Ellis and colleagues used the PARIHS framework to facilitate the description of the processes and outcomes of an evidence-based practice training programme. It appears that the authors used evidence, context and facilitation as a coding framework in the analysis of interview data, including the application of the high to low continuum to each element. The authors report that PARIHS was helpful in explaining the outcomes of the education programme.

Other examples of PARIHS being used as a conceptual framework include the following:

- Doran et al. (2007), who used the framework to develop and operationalise the development of an outcomes focused knowledge translation intervention. In this example, PARIHS was used to conceptualise the relationships among the factors that influence evidence-based nursing.
- Meijers et al. (2006) used the context element of the PARIHS framework to theoretically frame a systematic review of literature reporting the relationship between contextual factors and research utilisation. Their review successfully mapped to the dimensions of context (culture and leadership), but not onto the sub-element of evaluation.
- Coffey et al. (2007) applied PARIHS within a study that evaluated the context within which continence care is provided in rehabilitation units for older people. They used the dimensions of context to direct data collection activities and the high–low continuum as a way of assessing the 'state' or conduciveness of context for change.
- Conklin and Stolee (2008) used PARIHS to guide the evaluation of a health research transfer network and concluded that it had the potential to be used as a guide for evaluating other knowledge networks.
- Milner et al. (2006) used the PARIHS framework to inform the analysis of a systematic literature review of the research utilisation behaviours of clinical nurse educators. Essentially, they used the framework as a map to consider the sort of issues that were emerging from the review. They report that their findings did not map onto the context variables in PARIHS, but did for the evidence and some of the facilitation elements.
- Wallin et al. (2006), Estabrooks et al. (2007) and Cummings et al. (2007) report on a programme of work that used the context element of PARIHS as the basis for developing a derived measure of research utilisation, which was then used in multi-level modelling (structural equation modelling) to predict research utilization among nurses. Their work supports the importance of contextual factors to research utilisation. However, the role of facilitation was less clear as a predictor of research use and they also point out that much of the variance in their modelling was accounted for by individual factors.

Helfrich et al. (2010) provide a comprehensive review of how PARIHS has been previously used. Through a qualitative critical synthesis of peer-reviewed PARIHS literature (up until 2009), they found that, in general, it had been used as an organising framework for analysis within included studies. The authors of the review emphasise the potential of using PARIHS prospectively to guide implementation projects. This highlights the potential of embedding the framework within practice development activity from the outset, in a systematic and robust way.

SUMMARY AND CONCLUSIONS

Practice development activity depends on an ability to achieve significant and planned change involving individuals, teams and organisations. People are not passive recipients of evidence; rather they are stakeholders in problem solving processes, which are social and interactional. As I have shown here, PARIHS provides a helpful guide for navigating the complexities inherent in involving stakeholders in getting sound evidence into practice through practice development approaches, by alerting us to some key questions:

Evidence

- Is there any research evidence underpinning the initiative/topic?
- Is this research judged to be well conceived, designed, and conducted?
- Are the findings from research relevant to the initiative/topic?
- What is the practitioner's experience and opinion about this topic and the research evidence?
- Does the research evidence match with clinical, organisational and facilitation experience? If it does not, why might this be so?
- Do you need to seek consensus before it might be used by practitioners in this setting? How might you do this in your workplace?
- What is the patient's experience/preference/story concerning this initiative/topic?
- Does this differ from practitioners' perspectives?
- How could a partnership approach be developed?
- Is there any robust, local information/data about the initiative/topic?
- Would it be appropriate to develop a package, plan or learning resource that combines all these types of evidence of relevance to your context?

Context

- Is the context of implementation receptive to change?
- What are the beliefs and values of the organisation, team and practice context?
- What sort of leadership style is present (command and control – transformational)?
- Are individual and team boundaries clear?
- Is there effective team working (inter- and multi-disciplinary)?
- Does evaluation of performance rely on broad and varied sources of information?
- Is this information fed back to clinical contexts?

Facilitation

- Consider the answers to the evidence and context questions: what are the barriers and what are the facilitators to this initiative?
- What tasks/activities and processes require facilitation?

- Given the people and setting, what sort of skills and attributes will the person facilitating require to be effective in the role?
- Would it be appropriate to draw on the skills and knowledge of an external facilitator to work with internal facilitators?
- What role might the facilitator have in evaluating the outcomes of the project?

The development and refinement of the PARIHS framework will continue with further research and testing. In the meantime, as outlined here, PARIHS provides a parsimonious and flexible framework for you to include in your practice development toolkit.

REFERENCES

Brown, D. & McCormack, B. (2005) Developing postoperative pain management: utilising the promoting action on research implementation in health services (PARIHS) framework. *Worldviews on Evidence-Based Nursing*, **2** (3), 131–141.

Bucknall, T. (2011) Using evidence to improve patient safety and quality of health care. *Worldview on Evidence-Based Nursing*, **8** (1), 1–3.

Bucknall, T. & Rycroft-Malone, J. (2010) Evidence-based practice: doing the right things for patients. In: *Models and Frameworks for Implementing Evidence-Based Practice* (eds J. Rycroft-Malone & T. Bucknall), pp. 1–18. Wiley Blackwell, Oxford.

Coffey, A., McCarthy, G., McCormack, B., Wright, J. & Slater, P. (2007) Incontinence: assessment, diagnosis, and management in two rehabilitation units for older people. *Worldviews on Evidence-Based Nursing*, **4** (4), 179–186.

Conklin, J. & Stolee, P. (2008) A model for evaluating knowledge exchange in a network context. *The Canadian Journal of Nursing Research*, **40** (2), 116–124.

Cummings, G.G., Estabrooks, C.A., Midodzi, W.K., Wallin, L. & Hayduk, L. (2007) Influence of organizational characteristics and context on research utilization. *Nursing Research Supplement*, **56** (4), S25–S39.

Dopson, S. & Fitzgerald, L. (2005) *Knowledge into Action*. Oxford University Press, Oxford.

Dopson, S., Fitzgerald, L., Ferlie, E., Gabbay, J. & Locock, L. (2002) No magic targets! Changing clinical practice to become more evidence based. *Health Care Management Review*, **27** (3), 35–47.

Doran, D.M. & Sidani, S. (2007) Outcomes-focused knowledge translation: a framework for knowledge translation and patient outcomes improvement. *Worldviews on Evidence-Based Nursing*, **4** (1), 3–13.

Ellis, I., Howard, P., Larson, A. & Roberts, A. (2005) From workshop to work practice: an exploration of context and facilitation in the development of evidence-based practice. *Worldviews on Evidence-Based Nursing*, **2** (2), 84–93.

Estabrooks, C.A., Floyd, J.A., Scott-Findlay, S., O'Leary, K.A. & Gushta, M. (2003) Individual determinants of research utilization: a systematic review. *Journal of Advanced Nursing*, **43** (5), 506–520.

Estabrooks, C.A., Midodzi, W.K., Cummings, G.G., Wallin, L. & Adewale, A. (2007) Predicting research use in nursing organizations: a multi-level analysis. *Nursing Research Supplement*, **56** (4S), S7–S23.

Estabrooks, C.A., Squires, J.E., Cummings, G.G., Birdsell, J.M. & Norton, P.G. (2009) Development and assessment of the Alberta Context Tool. *BMC Health Services Research*, **9**, 234

Greenhalgh, T, Robert, G., McFarlane, F., Bate, P. & Kyriakidou, O. (2004) Diffusion of innovations in service organisations: systematic review and recommendations. *The Millbank Quarterly*, **82** (4), 581–629.

Grol, R. (2001) Success and failures in the implementation of evidence-based guidelines for clinical practice. *Medical Care*, **39** (8 Suppl. 2), 1146–1154.

Harvey, G., Loftus-Hills, A., Rycroft-Malone, J., Titchen, A., Kitson, A., McCormack, B. & Seers, K. (2002) Getting evidence into practice: the role and function of facilitation. *Journal of Advanced Nursing*, **37** (6), 577–588.

Helfrich, C.D., Damschroder, L.J., Hagedorn, H.J., Daggett, G.S., Sahay, A., Ritchie, M., Damush, T., Guihan, M., Ullrich, P.M. & Stetler, C.B. (2010) A critical synthesis of literature on the promoting action on research implementation in health services (PARIHS) framework. *Implementation Science*, **5**, 82.

Helfrich, C.D., Li, Y.-F., Sharp, N.D. & Sales, A.E. (2009) Organizational readiness to change assessment (ORCA): development of an instrument based on the Promoting Action on Research in Health Services (PARIHS) framework. *Implementation Science*, **4**, 38.

Kitson, A.L., Harvey, G. & McCormack, B. (1998) Enabling the implementation of evidence-based practice: a conceptual framework. *Quality in Health Care*, **7** (3), 149–158.

Kitson, A., Rycroft-Malone, J., Harvey, G., McCormack, B., Seers, K. & Titchen, A. (2008) Evaluating the successful implementation of evidence into practice using the PARIHS framework: theoretical and practical challenges. *Implementation Science*, **3**, 1.

Lomas, J., Culyer, T., McCutcheon, C., McAuley, L. & Law, S. (2005) Conceptualizing and combining evidence for health system guidance. Canadian Health Services Research Foundation (CHSRF). http://www.chsrf.ca/migrated/pdf/insightAction/evidence_e.pdf (Accessed 2 October 2012).

McCormack, B., Kitson, A., Harvey, G., Rycroft-Malone, J., Titchen, A., & Seers K. (2002) Getting evidence into practice - the meaning of 'context'. *Journal of Advanced Nursing*, **38** (1), 94–104.

McCormack, B., McCarthy, G., Wright, J., Slater, P. & Coffey A. (2009) Development and testing of the context assessment index (CAI). *Worldviews on Evidence-Based Nursing*, **6** (1), 27–35.

McGlynn, E.A., Asch, S.M., Adams, J., Keesey, J., Hicks, J., DeCristofaro, A. & Kerr, E.A. (2003) The quality of care delivered to adults in the United States. *New England Journal of Medicine*, **348** (26), 2635–2645.

Meijers, J.M., Janssen, M.A., Cummings, G.G., Wallin, L., Estabrooks, C.A., Y G Halfens, R. (2006) Assessing the relationships between contextual factors and research utilization in nursing: systematic literature review. *Journal of Advanced Nursing*, **55** (5), 622–635.

Milner, M., Estabrooks, C.A. & Myrick, F. (2006) Research utilization and clinical nurse educators: a systematic review. *Journal of Evaluation in Clinical Practice*, **12** (6), 639–655.

Morse, J.M., Hupcey, J.E. & Mitcham, C. (1996) Concept analysis in nursing research: a critical appraisal. *Scholarly Inquiry for Nursing Practice: An International Journal*, **10** (25), 3–77.

Rycroft-Malone, J. (2004) The PARIHS framework – a framework for guiding the implementation of evidence-based practice. *Journal of Nursing Care Quality*, **19** (4), 297–304.

Rycroft-Malone, J. (2008) Evidence-informed practice: from individual to context. *Journal of Nursing Management*, Special Issue, **16** (4), 404–408.

Rycroft-Malone, J., Harvey, G., Seers, K., Kitson, A., McCormack, B. & Titchen, A. (2004a) An exploration of the factors that influence the implementation of evidence into practice *Journal of Clinical Nursing*, **13**, 913–924.

Rycroft-Malone, J., Kitson, A., Harvey, G., McCormack, B., Seers, K., Titchen, A. & Estabrooks, C.A. (2002) Ingredients for change: revisiting a conceptual framework. *Quality and Safety in Health Care*, **11**, 174–180.

Rycroft-Malone, J., Seers, K., Titchen, A., Harvey, G., Kitson, A. & McCormack, B. (2004b) What counts as evidence in evidence-based practice. *Journal of Advanced Nursing*, **47** (1), 81–90.

Scott-Findlay, S. & Pollock, C. (2004) Evidence, research, knowledge: a call for conceptual clarity. *Worldviews on Evidence-Based Nursing*, **1** (2), 92–97.

Seers, K., Cox, K., Crichton, N.J., Edwards, R., Eldh, A., Estabrooks, C.A., Harvey, G., Hawkes, C., Kitson, A., Linck, P., McCarthy, G., McCormack, B., Mockford, C., Rycroft-Malone, J., Titchen, A. & Wallin, L. (2012) FIRE (Facilitating Implementation of Research Evidence): a study protocol. *Implementation Science*, **7** (25). http://www.implementationscience.com/content/pdf/1748-5908-7-25.pdf (Accessed 24 November 2012).

Squires, J.E., Estabrooks, C.A., Gustavsson, P. & Wallin, L. (2011) Individual determinants of research utilization by nurses: a systematic review update. *Implementation Science*, **6**, 1.

Stetler, C.B., Damschroder, L.J., Helfrich, C.D. & Hagedorn, H.J. (2011) A guide for applying a revised version of the PARIHS framework for implementation. *Implementation Science*, **6**, 99.

Wallin, L., Estabrooks, C.A., Midodzi, W.K. & Cummings, G.G. (2006) Development and validation of a derived measure of research utilization by nurses. *Nursing Research*, **55** (3), 149–160.

8 Working Towards a Culture of Effectiveness in the Workplace

Kim Manley[1], Annette Solman[2] and Carrie Jackson[1]

[1]Canterbury Christ Church University, Canterbury, UK
[2]The Sydney Children's Hospitals Network, Sydney, Australia

INTRODUCTION

This chapter provides a foundation and overview of an effective workplace culture, with a contemporary exploration of current theory and evidence about how to recognise and enable effective workplace cultures and how they positively impact on the outcomes of person-centred, safe and effective care. The chapter aims to enable the reader to critically apply theory to practice by including clear links to tools and frameworks that can be practically applied to the workplace, and incorporating some worked examples. Specific focus is given to the attributes and assessment of effective workplace cultures, their measurement and also how they are enabled through relationships, clinical leadership and facilitation.

The importance of understanding workplace culture and its impact on both patient and staff well-being, amongst other aspects, is coming into its own as, increasingly, examples of poor care become rife in local and national media, and national concerns about health care failures in delivery of essential care, dignity and human rights are the focus of patient organisation and government reports. The fundamental reason for these failures can be located within workplace culture. All cultures create social norms that frequently go unchallenged as people working in them take these norms for granted and rarely challenge them unless given an opportunity to reflect on and observe the workplace in a detached way. People exposed to toxic cultures for the first time often challenge pervasive assumptions and values, as workplace culture is most striking to newcomers and visitors. However, over time, if no change is achieved and individuals are not supported or listened to, these 'once new staff' often become accepting of the same social norms. Whilst many of these reports makes depressing reading, understanding the power of workplace culture to influence both good and poor care can help us grow, promote, recognise and replicate those aspects of effective cultures that enable the workplace to consistently achieve person-centred care and workplaces where everyone can flourish.

Central to practice development is understanding of effective workplace cultures, how they are developed, recognised and sustained. Driven by values and beliefs about person-centredness, ways of working and effectiveness, practice developers use the processes of collaboration, inclusion and participation (CIP) to transform workplace culture through achieving shared values and embedding these values into everyday practice and the workplace.

Practice Development in Nursing and Healthcare, Second Edition. Edited by Brendan McCormack, Kim Manley and Angie Titchen.
© 2013 John Wiley & Sons, Ltd. Published 2013 by John Wiley & Sons, Ltd.

CULTURE AND THE WORKPLACE

Culture is not about individuals but about the social contexts that influence the way people behave and talk, and the social norms that are accepted and expected. To transform how things are done at the practice level requires fundamental changes in mindsets, language and patterns of behaviour as it is these that manifest culture, reflecting the values, beliefs and assumptions held or accepted by staff in the workplace. Whilst culture is a not a tangible concept, practitioners often relate to Drennan's definition: *how things are done around here* (Drennan, 1992, p. 3), as it captures what culture means for most people and illustrates the influence that it has on individuals and their work.

More formally, Schein (1985) classically defines culture as 'a set of psychological predispositions called "basic assumptions" that members of an organisation (workplace) possess, which tend to cause them to act in certain ways'. Assumptions by definition are 'accepted truths' held by a social group that manifest themselves in deep rooted attitudes, values, beliefs and patterns of behaviour. Health care organisations have different cultures at different levels and within different departments and teams. There is interplay between corporate, organisational and local workplace cultures, each impacting on the other. Over the last decade, a particular focus has been given to organisational culture, linking it to performance (Mannion et al., 2005). This chapter focuses specifically on the local workplace culture defined as:

> *The most immediate culture experienced and/or perceived by staff, patients, users and other key stakeholders. This is the culture that impacts directly on the delivery of care. It both influences and is influenced by the organisational and corporate cultures with which it interfaces as well as other idiocultures through staff relationships and movement. (Manley et al., 2011b, p. 4)*

Manley et al. (2011b) argue that workplace culture represents the immediate culture impacting on both health care users and providers, and that this is different to the organisational culture. Idioculture is a preferred term rather than subculture as this challenges the assumption that 'subcultures' are derived from the organisational culture. Idiocultures interact with and influence each other, and from this emerges the organisational/corporate culture and vice versa (Bolan & Bolan, 1994). Whilst there may be many similar elements of effective cultures across different cultural levels, the workplace culture at the front line is the one experienced by patients and practitioners and therefore, the main focus of this chapter.

In the introduction, the potential consequences of ineffective and effective cultures on care experiences of patients and service users, and the work experiences of staff were highlighted. To summarise these consequences, workplace cultures impact on:

- the patient's experience and whether that experience is one of being treated in a person-centred way;
- quality of care (of which the patient's experience is part) in terms of coordination and continuity of care, access, waiting times and patient safety;
- health outcomes;
- staff well-being and commitment;
- how we learn in the workplace;
- how people work together and relate to each other;
- the use of evidence in the workplace;
- resources – with toxic and ineffective cultures wasting our valuable health care resources.

OUTCOMES OF EFFECTIVE WORKPLACE CULTURES IN HEALTH CARE

Research that aims to describe an effective workplace culture (Manley et al., 2011b), discussed later in more detail, identified three sets of consequences of such positive cultures that could be demonstrated in health care. These are outlined in Table 8.1, together with possible indicators or tools that could be used to demonstrate them.

Many of these concepts are further developed through the chapter and are incorporated into worked examples. The identified indicators provide useful potential for considering

Table 8.1 Consequences of effective workplace cultures together with potential measures/indicators to demonstrate them (after Manley et al., 2011b, with permission from IPDJ).

Consequence (C)	Potential indicators/tools
C1. Continuous evidence of the following: • Patients', users' and communities' needs are met in a person-centred way. • Staff are empowered and committed. • Standards, goals and objectives are met (individual, team and organisational effectiveness). • Knowledge/evidence is developed, used and shared.	• Qualitative 360-degree feedback; patient stories; patient feedback and satisfaction; compliments; person-centred key performance indicators (KPIs). • Staff stories, commitment/empowerment measures; retention, absenteeism and turnover, staff satisfaction. • Achievement of individual patients' goals and outcomes; achievement of individual practitioners' goals and outcomes; achievement of team action plans and objectives; achievement of organisational objectives. • National guidelines and standards are implemented in practice consistently; practitioner learning and inquiry as well as learning from patients/service users lead to demonstrable changes in practice. These changes are shared through internal and external networks, conferences, publications, and influence local and national policy
C2. Human flourishing for all	• Transformation, illumination, growth, connected energies, creating energy and freedom (Titchen et al., 2011) • Staff well-being
C3. Positive influence on other workplace cultures. . . . once an effective workplace culture is established; it is through the metaphorical flow of seeds to barren areas that other effective cultures can be grown, rather than rolling out a technically focussed cultural change programme across organisations. Cultural change programmes will therefore need to be 'enabling' and not 'prescriptive', cultivating the (bottom-up) growth of seeds rather than imposing ready-made carpets of grass. Through working with the enabling factors, values and attributes, other effective cultures can be nurtured.(Manley et al., 2011a, p. 16)	• Various cultural assessment tools • Leadership models

how data can be standardised at the end of practice development projects to contribute to an international database that can be built to demonstrate the achievement of effective workplace cultures through practice development (Manley et al., 2011a).

CHARACTERISTICS OF EFFECTIVE CULTURES

Over 10 years, researchers with expertise in practice development across different health care settings internationally, and as part of an international colloquium on theory in practice development, undertook a rigorous concept analysis to develop a framework that describes the characteristics of effective workplace cultures. The framework was intended to help others transform their workplace, at the front line, towards person-centred cultures that enable everyone to flourish (Manley et al., 2011b) and to directly and positively impact on patients, service users and staff. The research set out to answer three questions:

1. What are the characteristics of effective workplace cultures? Theoretically, these are often termed 'attributes'.
2. What are the enabling factors that help with developing effective workplace cultures?
3. What are the consequences you would expect of effective workplace cultures?

The resulting framework provides the key structure for this chapter, but in this section, the focus is on the defining attributes – those features that would be expected to be present within workplace cultures that are effective. The concept analysis identified five attributes of an effective workplace culture (Table 8.2). These attributes encompass the practice knowledge (know-how) required by practice developers.

The Attributes

The first attribute comprises ten values that are required to enable person-centred approaches where everyone can flourish. The other four attributes are features that enable these values and beliefs to be embedded into everyday practice to achieve sustainable person-centred experiences that integrate effective ways of working.

The ten values (attribute 1) are clustered into three groups (Figure 8.1). Person-centredness is the key value that underpins our relationships with patients and service users as well as with each other. The second value cluster is about how we work with each other and our stakeholders; this includes the three principles central to practice development: (1) collaboration, (2) inclusion and (3) participation (CIP; McCormack et al., 2006), as well as how we support and challenge each other to be effective, how we work as a team and how we develop our leadership potential. Leadership is a key influencing factor in developing and sustaining effective workplace cultures as it has an impact on whether and how people work together towards a shared purpose and vision. The third value cluster, around effective care, builds on the other two value clusters to include (1) how we use and develop evidence, learn in and from practice; and (2) how we enable others to positively engage with change to sustain effectiveness, and this also includes holistic safety.

Exploring one's own and others' values is often the starting point for practice development work (see Chapters 3, 5 and 6). Participating together with colleagues in making these explicit is a powerful strategy for developing a common vision and shared team purpose,

Table 8.2 Five attributes of effective workplace cultures related to the know-how required of the practice developer (after Manley et al., 2011b, with permission from IPDJ).

Five attributes (A) of effective workplace cultures	Know-how required of the practice developer
A1. Specific values shared in the workplace.	• To develop and identify shared values and beliefs in relation to team working and purpose and in relation to new initiatives and innovations.
A2. All the values are realised in practice, there is a shared vision and mission, and individual and collective responsibility.	• To help others understand what the values and beliefs mean for everyday practice and to make sense of these.
A3. Adaptability, innovation and creativity maintain workplace effectiveness.	• To work collaboratively, participatively and inclusively with all stakeholders. • To support others to work in this way and to develop their skills.
A4. Appropriate change is driven by the needs of patients/service users/communities.	• To facilitate and develop shared values and beliefs, shared visions and to develop strategic and operational plans from these
A5. Formal systems (structures and processes) enable continuous evaluation of learning, evaluation of performance and shared governance.	• To help others to investigate and recognise when there are contradictions between values and actions and how to act on these
	• To develop a culture that is safe and effective, which enables evidence use and development as well as ongoing learning in and from practice. One that enables informed risks, fosters creativity and imagination, and implements and evaluates innovation.
	• To support others in the development of this know-how.
	• To help others identify the needs of patients and service users and communities, evaluate person-centred care, and implement and evaluate the changes required.
	• To support others with the implementation of systems for ongoing evaluation and implementation of person-centred care, effectiveness and safety; formal participation of stakeholders in decision-making (shared governance); individual and team learning and inquiry into practice.

both generally and in relation to specific initiatives or innovations. Knowing and agreeing that everyone intends to go in the same direction is the second attribute. If there is a genuine shared approach then all individuals will share a collective responsibility to this end. Although, knowing and agreeing to a shared set of values is the first step towards an effective workplace culture, talking about the ten values and beliefs alone is insufficient, as the values need to be implemented and experienced by all in everyday practice and behaviours. Living and implementing these values in practice is often the start of a challenging journey towards transformation. To succeed requires attention to be given to how individuals work together, support and challenge each other in everyday work, and this includes how they give and receive feedback to one another (see Chapter 6). An example of these two attributes and their consequences are illustrated in Story 8.1.

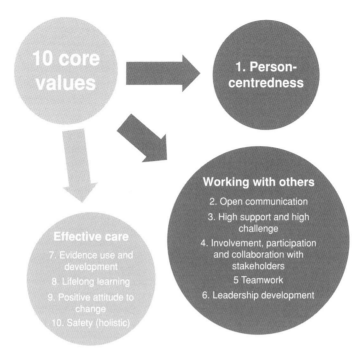

Fig. 8.1   Attribute 1 – the ten key values clustered into three groups (Manley et al., 2011b, p. 12, with permission from IPDJ).

Story 8.1: Example of using the CIP principles in practice and the outcomes

Within one large hospital, a ward managers' group from across the hospital met regularly to review the data that were collected to monitor and review performance around key indicators of effectiveness in their areas. At the first of six, 1-hour active learning sessions, staff expressed feeling demotivated, demoralised, dependent and feeling 'done to'. The facilitator started by working collaboratively, inclusively and participatively with the ward managers to identify where they were, negotiating areas to focus on, which would help the ward managers to share: how they supported and challenged each other and others; how they gave and received feedback to each other; and how they celebrated achievements. Eventually, the ward managers decided that they would like to explore their purpose and role in the data monitoring sessions as they had felt no ownership of this previously and this had led to the feelings of being undervalued and 'done to'. A values clarification exercise was used to develop a common purpose for both the sessions, their role and contribution. They recognised that there were other stakeholders involved with the meeting and so replicated the same exercise with these people so that everyone had the same vision. At the end of the six sessions, the ward managers argued successfully for their own peer support opportunity and demonstrated evidence of becoming self-directing, self-managing and taking responsibility for actions, as well as challenging senior colleagues they worked with to this end. Their enthusiasm and motivation was now palpable.

The remaining three attributes are about embedding the values and beliefs into every-day practice to ensure values are sustained even within changing contexts. New drivers to change will continue to be present as patients' and service users' expectations evolve and policies and new evidence become influential. Attribute 3, *adaptability, innovation and creativity maintain workplace effectiveness*, and attribute 4, *appropriate change is driven by the needs of patients/users/communities*, recognise that change is always a challenge to shared values and ways of working. Whilst core values around person-centredness and effectiveness would always need to be present, the values concerned with maintaining effectiveness, change and learning help us to positively respond to or anticipate changes in the external environment flexibility through adaptability, innovation and creativity. These processes help us find new or better solutions that enable core values to continue to be experienced. Attributes 3 and 4 would, therefore, be evidenced by staff attitudes, staff behaviour and social norms that:

- illustrate working together creatively to implement visions, find solutions and research practice;
- embrace change and proactively anticipate potential implications of external drivers that may influence practice;
- continually explore and evaluate patients and service users experiences, how these can be improved by finding creative and innovative solutions (see Chapter 11);
- demonstrate inquiry into individual and collective practice through critical dialogue and structured reflection and scholarly inquiry.

Finally, attribute 5, *formal systems (structures and processes) enable continuous evaluation of learning, evaluation of performance and shared governance*, is recognised by the formal structures that need to be implemented if the core values are constantly to be experienced in practice by all. It is these structures that embed the values so that they are authentically experienced by all and are not experienced as tokenistic/opportunistic.

Within one practice unit, this was achieved by enabling a matrix structure for key unit activities that reflected core values, for example, around learning and development, research and inquiry, supervision and mentorship, where every member of staff in every unit team was a member of one of the matrix teams and governance systems were established for each function.

Other examples of formal structures at a local level rather than an organisational level that exemplify this attribute include the establishment of reference groups/steering groups that include all stakeholders to provide ongoing feedback, support and challenge around development of practice and services; the establishment of supervision systems that include the periodic review and impact of reflective practice on patient and staff experience; the integration of 360-degree feedback into appraisal systems that include the patient/service users experience; and systems used to evaluate practice, teamwork, patient and staff experience.

Table 8.2 identifies the five attributes of an effective workplace culture and also the know-how required by practice developers to enable these attributes to become established. The remainder of the chapter will build on this know-how to include the tools that can be used to assess workplace culture, the enabling factors, including the facilitation skills that support the development of effective workplace cultures, and the role of leadership.

ASSESSING THE WORKPLACE CULTURE

We have demonstrated the relationship between workplace cultures and potential consequences, and emphasised the need to understand our workplace cultures and ensure that we invest in the development of effective cultures, particularly at the level of the patient/caregiver interface (Manley et al., 2011b, p. 2). To help you reflect on your own workplace culture and the experiences you have had working with different teams and in different wards/unit/organisations, consider the following questions:

- What was the lived experience of these different workplaces for you and your patients?
- What were the values and beliefs that you could identify as being present?
- How did these values and beliefs play out in the provision of teamwork and patient care?
- What are the practices that you experienced that supported a person-centred culture that you would like to emulate elsewhere?
- What were the practices that hindered person-centred care that you do not think support a person-centred culture?

Clarifying and knowing our own values and beliefs is an important piece of work to undertake for ourselves and a key starting point for many practice development activities (see Chapters 3, 5 and 6). We are all shaped by our lived experiences and have certain beliefs and values to which we aspire and to which we may react, rather than be responsive when these values are not present in the workplace. When a personal value is breached, if our emotional intelligence is not as well-developed as we would like, we can react to a situation rather than think through the situation and respond appropriately. Emotional intelligence is about recognising the emotion that is evoked when a value is not present and managing the emotion, thus leaving the emotion out of the communication. Goleman (1996) refers to emotional intelligence as self-awareness of our own emotional state, that is our mood and our thinking, to enable us to respond in a person-centred manner to address the concern/issue.

There are many approaches to understanding workplace cultures. Multiple approaches are used within emancipatory practice development work to gain a 'picture' of what is happening within a ward, clinical environment or organisation regarding the espoused values of, in this context, person-centred care. The following introduces approaches that you may consider, which are primarily organisational 'bottom-up' approaches to understanding a workplace culture. In practice, it is normal for a number of these strategies to be employed at different times with some occurring simultaneously. Please refer to original source for a detailed approach to the use of these tools.

Approaches for identifying workplace cultures

The resources identified in the following text will require support with their use if the reader is a novice practice developer.

Workplace Culture Critical Analysis Tool

The workplace culture critical analysis tool (WCCAT) is an observational tool that was developed to provide a framework and practical approach for staff when observing practice as a mechanism of informing a description of a workplace culture. This tool uses five phases as the process of creating a 'picture' of a workplace culture. The five phases as described by McCormack et al. (2009) are as follows:

1. *Pre-observation*: Preparing the staff and patients for the activity of observing practice within the care environment.
2. *Observation*: Actually undertaking the observations of practice within the work environment.
3. *Conscious raising and problematisation*: Checking out assumptions and areas of observation that are unclear, asking critical questions to gain a more in-depth understanding of data that were collected.
4. *Reflection and critique*: The observers meet and agree on the issues that will be feedback to the team from undertaking a comparison of each other's data sets. The observers facilitate an exploration of these issues, drawing attention to the espoused values by asking the staff the extent to which they align with the espoused values. Phase four includes the development of a practice development action plan and a staff development plan.
5. *Participatory analysis and action planning*: This phase engages the staff in the analysis and theming of the data that has been collected. It provides the staff with the opportunity to immerse themselves in the data to gain an in-depth understanding and ownership with a focus on impressions gained, feeling, metaphors, keywords and images.

The staff then work towards achieving the elements of the action plan and refining their work practices. The tool would be utilised at different points over time to identify changes that are occurring.

Nursing Context Index

The Nursing Context Index (NCI) was developed by Slater et al. (2009) to measure person-centred nursing practice, which in turn informs us about the culture of a given environment. The focus of this quantitative tool is to identify the extent to which a workplace is trending towards being person-centred. Specific measures were developed from an extensive literature review. A survey tool was then developed and tested for validation of the survey constructs. The tool can be administered either electronically or can be paper based. This tool is used in a number of organisations that are engaged in practice development, in addition to qualitative approaches to identifying and monitoring trends regarding the workplace culture. Nursing staff complete the survey, which is then analysed with the results communicated to staff using an empowering facilitated approach. The staff utilise this information to inform aspects of the workplace culture that are working well and seek to build upon these areas and to identify areas that would benefit from focused work to enhance the workplace culture.

Critical Incident Technique

A culture assessment approach known as the critical incident technique (CIT) is one approach built on the foundation work of Flanagan cited in Mallak et al. (2003). The CIT uses a bottom-up approach to ascertain a view of an organisations workplace culture. CIT produces categories from the data collection and uses these data to explore the extent to which the organisation's values are present within the workplace. The CIT method seeks staff stories of both positive and negative experiences, which they believe support or not the espoused values of the organisation (Mallak et al., 2010).

The CIT approach aligns closely to the quality and safety agenda, as the focus is on understanding a workplace culture to support the staff to build upon what is working well and to come up with solutions to address areas where improvements can be made. Ensuring a culture of quality and safety within patient care is being person-centred and links to the effective workplace cultural framework (Manley et al., 2011b).

Continuous Process Improvement

A central component of developing an effective workplace culture of being person-centred is the work of staff in undertaking continuous process improvement (CPI) and embedding this approach within their day-to-day work practices. Consumers have an expectation that the health care they receive is evidence based and of a standard of quality. Charmel and Frampton (2008, p. 83) identify that patients have the expectation of a service of quality and safety within their health experience. These authors identify that the shortage of health staff presents itself with challenges in recruiting and retaining staff if workplace environments are not reflective of a culture of caring with an agenda of quality and safety for both patients and staff. Castro et al. (2008) suggest that by focusing on leadership with clinicians there will be a positive impact on quality and productivity of health care provided by clinicians in the workplace.

Quality Improvement Activities

The data collection approaches, with examples cited earlier, to identify the workplace culture leads to a series of quality improvement activities (QIA), which is supported through transformational leadership with the clinical staff. It is our experience that when staff are involved in the data collection, analysis and theming, they take a higher level of ownership in developing and implementing the QIA. As there may be a number of areas that have been identified that the staff would like to focus on, it often becomes necessary to ask the staff to prioritise these activities and to commence with one or two.

When planning for QIA, the underlying principles of person-centred care need to be reflected in the approaches and evaluation strategies selected for the work. The action needs to be related to the issue or opportunity that presented itself through the data collection phase. There should be stakeholder involvement in the development of the QIA and then in the implementation and evaluation phase reflecting the principles of CIP and emancipation.

Important to all of the aforementioned approaches is ensuring that there is a focus on process as well as on outcomes. Processes and evaluation strategies need to support the intent of person-centredness. A review of processes as well as outcomes enables all to learn from their experience of what worked well, did not work well and could be done differently for the same or for a different outcome. PRAXIS is an evaluation framework that was developed by people involved in practice development work to support formative and summative evaluation of processes and outcomes (Wilson et al., 2008).

Sustainability of change and continuous improvement is critical to ensuring a workplace culture of effectiveness. Once strategies have been established to enhance the workplace culture, these strategies require monitoring for their sustainability and over time for their applicability to the current workplace context.

ENABLING EFFECTIVE CULTURES

The factors that support the development of an effective workplace culture are termed 'enabling factors' and these are classified as individual and organisational in their focus (Manley et al., 2011b). In order to maximise the potential of an organisation to learn and develop, there is need for support at both grass-roots level among front line staff and a strategic level. Developing meaningful relationships with patients, with each other, with teams and with the wider organisation, are an essential component of workplace culture. They are important interconnected parts of a functioning whole system that, when working in synch together, can learn, grow and flourish.

Individual enablers

In the workplace, individual practitioners who are aware of their own values, beliefs, strengths and limitations are central to an effective workplace. Manley (2004) makes a strong case for working with values and beliefs in order to understand and transform workplace culture. As individuals, our actions and reactions are influenced by personal values, beliefs and experiences, which in turn influence our way of being, decision-making and behaviour in the workplace. Individual self-awareness is an important foundation block for life-long learning. Practitioners therefore need to be supported to develop self-awareness through a process of critical review and self-reflection, rather than continued reliance on practice that is ritualised, accepted uncritically, taken for granted or viewed as 'common sense'. Once there is an awareness of what constitutes best practice, it is the mechanisms of support, feedback, evaluation and clinical supervision that enable the individual and the wider team to become aware of, and motivated to change, attitudes and behaviours.

In effective workplace cultures, the presence of strong transformational clinical leaders, skilled facilitation and role clarity are essential. Transformational leadership is key to cultural change and is discussed later in the chapter. It is important to note here that effective transformational leaders focus on the development of their workplace culture, role-modelling shared values and achieving a common vision to engage the hearts and minds of colleagues in the workplace. Ensuring clarity of professional roles, with clearly defined expectations of the contribution an individual can make to the work environment, creates a sense of purpose, self-worth and motivation, as well as empowers individuals to be accountable and responsible for their behaviours and actions.

Qualitative 360-degree feedback has been the most frequently tested strategy for achieving role clarity, and is based on the systematic collection and feedback of performance information on an individual or group, derived from a number of the stakeholders (Ward, 2002). The group of stakeholders may be the practitioner's role set (those people in the team they work most frequently with, usually no more than ten). However, it can also include feedback from patients and service users and evidence from appraisal and staff interviews, patient and staff stories. In a transformational relationship, focus is on giving and receiving regular feedback that provides high support and high challenge in the workplace. This is discussed in more detail in the Section 'The Role of Facilitation in Developing Effective Workplace Cultures'.

Organisational enablers

In effective workplace cultures, the organisation will demonstrate a consistent and sustainable commitment to providing care that is person-centred, evidence-based and continually modernising, where everyone can flourish (Manley, 2004; McCormack & Titchen, 2006). A transformational organisational culture is synonymous with the characteristics of effective workplace culture because they are composed of a number of interrelated factors that impact on the way individuals and teams work. A transformational culture is one where adapting to change has become a way of life for all members and it continues to develop a quality of service that is owned by all (Manley, 2004).

Enabling organisations have a flattened and transparent management system, which devolves responsibility across the organisation with an enabling approach to leadership and decision-making at all levels. Practitioners are viewed as 'partners in a solution', not a 'problem', and the organisation is underpinned by a supportive human resource department. Human resource departments are highly influential because they are responsible for both maintaining the organisation's values, particularly in relation to recruitment and selection, staff expectations and performance, as well as being responsible for enabling organisational learning and development (Manley, 2001).

An organisational readiness and commitment to readily share knowledge and learn both for itself and for its workforce enables an organisation to adapt more readily to the changing needs of society (Jackson, 2010). A learning organisation demonstrates a shared vision and collective goals for development across the whole organisation and provides the conditions that empower staff to learn, develop and be involved in or drive the change process and embed values in practice. This in turn creates a greater sense of staff well-being and commitment to delivering organisational goals as partners in the process. Research from Magnet Hospitals (deemed learning organisations) shows that learning organisations report greater staff job satisfaction and staff retention with better outcomes for patient care and patient safety, as well as greater commitment by employees to the organisation's goals. (Moss et al., 2008; Manley et al., 2011b).

Organisations can support the development of effective workplace cultures through the development of both, transformational leadership and facilitation skills, supervision, support and peer review for clinical leader roles, such as, those facilitating the development of practice. Skilled facilitation of others' effectiveness through learning in and from practice, inquiry and evaluation, evidence use and implementation within the workplace is crucial to enabling effective workplace cultures and achieving sustainable change (Manley et al., 2011a). Crucial to organisational success is role negotiation and clarification consistent with purpose, together with workplace culture development (linked with evaluating and improving patient, user and staff experiences) being included in job descriptions, to prevent it being lost in the daily challenges of operational issues and the pressure of service delivery (McCormack et al., 2006).

THE ROLE OF RELATIONSHIPS IN DEVELOPING EFFECTIVE WORKPLACE CULTURES

Story 8.2 illustrates the role of relationships in growing practice development capacity and direction in tandem to developing person-centred culture of effectiveness. It provides an example from practice within an Australian children's hospital for which Annette, one of the chapter's contributors, is the Director of Nursing.

Story 8.2: The role of relationships

A strategic vision and plan for the organisation was developed that supports the implementation of cultures of person-centredness. The strategy was developed working in partnership with the corporate strategy, the executive team, and with the wards/units. It is ward and unit staff who realise the vision of person-centredness within the patient care/delivery interface that underpins the essential relationship that needs to exist to achieve cultures of person-centredness. Within the corporate strategy of a large hospital in New South Wales, Australia, there is a strategic plan for practice development. This plan was developed with stakeholder input and is readily available on the hospital intranet for staff to access and contribute their thinking. A component of the strategy is to build capacity across the organisation in relation to practice development knowledge and skills. The nursing executive team have all attended the International Practice Development School, with some of the executive team now being facilitators of the schools within Australia. A number of clinical nurses and others are supported each year to attend these schools. This approach is about building capacity within the organisation to realise the strategic vision for a culture of person-centred care. In addition, the hospital nurses are encouraged to participate in improving their immediate ward/unit and hospital workplace culture. As part of the corporate strategy, the hospital invests in a Nursing Research and Practice Development Unit with a Clinical Nursing Professor to support this important work.

The focus of the work is identified by the clinical team by using a range of strategies that includes the NCI; this survey is undertaken annually and the results are provided back to the ward/unit. As this piece of work occurs annually, the clinical team can review how they are doing using these results over time. The WCCAT is used within each of the wards/units along with a range of other quality improvement approaches to build up levels of data to describe the current workplace culture. Other sources of data include compliments, complaints, critical incidents, sick leaves and attrition of staff, patient stories, family stories, staff stories and QIA processes and outcomes.

Within the ward/unit, the workplace culture work is identified by the staff (supported by an internal facilitator and an external facilitator) and processes are put in place to create a culture of quality improvement, learning and feedback. Giving and receiving feedback from one another is important in establishing a culture of effectiveness in the workplace. The purpose of the feedback aligns with Schlecht's (2008, p. 68) 'intent to influence, reinforce, change behaviour, concepts, or attitudes'. Often, we see things from our own perspective and do not recognise how our own behaviours and language impact on our co-workers, patients and their families, and may be incongruent with the team's espoused values and our beliefs. In the provision of providing feedback, we have found it is more effective when there has been a process in place where staff are encouraged to provide each other with high challenge in the provision of feedback within an environment of high support for the individual and team. These skills have been achieved within the hospital through effective role-modelling by the facilitators and the leaders within the broader organisation and supported by practical processes such as giving and receiving feedback workshops. We have in place action learning sets, clinical supervision and active learning groups to support the giving and receiving of feedback and in the further development of emotional intelligence that is critical to this process.

There are, in addition, supportive educational leadership development opportunities to enhance the development of staff to that of transformational leadership.

Outcomes from this work have included clinical re-design activities and quality improvement projects. We have experienced a decrease in staff vacancies and have in place effective mechanisms to enable us to track our ability in creating and sustaining workplace cultures of effectiveness. A number of staff have presented the team's work at local, state, national and international conferences, sharing their journey and lessons learned. We have moved to a performance review system of seeking feedback from colleagues as part of the process. There have been improvements to our workforce practices as well as to our leadership and management development capabilities in the giving and receiving of feedback. We are seeing an increased focus of staff education and learning in the workplace. Patient and family input are integral to our processes of care. We are currently implementing the strategic plan for person-centred care – cultures of effectiveness – and know that we have made significant progress; however, there is much work to be done to embed this work within all areas of the wards/units of the hospital.

Organisational cultural change requires a transformational leadership approach to achieve a culture of effectiveness in person-centred care. Transformational leadership is congruent with the intent, processes and desired outcomes of organisational change using practice development approaches.

THE ROLE OF LEADERSHIP IN DEVELOPING AN EFFECTIVE WORKPLACE CULTURE

Leadership and culture change in practice

There has been a plethora of literature regarding a range of leadership styles over the last decade, highlighting the strengths or otherwise of these different leadership approaches (Kleinman, 2004; Murphy, 2005; Robins & Davidbizar, 2007; Snodgrass & Shachar, 2008; Solman & FitzGerald, 2008). A transformational leadership style supports the work of practice development as it is about working with people to move towards person-centred care practices. Transformational leaders inspire a shared vision and work with staff to achieve this vision through enabling others to take action and to maximise their leadership and teamwork potential. Bass and Reggio (2008) highlight the importance of transformational leadership in encouraging intellectual stimulation (through challenge and supportive mechanisms) towards ethically inspired goals resulting in a high level of performance.

The capabilities of a transformational leader are many and include the ability to inspire a shared vision, work in an ethical manner, support progression of patient-centred care practice, invest in staff development, inspire others to reach higher than they thought was possible and work in a constructive and positive way with the team enabling others to take the lead where possible. It is important to note here that effective transformational leaders focus on the development of their workplace culture, role-modelling shared values and achieving a common vision to engage the hearts and minds of colleagues in the workplace (Binnie, 2000; Davies et al., 2000; Haworth, 2000; Jones and Redman, 2000; Manojlovich and Ketefian, 2002; Bevington et al., 2004a, 2004b).

The learning and the sustainability of process and practice change that occurs through practice development work regarding the workplace culture and care practices are enhanced when transformational leadership is present. Transformational leaders support and encourage dedicated work to exploring the values and beliefs of staff and how these translate or not into the workplace and to achieving the vision for the service. A transformational leader encourages and supports these activities and the use of evidence to inform practice, focuses on staff development, and reviews processes and systems to maximise their potential in improving information and work practices (Solman, 2010).

A transformational leader has insight into personal drivers that influence their thinking, work ethics, practices and their personal values, and how this shapes their world view and assumptions. To support others as a leader requires this level of self-understanding, as conflict in the workplace from our experience, is most often associated with an actual or potential breach of values. The leader needs to be able to separate out their own feelings and values to truly listen and understand another's perceptive. Kouzes and Posner (2007) support the importance of understanding core values and those of others, as they are central to who we are as human beings and how we respond or react to circumstances.

Transformational leaders support staff to work through opportunities upon which to maximise challenges and crisis. Support in this way can result in enlightenment by team members about factors that contributed to the situation they are experiencing. This in turn leads to emancipation from the patterning of old thinking and practices from this new understanding of a situation. A transformational leader encourages staff to acknowledge and celebrate each other's and team's achievements. Celebration of achievements is important in acknowledging progress with the work, valuing the contribution of others and creating energy and pride within the team.

Situational leadership is a framework that can be used to support staff development throughout practice development. Transformational leaders using this approach would discuss the areas of strengths and less developed areas with the staff member; the intent of supportive development is to further the staff members capabilities. Touchstone (2009) suggests that the situational leadership framework supports individual staff development through the use of reflective practice strategies. Strategies may include coaching, clinical supervision, active learning, action learning sets, claims concerns and issues evaluation. Reflective practice strategies are used by transformational leaders to work with individuals and teams to learn from the experience. This learning informs their thinking, challenges assumptions, illuminates their strengths and identifies areas for development work into the future. Reflective practice approaches support an enhanced understanding of the situation, what/who contributed to the situation and the place of self within the situation, and has been documented within the practice development literature (Dewing, 2008; Solman & FitzGerald, 2008). See Touchstone (2009) for further information regarding the use of situational leadership in your work practices.

THE ROLE OF FACILITATION IN DEVELOPING EFFECTIVE WORKPLACE CULTURES

Facilitation is described as 'a helping relationship, essentially one of enabling others and consequently self, through transition to achieve growth/development and ultimately self-actualisation' (Mayeroff, 1971).

In an effective workplace culture, positive nurturing relationships are key to transformation and human flourishing. Facilitation focuses on the development of enabling relationships that are mutually beneficial to the parties concerned as they provide opportunities to share learning, give and receive feedback in a supportive environment and really get to know the persons in the relationship and the context in which they work. Facilitation can help to (1) illuminate the nuances of everyday practice that we often ignore; (2) help us to reframe the values, beliefs and assumptions we make about problems or issues we face so that we can find alternative solutions; (3) develop our own self-awareness of how our actions, behaviours and feelings impact on our own and others' practice; and (4) critique the history, policy and practice contexts and evidence base that underpins it to make sense of our workplace culture.

In an effective workplace culture, skilled facilitation is woven into the fabric of the team and highly valued as a way of role-modelling leadership behaviours and communication styles that underpin person-centred ways of working, with all team members taking responsibility for the delivery of the shared vision and common purpose. All members of the health care team are actively encouraged to participate in processes and practices that create an empowering work environment to enable the transfer of knowledge into practice and effective use of the resources of the team. It is important that individual roles and responsibilities within a team are clearly identified to promote shared accountability for decision-making. A skilled facilitator models critical thinking and reflection on action to help the team to improve their capacity to find innovative solutions to practice problems, and draw upon a range of evidence to support decision-making, using a range of skills including:

- working with values, beliefs and assumptions;
- challenging contradictions;
- developing moral intent;
- focusing on the impact of the context of practice, as well as practice itself;
- enabling others to 'see the possibilities';
- using self-reflection and fostering reflection in others;
- fostering widening participation and collaboration by all involved.

In many practice situations, facilitation enables health care professionals to develop awareness of the need for change by identifying contradictions between what is believed to be happening and the actual realities of practice. The following example demonstrates how skilled facilitation can help to develop a common vision and framework for action when teams experience difficulty in changing practice (Story 8.3). In this example, the facilitators worked with a team to help them to analyse and change current ways of working. The model of external–internal facilitation, where facilitators from outside the work setting work with identified internal facilitators using a range of support and supervisory methods, enabled not only the development of a common vision and framework for action but also the development of the internal facilitator's own skills and knowledge in managing change. An enabling facilitator is one who seeks to explore and release the inherent potential of others. The facilitators created the conditions whereby reflection, critique, collaboration, high challenge with high support and active learning can be sustained as integrated components of practice and which collectively bring about changes in the practice culture.

Story 8.3: Example of using skilled facilitation to develop a safeguarding vision/purpose, strategy and governance framework for a large teaching hospital

In a large teaching hospital, the Safeguarding Governance Group had responsibility for delivering the organisational strategy for managing risk and identifying the impact of strategies to safeguard vulnerable patients and service users. Although the group had been established for some months with Terms of Reference for its work, it was finding it difficult to establish a clear action plan for how it would deliver the strategy. There was a clear dissonance between what the group believed it was set up to achieve, and the reality of how difficult this was to deliver in practice.

A 2-hour team workshop was facilitated by external consultants using a structured programme of activities aimed at enabling governance group members to identify their common purpose, strategic objectives, roles and responsibilities of the governance group and individuals within the organisation for delivering the safeguarding strategy. The facilitators used a values clarification activity, to enable the steering group to identify their shared vision by using the following statements:

I/we believe the ultimate purpose of safeguarding is. . . .
This purpose can be achieved by. . .
Safeguarding is recognised as happening when. . .
The enablers and inhibitors to safeguarding are . . .
The difference between adult and children safeguarding is. . .
The responsibilities of every staff member (individual) in the organisation for adult
    safeguarding are. . .
The hospital's responsibilities for safeguarding are. . .
The responsibilities of the Safeguarding Governance Group are. . .

The themes distilled from this activity were used to identify a shared ultimate purpose, namely: safeguarding is to protect and avoid harm to the patients/service users, promote recovery and well-being, whilst being compassionate and fair. The steps identified by the group for how this could be achieved were by:

- providing good leadership and role models for safeguarding;
- taking individual and collective responsibility and holding our staff to account;
- having good communication, protocols, procedures assurance and governance systems;
- encouraging and working together in partnership;
- learning from experience, building expertise, providing education and training;
- reducing complaints;
- complying with the law;
- understanding the differences between safeguarding for adults and children.

The workshop enabled the participants to identify the roles and responsibilities of the Safeguarding Governance Group and individual health care professionals within the organisation (every staff member) and a number of strategic objectives were formed from the themes distilled as follows:

1. To enable individuals to take responsibility and be accountable for safeguarding through learning, education.
2. To develop assurance systems that comprises communication mechanisms, protocols, procedures and governance.
3. To build organisational capacity and expertise around safeguarding through leadership.
4. To manage organisational risks in relation to safeguarding.

Each of the strategic objectives required further development to create a number of SMART (Specific, Measurable, Achievable, Realistic, Timed) operational objectives and a work plan. This work plan will be overseen by the Safeguarding Governance Group and will constitute the key work of the group. The enablers and inhibitors identified in the values clarification activity have been used along with indicators of success to provide a hospital framework for safeguarding that can guide the work of the organisation and enable a joined up approach in its implementation and evaluation. Its role will be to guide the implementation of the strategy as well as potentially be the basis of an audit/observation tool with regard to the attributes. It will also be used as a project in the hospital leadership programme to test out an approach around the attributes.

This workshop enabled a key organisational team who were 'stuck' in its thinking, to develop a shared common vision for its roles and responsibilities for delivering a hospital-wide strategy for safeguarding and to generate a measurable framework to demonstrate impact of its intervention work for the future. It demonstrates what can be achieved in a short space of time through skilled facilitation, which focused critical thinking, reflection in and on action and active learning to develop a common vision for adult safeguarding and operationalisation of a safeguarding strategy and framework. Participants described the workshop as thought provoking, challenging, and were surprised at what could be achieved through focused activity in a short period of time and a great deal of satisfaction with their creative outcomes.

In an effective workplace culture, identifiable systems are in place to promote learning and development for individual health care professionals as well as teams. This may take the form of clinical supervision, mentorship, coaching, critical companionship, communities of practice, and action learning sets. Most readily identifiable in the culture is a commitment to develop colleagues to be the best they can, by enhancing their capacity to learn at, through and from work, and helping to support the development of their self-awareness, knowledge and skills to become effective leaders and to respond flexibly and creatively to practice problems and issues. An effective facilitator will role-model how to ask effective questions, provide high challenge and a high degree of support, as well as model how to give and receive feedback, encouraging colleagues to develop and use these skills in their everyday practice using active learning as a critical reflection activity.

Titchen's (2000, 2004) critical companionship model emphasises the importance of facilitating learning from practice, and the co-creation of new knowledge through critical reflection and dialogue between the practitioner (or learner) and an experienced facilitator (the critical companion). Critical companions are partners who act as a resource on a journey of discovery – someone who can be trusted, a supporter who has a genuine interest in development and growth through providing high challenge and high support. The role of the companion is to help others develop theoretical insights to transform self, identify issues that hinder improvements in practice and develop strategies to overcome these. Story 8.4 demonstrates the impact of a critical companionship journey on the career aspirations of a colleague.

Story 8.4: An example of how critical companionship has helped to transform the leadership potential for a colleague

I was recently approached by a colleague who asked for my support as a critical companion to help them to make sense of recent experiences that were troubling them. The colleague was frustrated by their inability to comprehend why they had not been promoted to a more senior level within their organisation. In a series of meetings over an initial 6-month period, we worked together to identify and develop critical insight into the issues that were hindering her aspirations. Key to our relationship was the importance of providing a safe environment to enable her to open up and share her experiences, problems, issues and aspirations and that we were able to explore these together in a mutually respectful shared learning experience.

In our first meeting, we established ground rules for working together, outlining our expectations of each other in the relationship and agreeing our ways of working. We undertook a claims, concerns and issues activity to explore what factors had been helping or hindering her development in order to tease out the priorities for action. Between our first and second meeting my colleague attended a Leadership Development Centre that enabled her to gain 360-degree feedback from an identified role set on her skills, abilities, strengths and areas for development. The 360-degree leadership tool provided her with feedback from a range of colleagues who work with her on a regular basis. In our second meeting, we explored the strengths and areas for development, drawing up a personal development plan and strategies for developing her knowledge and skills further, including the resources that would be required to achieve a series of SMART objectives.

Drawing on the principles of high challenge and high support we were able to identify that there were several areas of her practice that she had previously thought she shone at, but which were in fact perceived to be areas for further development by the role set who had provided feedback. The resultant action plan enabled us to focus on these areas and to prioritise these as areas for development.

Moving her beyond her comfort zone, we were able to identify new areas of practice that required her to develop her leadership skills. In the subsequent meetings, we explored critical incidents in which she had taken on new areas of responsibility to develop her skills, and underpinned this critical reflection with exploration of relevant theories and strategies to raise her awareness of how to capitalise on successes, and how to overcome problems or issues in practice that were more complex. By the sixth meeting, she had begun to add a new range of skills and strategies to her workplace toolkit in order to help her make the most of learning in and from practice. I encouraged her to join an action learning set that was focused around a new area of leadership that she was developing so that she could work with a team of colleagues to develop the insight and skills to lead workplace innovation and management of change. Twelve months into the critical companionship relationships, she has applied for and been successful in her promotion, is now coaching other colleagues in her team, role-modelling the skills that she has learned, and we continue to meet on a regular basis to test out and reflect on her achievements and issues that arise in practice. She reports to have developed a great sense of awareness of how she behaves and the impact it has on others, pride in the skills she has developed in supporting the development of others, a sense of achievement in managing complex practice innovation and a thirst for new knowledge and aspirations for her career development for the future.

This example demonstrates that a critical companionship relationship should be open and supportive, and develop the self-confidence of the practitioner, helping them to think laterally about situations and experiences. Being non-judgemental, approachable and reliable are key skills for the critical companion to possess. Getting to know them as a whole person as well as a colleague is important, as is ensuring that the giving and receiving of feedback, support or challenge is undertaken in a mutually collaborative way and in a safe environment.

Critical companionship and skilled facilitation then is key to the development of effective workplace cultures because it focuses on enabling and empowering individuals to grow, develop and to be the best they can be, underpinned by structured frameworks and models that promote raised self-awareness and the potential for learning and development. Alongside this is the importance of using structured models and processes to evaluate learning so that its impact on individuals, patients, teams and organisations can be evidenced. This may range from using mechanisms such as patient stories, reflective reviews in the form of personal narratives, 360-degree questionnaires to provide feedback on performance, annual appraisal documents, team action plans and observations of care, to name a few.

How would you recognise that facilitation has impacted positively on your workplace culture?

For practitioners and clinical leaders aspiring to develop their facilitation skills, there are some important indicators and standards you can use to demonstrate the impact that facilitation can have on the development of an effective workplace culture where everyone can flourish. The key question is how would you recognise that facilitation has contributed to transforming the workplace culture? In addition to the outcomes identified earlier in the chapter, some examples you might expect to see include the following:

- The team recognises and values the contribution that all members make in their roles of delivering high-quality person-centred, safe and effective care in the workplace.
- There is open, honest and clear communication and good working relationships among the team.
- The workplace fosters and experiences a culture of high support and high challenge using recognised systems of facilitation in their daily work enabling and supporting members of the team to be the best they can be.
- Team members demonstrate an enhanced ability for critical self-reflection and appraisal, through experiencing the giving and receiving of structured feedback.
- The team demonstrates an improved ability to link theory with practice through reflective conversations and can articulate how evidence informs their practice.

- There are mechanisms in place to help the team to deconstruct and reconstruct experiences, for example action and active learning, mentoring, coaching, critical companionship, journal clubs, and critical incident analysis.
- The team are able to describe positive learning experiences through a supported and facilitated, transformational journey of discovery.
- There are formal structured mechanisms, frameworks and processes in place to facilitate life-long learning. (Manley et al., 2001; Manley et al., 2008).

The Facilitation and Workplace Standards included in the RCN's Workplace Resources for Practice Development (RCN, 2006) provide an invaluable framework for assessing and signposting the essential components of an effective workplace culture and provide benchmark facilitation standards by which individuals and teams can assess and reflect upon their level of competence in their developmental journey. The four main standards are as follows:

1. Developing person-centredness.
2. Developing individual, team and service effectiveness.
3. Developing evidence-based health care including knowledge utilisation, transfer and evidence development.
4. Developing effective workplace culture.

An effective transformational workplace culture is recognised by the presence of (1) practice development with a focus on person-centred, evidence-based care; (2) staff empowerment; (3) shared values and practices; (4) adaptability internally and externally reflected by a learning culture; (5) services that match needs; (6) valued stakeholders; and (6) leadership that is valued and its potential developed at all levels. You may wish to use this framework to evaluate your own workplace culture.

CONCLUSION

This chapter has set out to help the reader recognise the central importance of workplace culture in enabling person-centred care to be experienced by patients and service users as well as the role of culture for staff well-being and enabling everyone to flourish. The culture we have specifically focused on is experienced at the interface between patients, service users with staff, although organisational culture is an enabler to this.

Through developing insights into effective workplace cultures, how they are recognised, their enabling factors and consequences, we hope the reader will be encouraged to ponder their own workplace culture using the reflective questions we have presented throughout the chapter. Whilst as an individual, it is sometimes difficult to grasp how one person can impact on any workplace culture, we have identified a number of strategies that enable such a journey to commence at any level, be that through relationships, such as critical companionship; leadership, particularly transformational leadership; and finally through skilled facilitation of others. Many of the skills required are reiterated throughout this book as are stories that demonstrate its achievement.

REFERENCES

Bass, B. & Reggio, R. (2008) *Transformational Leadership*, 2nd edn. Taylor and Francis e-Library. www.eBookstore.tandf.co.uk (Accessed 8 October 2012).

Bevington, J., Halligan, A. & Cullen, R. (2004a) Culture vultures. *Health Service Journal*, **114**, 30–31.

Bevington, J., Halligan, A. & Cullen, R. (2004b) Pass it on. *Health Service Journal*, **114**, 28–29.

Binnie, A. (2000) Freedom to practice: changing ward culture. *Nursing Times*, **96** (6), 41–42.

Bolan, D.S. & Bolan, D.S. (1994) A reconceptualization and analysis of organizational culture: the influence of groups and their idiocultures. *Journal of Managerial Psychology*, **9** (5), 22–27.

Castro, P., Dorgan, S. & Richardson, B. (2008) A healthier health care system for the United Kingdom. *The McKinsey Quarterly, February*, 1–5.

Charmel, P. & Frampton, S. (2008) Building the business case for patient-centred care. *Healthcare Financial Management*, **62** (3), 80–85. ABI/INFORM Global.

Davies, H., Nutley, S.M. & Mannion, R. (2000) Organisational culture and quality of health care. *Quality and Safety in Health Care*, **9** (2), 111–119.

Dewing J. (2008) Becoming and being active learners and creating active learning workplaces; the value of active learning in practice development. In: *International Practice Development in Nursing and Healthcare* (eds K. Manley, B. McCormack & V. Wilson), pp. 260–272. Blackwell Publishing Ltd., Oxford.

Drennan, D. (1992) *Transforming Company Culture*. McGraw-Hill, London.

Goleman, D. (1996) *Emotional Intelligence - Why It Can Matter More Than IQ*. Bloomsbury Publishing Plc, London.

Haworth, S. (2000) New management culture in the NHS. *Nursing Management*, **7** (3), 16–17.

Jackson, C. (2010) How does learning happen in the workplace? In: *Workplace Learning in Health and Social Care: A Student's Guide* (eds C. Jackson & C. Thurgate), pp. 12–21. McGraw-Hill, London.

Jones, K. & Redman, R. (2000) Organizational culture and work design: experiences in three organizations. *Journal of Nursing Administration*, **30** (12), 604–610.

Kleinman, C. (2004) The relationship between managerial leadership behaviors and staff nurse retention. *Research and Perspectives on Healthcare*, **82** (4), 2–8.

Kouzes, J. & Posner, B. (2007) *The Leadership Challenge* (Revised), 4th edn. Jossey-Bass, San Francisco, CA.

Mallak, L.A., Lyth, D.M., Olson, S.D., Ulshafer, S.M. & Sardone, F.J. (2003) Diagnosing culture in health-care organizations using critical incidents. *International Journal of Health Care Quality Assurance*, **16** (4), 180–190.

Mallak, L., Lyth, D., Olson, S., Ulshafer, S. & Sardone, F. (2003) Diagnosing culture in health-care organisations using critical incidents *International Journal of Health Care Quality Assurance*, **16** (4), 180–198.

Manley, K. (2001) *Consultant Nurse: Concept, Processes, Outcomes*. Unpublished PhD thesis, Manchester University/RCN Institute, London.

Manley, K. (2004) Transformational culture: a culture of effectiveness. Chapter 4. In: *Practice Development in Nursing* (eds B. McCormack, K. Manley & R. Garbett), Blackwell Publishing Ltd., Oxford.

Manley, K., Crisp, J. & Moss, C. (2011a) Advancing the practice development outcomes agenda within multiple contexts. *International Practice Development Journal*, **1** (1), Article 4.

Manley, K., McCormack, B. & Wilson, V. (eds.) (2008) *International Practice Development in Nursing and Healthcare*. Blackwell Publishing Ltd., Oxford.

Manley, K., Sanders, K., Cardiff, S. & Webster, J. (2011b) Effective workplace culture: the attributes, enabling factors and consequences of a new concept. *International Practice Development Journal*, **1** (2), Article 1. http://www.fons.org/library/journal/volume1-issue2/article1 (Accessed 8 October 2012).

Mannion, R., Davies, H. & Marshall, M. (2005) Cultural characteristics of 'high' and 'low' performing hospitals. *Journal of Health Organization and Management*, **19** (6), 431–439.

Manojlovich, M. & Ketefian, S. (2002) The effects of organisational culture on nursing professionalism: implications for health resource planning. *Canadian Journal of Nursing Research*, **33** (4), 15–34.

Mayeroff, M. (1971) *On Caring*. Harper and Row, London.

McCormack, B., Dewar, B., Wright, J. Garbett, R., Harvey, G. & Ballantine, K. (2006) *A Realist Synthesis of Evidence Relating to Practice Development: Final Report to NHS Education for Scotland and NHS Quality Improvement Scotland*. NHS Quality Improvement Scotland, Edinburgh.

McCormack, B., Henderson, E., Wilson, V. & Wright, J. (2009) Making practice visible: the workplace culture critical analysis tool (WCCAT) *Practice Development in Healthcare*, **8** (1), 28–43. Published online in Wiley Interscience. www.interscience.wiley.com(Accessed 1 June 2012).

McCormack, B. & Titchen, A. (2006) Critical creativity: melding, exploding, blending. *Educational Action Research*, **14** (2), 239–266.

Moss, C., Walsh, K., Jordan, Z. & Macdonald, L. (2008) The impact of practice development in an emergency department: a pluralistic evaluation. *Practice Development in Health Care*, **7** (2), 93–107.

Murphy, L. (2005) Transformational leadership: a cascading chain reaction. *Journal of Nursing Management*, **13**, 128–136.

Robbins, B. & Davidhizar, R. (2007) Transformational leadership in health care today *Health Care Manager*, **26** (3), 234–239.

Royal College of Nursing (RCN) (2006) *Workplace Resources for Practice Development*. RCN, London.

Schein, E.H. (1985) *Organizational Culture and Leadership*, 2nd edn. Jossey-Bass, San Francisco, CA.

Schlecht, K. (2008) Feedback international. *Anesthesiology Clinics*, **46** (4), 67–84.

Slater, P., McCormack, B. & Bunting, B. (2009) The development and pilot testing of an instrument to measure nurse's working environment: the Nursing Context Index. *Worldviews on Evidence-Based Nursing*, **6** (3), 173–182.

Snodgrass, J. & Shachar, M. (2008). Faculty perceptions of occupational therapy program director's leadership styles and outcomes of leadership. *The Journal of Allied Health*, **37** (4), 225–235.

Solman, A. (2010) Director of nursing and midwifery leadership: informed through the lens of critical social science. *Journal of Nursing Management*, **18**, 472–476.

Solman, A. & FitzGerald, M. (2008) Leadership support. In: *International Practice Development in Nursing and Healthcare* (eds K. Manley, B. McCormack & V. Wilson), pp. 260–272. Blackwell Publishing Ltd., Oxford.

Titchen, A. (2000) *Professional Craft Knowledge in Patient-Centred Nursing and the Facilitation of its Development*. D. Phil thesis, Linacre College Oxford. Ashdale Press, Tackley.

Titchen, A. (2004) Helping relationships for practice development critical companionship. In: *Practice Development in Nursing* (eds B. McCormack, K. Manley & R. Garbett), pp. 148–174. Blackwell Publishing Ltd., Oxford.

Titchen, A., McCormack, B., Wilson, V. & Solman, A. (2011) Human flourishing through body, creative imagination and reflection. *International Practice Development Journal*, **1** (1), Article 1. http://www.fons.org/library/journal.aspx (Accessed 1 October 2012).

Touchstone, M. (2009) The Supervisor as coach. *EMS Professional Development*, **6**, 64–66.

Ward, K. (2002) A vision for tomorrow: transformational nursing leaders. *Nursing Outlook*, **50** (3), 121–126.

Wilson, V., Hardy, S. & Brown, B. (2008) An exploration of practice development evaluation: unearthing praxis. In: *International Practice Development in Nursing and Healthcare* (eds K. Manley, B. McCormack, & V. Wilson), pp. 126–146. Blackwell Publishing Ltd., Oxford.

9 Evaluation Approaches for Practice Development: Contemporary Perspectives

Sally Hardy[1], Val Wilson[2] and Tanya McCance[3]

[1]City University, London, UK
[2]University of Technology, Sydney, Australia
[3]Belfast Health and Social Care Trust, Belfast, UK

INTRODUCTION

Within this chapter, we explore a variety of approaches to evaluation used within practice development. The aim is to provide a practical and theoretical discussion for the reader to consider when using evaluation within their practice settings. Alongside this, we aim to foreground the importance of evaluation as an effective means to further inform the international agenda on the significance of practice development, as a methodology and complex intervention, contributing to global transformational health care.

We suggest there are three main reasons for undertaking evaluation. These are to:

1. demonstrate impact and outcomes of a specific/locally delivered practice development project or programme of work;
2. obtain evidence that further informs and influences organisation-wide strategic transformational change;
3. generate new knowledge that can contribute to the evidence base.

We aim to show how integral complexity is within evaluation and how this complexity can be capitalised upon, understood and then utilised to inform and expose both process and outcomes of practice-based transformation. Rather like strata that make up the earth's crust, there are many layers to evaluation. Some evaluation approaches allow a deep exploration into the inner core of an organisation, whilst others aim to and can effectively work with more prominent surface layers, where rich and fertile soil is available to plant and nurture growth.

The evaluation chapter in the first edition of this book introduced the concept of evaluation in practice development work and outlined evaluation methodologies in common use that share theoretical principles, ontological values and emancipatory intent within a practice development approach. Within this chapter, we build on this through an evolving understanding of the evaluation of practice development programmes. We offer a range of evaluation approaches that will enable practice developers, at different levels of experience, to engage in rigorous and systematic evaluation activity, sharing working examples from our personal experiences. Our objective is to help reveal the importance of using collaborative

Practice Development in Nursing and Healthcare, Second Edition. Edited by Brendan McCormack, Kim Manley and Angie Titchen.
© 2013 John Wiley & Sons, Ltd. Published 2013 by John Wiley & Sons, Ltd.

and inclusive systematic approaches to evaluation, and the practical strengths and limitations of these are discussed.

Major methodologies, such as action research, realistic evaluation (RE) and fourth generation evaluation, are highlighted first as influential methodological frameworks that underpin evaluation approaches used to further influence social change and human flourishing. We then move to present more specific and potentially sophisticated approaches that have been devised specifically to capture the complexity and inclusive approaches suitable for evaluating both processes and outcomes of transformational practice development activity.

BACKGROUND

If you keep on doing what you've always done, you'll keep on getting what you've always got.
(Bateman, 1824–1903)

Within the evidence-based health care arena, it remains a 'gold standard' approach that experimentation through randomised controls are considered the best enquiry approach to measure, monitor and predict outcomes. However, when approaching health care outcomes from a critical perspective, social democratic evaluation approaches provide a counter argument to relying solely on scientific objectivity, claiming such objectivity removes and reduces opportunity for new insight, understanding and innovation to occur (Guba & Lincoln, 1989; Stake, 1994; Simons, 1996; Pawson & Tilley, 1997; Kushner, 2000); let alone consider how best to reflect the range of stakeholder values implicit and explicit in an evaluation.

For an evaluation to be comprehensive, logical, inclusive, rigorous, and meaningful, evaluation design needs to embrace a range of methods, working with the strengths of quantitative data sets and complementing these with sensitive, robust forms of qualitative evidence. A mixed methods approach is often used in practice development evaluation and allows methods to be dictated by the issues under investigation. Increasingly important is the very process through which an inclusive (i.e. broad stakeholder representation) evaluation team is brought together and supported to make informed decisions as to which are the best approaches to be used that can adequately answer the critical evaluation questions posed (exposing any assumptions, preferred ontology, or potential prejudices).

According to Owen and Rogers (1999), a programme's worth is judged on the quality of evidence produced, and whether that evidence is able to answer the evaluation questions posed.

We add that effective evaluation will also provide opportunity to further expose reflexive questions (where reflexivity is a process of critical reflection that informs and exposes values, and any potential bias that might affect actions). These additional 'new insight'-based questions can then be used to further inform transformational intent and practice innovation. As greater understanding and awareness of stakeholder perspectives are revealed, there will also be greater opportunity to focus on potential impact within the evaluation. Quinn-Patton (1997) presents a detailed approach to what he terms *Utilisation-Focused Evaluation*. He argues that the worth of any evaluation activity is the utility of the results to 'real people in the real world'.

Quinn-Patton (1997, p. 20) asserts that '. . . evaluations should be judged by their utility and actual use; therefore, evaluators should facilitate the evaluation process and design any evaluation with careful consideration of how everything that is done, from beginning to end, will affect use'.

EVALUATION AND PRACTICE DEVELOPMENT

Complexity in global population health is being reported through an increased ageing population and a rapid introduction of highly technologically advanced interventions, all of which requires an integrated approach to health care delivery (Benatar & Brock, 2011), improved use of information (Black et al., 2011), quality data management (Reynolds & Wyatt, 2011) and a workforce fit for purpose (Macfarlane et al., 2011). At the same time, there has been increased level of pressure on practitioners to deliver care that patients feel is right for them, with a resultant increased risk of complaints, litigation claims and media attention aiming to expose 'failing' health care institutions. A key component of global health care practice, therefore, is an ability to evaluate the effectiveness of health care delivery.

The development of an appropriate evaluation framework for a practice development programme, however, rests on a clear sense of expected outcomes, and indeed how these outcomes can be evidenced. Kirkpatrick (1994) provides a simple four level taxonomy for evaluating training programmes, used widely for its simplicity, yet many have taken his taxonomy further in the realisation that there are complex inter-relational aspects that need to be captured to fully understand what contributes to a programme's outcomes. Complexity also increases when expected outcomes are related back to different stakeholder group perspectives, that aim to incorporate, represent and accurately reflect individual, team and organisational perspectives. These anticipated outcomes will influence the kind of evaluation questions that need to be asked, which in turn will inform the methods to be used. This is illustrated in Figure 9.1.

There is a range of evaluation tools that can be used to collect data to evidence outcomes expected through the delivery of practice development programmes. Evaluation tools such

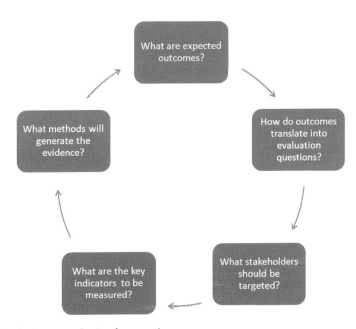

Fig. 9.1 Developing an evaluation framework.

as 360-degree feedback, reflective accounts and other self-assessment tools can be used to evidence individual outcomes.

Evidencing outcomes that reflect team effectiveness and the development of effective workplace cultures rely on tools such as *Claims, Concern and Issues* (Guba & Lincoln, 1989), focus group interviews and the use of specifically designed instruments for practice development evaluation, such as the Context Assessment Index (McCormack et al., 2009) and the Person-Centred Nursing Index (Slater, 2006). Evidencing outcomes for patients and clients tends to focus on the use of tools that enable patient feedback, such as patient stories. There are, however, other tools emerging that are beneficial in this context, such as the use of emotional touch points (Dewar et al., 2009).

We would argue that approaching evaluation in this inclusive way could be applied to any development or innovation in any practice setting, reflecting the potential to evidence the impact of a range of development activities. This debate reflects work undertaken in Northern Ireland by the Research & Development (R&D) sub-group of the Central Nursing Advisory Committee (CNAC R&D, 2012), the aim of which was to define the term 'development' and clarify where such activities sit on the R&D continuum. This was an attempt to frame how nurses and midwives are enabled to use evidence in practice that contributes to improvements in quality of patient care through approaches such as practice development. A participatory, critical and creative approach to clarifying the concept of 'development' was undertaken, which involved engaging with a range of stakeholders who were familiar with the concept in their everyday work. The process sought to uncover knowledge embedded in everyday practice, in an endeavour to bring clarity to the concept. This resulted in an agreed definition for 'development' in the context of R&D, and a conceptual framework that can illustrate the spectrum of activity that constitutes R&D and their interconnectedness.

The framework is presented in Figure 9.2 and illustrates activities that:

1. represent research, defined as 'the search for new knowledge using scientific methodologies and approaches' (R&D Office, 1999, p. 27);
2. represent 'development', defined as those activities that 'focus on creating the conditions for evidence utilisation to systematically innovate or improve practice, including integrated evaluation that demonstrates effective processes and outcomes and has the potential to generate new knowledge' (CNAC R&D, 2012);
3. could be described as precursors to development, in that they have the potential to inform developments in practice, but have not yet impacted on practice, such as service evaluation;
4. meet the criteria for both research and development.

Practice development represents activity that can fall into the fourth category, which on the one hand can be focused purely on bringing about changes in practice, but on the other has potential to generate new knowledge when a robust methodological evaluation framework is integral to the activity. Therefore, the level of evaluation is the defining feature that enables practice development, not only to evidence changes at organisational, service, team or individual level, but also to add to the evidence base. The key message, however, is the importance of evaluation as integral to practice development, irrespective of whether it demonstrates changes from a specific project at local level (denoted by a practice development with a small 'd') or a research endeavour that will contribute something new to the evidence base (denoted by practice Development with a capital 'D'). The evaluation approaches

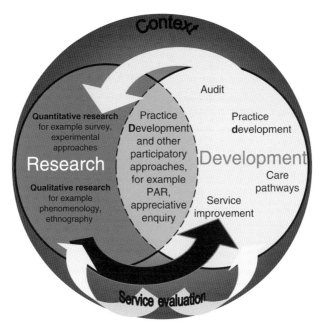

Fig. 9.2   Conceptual framework (CNAC R&D, 2012).

discussed in the following section can contribute to practice development across the spectrum of R&D, which of course is dependent on how the evaluation is planned and executed.

However, being clear about the transformational intent of an evaluation also highlights tensions that can exist between what constitutes practice development and evaluation, with a particular concern centred on a dissonance between what practitioners and researchers understand to be effective evaluation processes (Carr et al., 2008). Yet, the very existence of these tensions can provide a starting point for introducing an integrated evaluation approach that captures, exposes and tackles stakeholder convergence and divergence when it comes to expectations, experience and outcome measures for high-quality health care delivery. Practice development engages with and works alongside stakeholder groups, working from a starting point of identifying shared values, principles of meaningful engagement and an ethos of inclusive participation. These elements can all be utilised within evaluation to further expose and clarify a workplace culture of effectiveness; where all are aware of their contribution, roles and responsibilities, implications and consequences of actions, behaviours and practices, working towards a clearly articulated shared vision and promoting practice expertise.

As outlined above, working with evaluation provides the conditions for focusing activity on evidence utilisation that promotes innovation, and practice improvements. Chin and Hamer (2006) reported a critical evaluation undertaken to measure the effectiveness of a practice development approach across three NHS organisations and to monitor the impact of the programme on improvements to patient care. Findings revealed that practitioners improved their level of confidence when focusing attention on clinical initiatives, which led to improved understanding of what strategic organisational transformation entailed. However, direct impact on patient care was not achieved, which may well have been due to the evaluation design concentrating on practitioner-based feedback. Coster et al. (2006) reported an evaluation study that aimed to capture perceived impact of the consultant nurse role on service and patient care delivery using a multi-method evaluation. Results concluded that 71% of consultant nurses self-reported that they felt they did impact on service improvements after being in post for 2 or more years, whilst their major impact was identified as supporting other staff and reducing service expenditure.

Engaging practitioners in a process of evaluation can provide a peer review mechanism that promotes individual thinking (Chin & Hamer, 2006), improved patient experience (Coster et al., 2006), alongside significant patient health outcomes through innovative service changes (Tolson, 1998), through to potential influence on policy makers. We would propose that working with evaluation within the context of practice development enables not only the potential to expose, capture and utilise evidence of workplace complexity, but can also act as a process that creates the conditions for transformation. Working with an integrated evaluation approach enables practitioners to demonstrate the effectiveness of processes and outcomes, and how these can then be integrated into the generation of new knowledge and sustainable practice improvements.

EVALUATION APPROACHES

Outlined above is a background rationale for utilising evaluation in all practice development work and explanation of where and how evaluation fits with practice development principles, values and a transformational intent. Attention is now turned to present different evaluation approaches for achieving transformational intent associated with practice development. This is by no means a comprehensive or exhaustive review of evaluation per se; it is offered for the purpose of providing an overview of a number of different frameworks and models that are being used in evaluating both process and outcomes of practice development work. We are not advocating any one approach, but present here examples to enable practitioners to make informed choices in designing and negotiating their own evaluation framework or programme. To begin, an overview of three key overarching methodological approaches (action research, fourth generation evaluation and RE) is presented. More specific examples of practice-focused evaluation, suitable for capturing and working with transformation, are provided to expose the practical strengths and limitations of each approach discussed.

Participatory action research

Participatory action research (PAR) is a commonly used research approach in practice development work that involves research participants as co-constructors and co-investigators of the evaluation process through reflective cycles that lead to action-orientated change. PAR involves spirals or cycles of critical reflection, with each step of a project or programme being taken through a process of evaluation and review as the process continues (Kemmis & McTaggart, 2005). As a research approach, PAR has been extensively used within education, health and social care to simultaneously develop, implement and evaluate a wide and diverse range of initiatives. For example, a community programme to help young pregnant smokers to quit (Bryce et al., 2009), facilitating changes to the provision of dementia care (Chenoweth & Kilstoff, 1998), a cardiac rehabilitation programme (Davidson et al., 2008), a violence prevention programme for emergency departments (Gates et al., 2011), an obesity prevention programme (Reifsnider et al., 2010), an osteoporosis education programme (Whitehead et al., 2004) and change to handover practice (Wilson et al., 2007), to name but a few.

PAR project example: changing handover practice project (Wilson et al., 2007)

In this study, the process of undertaking PAR was supported by a simultaneous action learning (AL) group (McGill & Beaty, 2001). The AL group members supported but also posed critical challenges to the PAR project team as the study progressed. Taking time to stop and reflect upon what was happening within the study enabled members of the project team to continuously evaluate the process of the project, whilst at the same time introduce and make changes to activity in light of what was being uncovered. An example of this related to the evaluation mechanism of seeking staff feedback during the trialling of the intervention. Feedback was initially fairly negative, with staff complaining about a range of things, including an increase in their perceived workload (having to input data onto the handover system), wasting resources (new tool required in each shift, thereby seen as wasting paper) and potential disclosure of confidential information (the handover sheet being left around the clinical area). Whilst these 'issues' may seem minor, they had the potential to negatively impact on the uptake of the intervention (using the newly devised handover tool). By collecting evaluation data, the project team were not only kept abreast of what was happening for staff, they were also able to critically review the issues and alter the intervention as and when required. For example, the project team discussed *confidentiality* with staff and highlighted that much of the information they work with everyday (about patient care) needs to remain confidential and therefore the handover tool was merely another component of that. To alleviate issues such as accidentally leaving the completed handover tool around the practice environment, it was agreed to introduce a confidential waste recycle box where staff could insert the handover forms at the end of their shift. Numerous programme changes arose as a result of continual stakeholder feedback and evaluation at each of the five phases of action research (Figure 9.3), as outlined by Wilson et al. (2007). As a result of the handover project, staff not only changed handover practice, they used this to also change the way they planned and delivered care; they involved medical staff in changing their handover mechanisms

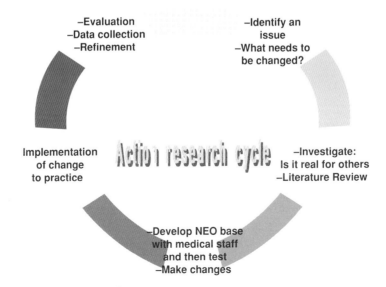

Fig. 9.3   Research cycle for handover project.

(although this had not been the original intent), and this resulted in the multi-disciplinary team all using the same approach to handover.

Utilising a PAR approach brings together action, reflection, theory and practice in a systematic way in order to create practical knowledge that is of value to those involved in the focus of the research (Reason & Bradbury, 2006). PAR allows knowledge development, which can be applied back to the practice area from which it was created (Roulin et al., 2007); staff in the unit were developing their understanding of research and evaluation as well as their knowledge about handover practice. An advantage of a PAR approach is the collaborative relationship between the researchers, staff and, where applicable, patients in the clinical setting that can enable sustainable changes to patient care and the work environment (Soh et al., 2011).

As can be seen from the example provided, PAR is an approach to research with an in-built continuous evaluation mechanism. It not only encompasses the collection and review of data systematically, but also has the intent to act upon findings as it moves through each cycle of the PAR process. This approach has meaning for those involved in practice development work as it enables participants to look at the reality of their practice world, it engages practitioners in researching their own practice, in developing ideas for changing their practice and ways in which they can implement and evaluate both the processes and the outcomes of such change.

Fourth generation evaluation

Fourth generation evaluation (Guba & Lincoln, 1989) has been a methodology of choice for evaluating the processes and outcomes of practice development activity through projects such as the RCN Expertise in Practice Project (Manley et al., 2005; Hardy et al., 2009) and the Consultant Nurse project (Manley & Titchen, 2012). As an approach derived from a PAR tradition, fourth generation evaluation uses concerns, claims and issues to capture stakeholder opinion, and then uses these to construct a developing consensus for ongoing project activity. Guba and Lincoln (1989) outline 12 steps in the evaluation process, although not to be taken as a linear staged process, engaging in each of these steps (see Box 9.1) helps formulate a robust and systematic approach to evaluation.

The underlying values of fourth generation evaluation are about sharing power through a process of enlightenment and empowerment with the ultimate goal of emancipatory practice changes.

Fourth generation evaluation example: an organisation-wide modernisation programme (Hardy et al., 2012)

Working with health care teams in Victoria, Australia, a small team (consisting of practitioners, academics and researchers) met regularly to evaluate the impact of practice development approaches being implemented across several tertiary health care sites. Identifying the tools and measures to capture, implement and continue to critically review complex environments (such as extraneous activities of organisational modernisation), and provide practitioners with high support amidst the challenges of strategic organisational change was achieved through framing the programme within a fourth generation evaluation approach (Guba & Lincoln, 1989). Individual practitioners, clinical teams, managerial groups and senior executive teams were all engaged as participants involved in project development, implementation and evaluation strategies. The extent to which change was being achieved was captured using

---

Box 9.1: 12 steps in fourth generation evaluation.

1. **Contracting**, or identifying who is the sponsor/client and then clarification of purpose with identified agreement between contributors
2. **Transparent approach** to how the project will be conducted, including technological requirements, selection and engagement of participants and working contracts
3. **Identification** of additional stakeholders, those for whom the project will be used, those for whom the project may benefit and those for whom the project may negatively impact (i.e. agents, beneficiaries and victims)
4. **Development** of the project group construction
5. **Broadening** or enlarging of the stakeholder constructions, which is achieved through focus groups, project steering and or advisory groups
6. **Identification** and sorting out any resolved claims
7. **Consideration** of unresolved claims, in order to maximise clarity, expectations and shared understanding of issues
8. **Collection** of information/data to support or discredit claims, moving and adding elements as a level of sophisticated understanding arises
9. **Renegotiation** of activities
10. **Informing** agendas for ongoing change
11. **Dissemination** and reporting more broadly
12. **Recycling**, where ongoing new learning can be used to commence another cycle of evaluative activity

---

different tools such as the Person Centred Nursing Index (PCNI; Slater, 2006); values clarification (VC; Warfield & Manley, 1990); non-participant observations; unit/team-based action plans; AL sets; patient, family and staff satisfaction surveys; audit data; narratives (including photographic diary entries); workshops; seminars; individual supervision; critical companionship (Titchen, 2000); coaching sessions and critical steering group meetings. Therefore, a variety of tools were applied, reviewed and utilised to map, monitor and evaluate impact of organisational change. Working within the fourth generation evaluation framework enabled the evaluation team to integrate a number of different approaches. As each event, situation or circumstance emerged, its emergent evidence and impact was harnessed, reviewed and integrated into the evaluation approach. Outcomes of this 3-year project are still forthcoming, currently being reported and continue to be integrated into organisational modernisation plans. Enormous data sets have resulted, which is a potential strength and a challenge to working on such a large-scale programme. Therefore, a transparent dissemination strategy is required to convey goals and outcomes achieved, rather than leaving the team feeling swamped under the weight of information/evidence available.

Realistic evaluation

Pawson and Tilley (1997) developed RE in response to a dominance of approaches that aim to establish causal relationships between systems/processes and outcomes (Kirkpatrick, 1994). Pawson and Tilley (1997) argue that evaluation should be based in philosophical realism, which attempts to account for explanatory elements in the social world that are often overlooked by experimental approaches, such as a traditional randomised control trial (RCT).

Pawson and Tilley (1997) argue that essentially an evaluation is an evaluation of a social system. Social systems consist of interplay between individuals and institution, of agency and structure and of micro and macro social processes. The methodology of RE operates within five key concepts:

1. *Embeddedness*: There are in-built assumptions around a wider set of social rules and institutions that underpin social actions. Using a statutory training activity (e.g. drug administration) as an example; the training activity equates to being understood as a social rule, in that it becomes taken for granted that drug administration has a significant place within the social organisation of a hospital where treatment invariably includes medication.
2. *Mechanisms*: Social interventions occur not as isolated 'variables' but through a weaving together of resources (such as expert facilitation amalgamated with expert clinical reasoning to inform and embed sustainable practice change) to become an integrated process of shared decision-making rather than viewing them as isolated/separate independent variables.
3. *Contexts*: All social interventions have prevailing contextual conditions. These contextual conditions are crucially important when explaining the initiation, implementation and successes and/or failure of socially orientated change programmes. Context does not simply mean geographical, spatial or institutional location, but includes established socially constructed rules, norms, values and inter-relationships that influence (enhance or inhibit) a social programme.
4. *Regularities*: Regularities are explained as the relationship between mechanisms and contexts and their impact on the goal of a social programme.
5. *Change*: The way in which social programmes develop is determined by the inter-relationship between regularities, mechanisms and contexts (as outlined above). For example, people in an organisation may have limited knowledge about the context (e.g. decision-making structures) and regularities (e.g. code of professional conduct) within which a social intervention (e.g. a medication management programme) works in practice.

Evaluation programmes adopting a 'realist' methodology (e.g. Tolson, 1998) operate within 'the realist evaluation cycle' where there is interplay between theory generation, hypothesis testing, observation and programme specification. Working with a RE cycle enables the development of an evaluation framework that moves from describing the elements of the programme in detail towards creating a 'hypotheses' that can then be tested through an evaluation.

Realistic evaluation example: evaluating the Nursing Research and Practice Development Unit

A VC process is commonly used when working with teams to identify shared concepts and their meaning. In the first phase of the RE, focus is centred on describing the answers to the following questions:

- **What** are the relationships between mechanisms for change (i.e. using a VC)? Identifying the key elements of context that might impact on any developmental activity (i.e. where and for whom the VC process was being used (in this case a multi-disciplinary team in X ward)).

- **Why** VC was being used (to develop a shared vision for delivery of care to patients on X ward)?
- **How** VC is used (seven-step process to VC as outlined by Wilson, 2005)? Supporting the staff to participate in the process (agree time for staff to attend sessions) and explaining the relationships between patterns and associations in the programme and the subsequent outcomes that are then realised.

This early stage of the evaluation aims to explain the relationship between mechanisms and contexts and their impact (outcomes) on the goal of the social programme (in this case, the VC work undertaken by the Nursing Research and Practice Development Unit (NRPDU) in ward X) in order to predict 'what *might* work for whom and in what circumstances', that is hypothesis generation. The identification of these hypothesis forms the agenda for stage 2 of the evaluation cycle, whereby the use of multi-methods of data collection enables the testing out of the hypothesis in order to identify *what works for whom and in what circumstances*.

In the case of the NRPDU evaluation (Wilson et al., 2011), data collection was gathered from a broad range of teams being supported to undertake a VC process, applying the mechanisms in a variety of contexts, and from a range of perspectives (i.e. those involved in the VC process, other staff who interact with the team and patients) using a variety of data collection processes (i.e. team meeting notes, staff interviews, observations of practice and patient stories) to highlight the outcomes (i.e. if the values of the team were evident in everyday practice). This broad-spectrum approach resulted in uncovering what was working and not working in the VC process, for whom it was working or not working and in what circumstances it was working (or not working; i.e. when teams engaged with the VC process as a 'task', it resulted in difficulty translating values into practice change).

This second phase is described as 'programme specification': a detailed description and analysis of the programme that includes details of the relationships between mechanisms, context and outcomes.

Working with RE then provides a structured process from which to understand and dig deeper into what can become mechanistic behaviours, and provides a process through which practitioners/individuals can then begin to understand how their interactions impact and influence their working practices. However, some would argue that working from a RE perspective merely replicates a technological approach to understanding a programme, and has little impact on transformative change. Porter and O'Halloran (2012) argue that the limitations of working with RE is that its fundamental assumption centres on realism, which omits potential for a more postmodern understanding of what constitutes reality, overlooking what can be accepted or challenged in terms of dominant discourses[1].

Limitations of working with action research and fourth generation evaluation is the potential for the action cycles to become lengthy and time consuming, making this approach potentially problematic for short-term programmes and projects. Despite this, all three core frameworks provide robust, systematic approaches to evaluation. For some, all social change programmes have an inherent potential for transformation, whilst others would argue transformative intent is a utopia that is unattainable and unrealistic in the changing world of

---

[1] A dominant discourse is created by those in positions of authority and power, and are often the most common and accepted way of looking at or speaking about a particular subject or issue.

health care and social reformation. We move now to consider more specific models of evaluation that have emerged from the desire to produce rapid response to contemporary complex settings.

The 'CIPP' Model (Stufflebeam et al., 2000)

Much of practice development work focuses on the development and implementation of interventions, used to enable staff to learn how to improve practice, either through informal learning opportunities (e.g. in-service training programmes, work-based learning or bedside teaching) to more formal learning opportunities (e.g. short courses, workshops and AL groups). In education, an evaluation focus is often limited to one of the following approaches:

1. Stakeholder focused – data collected from consumers/beneficiaries.
2. Values focused – does the programme meet the values of society?
3. Continuous quality improvement (CQI) focused – systems analysis (i.e. structures, processes and outcomes).

Education evaluation often focuses on just one of these aspects of evaluation, such as participant learning is illustrated in the example in Box 9.2, the mechanisms to evaluate this can prove to be problematic.

Box 9.2: Common evaluation design limitations

Evaluation of a 1-day conference on medication safety

The evaluation mechanism chosen is a participant survey given to individual participants and then collected at the end of the day. The survey has a five-point scale measuring satisfaction with the content and delivery mechanisms used that day. Whilst the survey may report something about how satisfied participants are, it reveals little about the learning achieved or whether individuals increased their confidence with medication safety, neither will it identify the cost effectiveness of the day, or what the impact might be on practice, individual participant competency levels with medication safety, how learning is shared back in the clinical area, what information the educators/facilitators need to improve future programmes and so on.

Pross (2010) argues that evaluation plans are largely incorrect, insufficient or unreliable in gathering the right data to be used to base future decisions.

One model that does take into account multiple perspectives and integrates each of the three above approaches into a single evaluation framework is the context, input, process, product (CIPP) evaluation model developed by Stufflebeam et al. (2000) (see Figure 9.4).

The CIPP model can be used by facilitators of learning in developing and implementing evaluation plans that not only take into account the needs of multiple stakeholders and their perspectives but also guide the evaluator in the collection of data that is meaningful in terms of how best to inform future decisions about education and learning programmes.

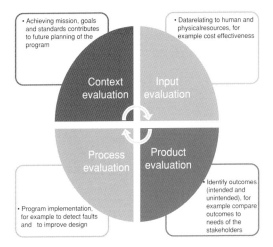

Fig. 9.4   *The CIPP Model: Diagram adapted from Stufflebeam et al., 2000.*

CIPP example: evaluating the impact of clinical supervision

This example outlines how the CIPP model is being utilised in the evaluation of clinical supervision in one organisation. The intent of the clinical supervision programme in the organisation was to ensure that nurses and allied health professionals had access to ongoing opportunities to enhance their professional development and clinical skills within a facilitated confidential environment (e.g. Hardy & Park, 1997). The main goals of clinical supervision are to:

- develop professional practice through reflection;
- support learning and effective clinical decision-making;
- facilitate role development through reflection;
- ensure safe, ethical and professional standards of practice;
- provide professional and peer support.

The programme has been implemented for a number of years, providing opportunities for people to both undertake clinical supervision training in order for them to become clinical supervisors, as well as experience clinical supervision as an individual practitioner or as part of a group. The evaluation of the programme lends itself to the CIPP model as a wide range of evaluation perspectives need to be taken into account. The evaluation model is presented in Table 9.1. For ease of reading, it is presented as linear but in reality, the different components of the evaluation occur alongside one another. The stakeholders for this evaluation are identified as the people undertaking clinical supervision, those providing clinical supervision and clinical supervision training, the sponsors (champions) and the teams in which clinical supervision is being utilised (including managers and educators of those teams who more broadly reflect organisational stakeholders). The outcomes of this evaluation will inform ongoing development and support of the clinical supervision programme and will be presented through reports (in the organisation) and disseminated externally via publications.

Table 9.1 CIPP (context, input, process, product) evaluation in clinical supervision (CS) project.

	Evaluation question(s)	Informants	An examples of data (these are really methods that generate data)
Context	Have the aims (see Section 'CIPP example: evaluating the impact of Clinical Supervision) of the CS programme been achieved?	• Sponsors and champions • CS trainers and staff who have received CS training	Interviews with key stakeholders
Input	How many staff have: 1. undertaken CS training – which includes session offered, attendance, follow up etc.? 2. delivered CS to individuals and groups – including frequency and time allocated? 3. participated in CS – including frequency and time allocated?	• Sponsors and champions • CS trainers • Those who provide and undertake CS	Staff engagement (attendance) and the resource implications including direct (i.e. cost of trainer) and indirect (i.e. staff release)
Process	Does the CS training meet: 1. the learning needs of staff intending to become CS? 2. the needs of the organisation in providing access to CS training? Is the implementation of CS meeting the needs of those who want to provide supervision and those who wish to receive (or support their staff to receive) supervision?	• Sponsors and champions • Those who provide and undertake CS • Managers, educators and other relevant support staff	Learning outcomes obtained from the completion of training courses How were these determined?
Product	What outcomes have been achieved by the provision of CS and CS training for the organisation, for staff who have trained as CS, for staff receiving CS and for staff who work in teams where CS is being used as a mechanism for professional development?	• Sponsors and champions • CS trainers and staff who have received CS training • Those who provide and undertake CS • Managers, educators and other relevant support staff	Survey of all staff involved with CS (including outcome indicators and feedback processes)

PRAXIS evaluation

PRAXIS evaluation (Wilson et al., 2008; Hardy et al., 2012) aims to provide an innovative approach to evaluation that captures and utilises the dynamic subtleties of individual, team and organisational transformation. The approach was developed from working within the complexity of contemporary health care contexts to initiate, map and progress transformative action. More recently, PRAXIS evaluation has also been employed in education settings as well as health care. PRAXIS evaluation offers a collaborative process for evaluating practice-based change, taking into consideration issues of effective workplace culture (Manley et al., 2011). First comes a collaborative clarification of the project's *P*urpose, then *R*eflexivity as a process of identifying the key critical questions. Third is the issue of choosing appropriate *A*pproaches to gathering evidence, alongside consideration of the conte*x*t within which the work is taking place. Fifth is the notion of *I*ntent, which overarches purpose and links with reflexivity to inform choice of approaches, and further influences the potential outcomes of the entire work being undertaken. Finally, the sixth element is the processes for inclusion and participation with *S*takeholders. However, these six core elements of evaluation do not work well as a linear process as outlined above, but are best used creatively, interwoven to provide a contemplative consideration and spatial mapping of the process of participation, project planning and data collection that integrates evidence into transformative action, all achieved through the mnemonic tool 'PRAXIS'.

One intention of the PRAXIS evaluation framework is to inform and stimulate knowledge co-creation with stakeholders, alongside the operational management of an evaluation project. Working in an inclusive and reflexive manner enables progress towards transformation as critically informed and considered practical action, defined as 'PRAXIS'. PRAXIS (as critically informed, emancipated action) is the ultimate purpose of this evaluation approach. By paying attention to both the process and the outcomes of evaluation data, which is critically co-created and explored in an eclectic, collaborative way, PRAXIS evaluation aims to promote transformation. PRAXIS evaluation also aims to expose, critically consider and utilise multiple issues, often hidden or taken for granted in complex clinical practice settings, in a systematic way that can capture influential elements of health care transformation at the same time as capturing significant outcomes. Figure 9.5 captures the key aspects of the PRAXIS evaluation approach.

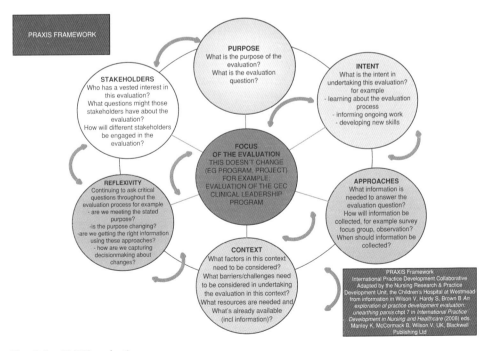

Fig. 9.5 PRAXIS evaluation.

Whilst the evaluation focus remains the same (captured in the inner circle), for example, evaluation of a leadership programme, the other five elements provide a dynamic and evolving process that inform and interconnect with the ongoing evaluation (see Wilson et al., 2008 for further details).

A potential limitation of the model is that conventional thinking promotes a linear approach to project development, lines of enquiry and learning approaches, whereas working with PRAXIS can mean that multiple spirals of activity occur at any one time. Facilitation of the process is a key role, to ensure that participants do not become muddled, confused or disorientated in terms of what the next stages of activity ought to be.

PRAXIS evaluation example: implementing evidence-based practice

Working with practitioners to consider how best to implement evidence-based practice within their workplace environment led to a small project team being developed, who worked through the PRAXIS framework, to identify and initiate an evaluation project suitable to their local context needs. Staff were reluctant to engage with *yet another* initiative that they felt was taking them away from their clinical priorities. However, once some initial observations of workplace culture had been achieved, using the workplace cultural critical analysis tool (WCCAT; McCormack et al., 2009) and staff meetings held to identify what were the specific concerns, claims and issues staff were tackling (an approach used in fourth generation evaluation as outlined earlier), it soon became evident that there was a disparity between what staff felt they were achieving as a cohesive team and what was in reality being experienced by more junior staff in particular. The ward was arranged across two ends, one end for more acutely ill patients, whilst the other end was used for patients nearing discharge. The more junior staff were most frequently allocated to the less acute end, making them feel excluded from the enormous learning potential they craved (i.e. to be working alongside a more senior practitioner at the acute end of the unit). Through using the PRAXIS tool, and reviewing each element individually with a shared collective of stakeholders, unrecognised issues began to surface. Staff were quick to challenge that excluding students was not the intention, so additional time was spent considering and clarifying what was the *I*ntent to the evidence-based practice project, rather than focusing on project *P*urpose. As a consequence of this reflexive debate, stimulated through undertaking the PRAXIS framework, and despite initial reservations, the nurses introduced team nursing, allocating more junior staff to work alongside more senior clinicians, and gain experience and confidence in patients with more complex needs. Subsequently, the need to facilitate learning at the bedside emerged as a key challenge for evidence-based health care to be implemented. Once this barrier had become identified, overcome and evaluated, improved staff engagement prepared the path to implement the more ambitious programme of evidence-based practice.

From a consideration of the evaluation frameworks and models explored in this section, there are a number of similarities. All are action orientated in nature and involve the engagement of multiple stakeholders to develop, undertake, inform and make sense of the evaluation process alongside the achievement of evaluation outcomes. Each approach advocates evaluation as an integral part of the work being undertaken. Greater level of potential impact is achieved within the planning stages of an evaluation, rather than leaving consideration of evaluation until near the closure or completion of a project or programme.

Evaluation is presented as a continuous process that informs ongoing action. Failure to evaluate is therefore a missed opportunity to build on valuable information and gain new insights and new knowledge to inform future critically informed actions (as a process of PRAXIS innovation). Each evaluation approach presented focuses on both the outcomes of the programme or project *and* the processes that enable outcomes to be or not to be achieved. Such fluidity benefits evaluators through the broader application and learning that results. Integrated learning matches the intent of practice development to be transformative in relation to people, processes and the systems practitioner's work.

PRACTICAL ISSUES

This final section provides a brief overview of some of the methods, mechanisms and principles used in practice development evaluation and why, when and how these might be used.

A range of methods, mechanisms, principles and issues are used to inform and support practice development work and its evaluation. Drawing from the methodologies and approaches presented in this chapter, evaluation in practice development encompasses:

- processes and principles by which participants are engaged in practice development work and in creating meaning, providing evidence about the practice context (including baseline, pre- and post-'measures');
- issues related to capturing outcomes of practice development work (for patients, families, staff and organisations);
- activities from which data is derived.

We have collated what we term, an 'evaluation checklist', based around a number of headings such as *evaluation purpose, stakeholders, information sources/evidence, processes and outcomes* (Table 9.2). As particular methods, mechanisms and principles can be used within all areas, it will be important to view the table as a matrix. VC, for example, may be an evaluation tool used to highlight dissonance in the current context and then to test espoused notions of practice against what actually happens in reality. VC can be used as a method for engaging people in transformational work. It may also be used as a process for capturing the ideas of practice in context that may be used to inform, for example, the development of a new model of care, roles and responsibilities of staff, staff appraisal, change projects, and to measure practice change over time. As with all tools, an issue that may arise with the VC process is how and why it is used and what then becomes of the data collected within the process. All too often, complaints are received from staff when they have put a lot of time, work effort and disclosed something of themselves in the process, only to find later that the product (outcome) of the VC process is lost in translation.

In summary, an effective evaluation is one that:

- recognises, exposes and engages with the influence of context (in all its complexity);
- is able to negotiate inclusion of a broad range of stakeholder perspectives;
- works with critically reflexive (multiple) approaches to evidence gathering;
- produces meaningful insights that then can be utilised to further stimulate transformation.

Table 9.2 Evaluation checklist.

An evaluation checklist: clear evaluation purpose	Stakeholder engagement	Information required/ evidence sources	Suitable approaches	Process measures	Outcome measures
What do you want to be able to achieve as a result of the evaluation? *Decide whether an internal or external evaluator is required to achieve the purpose?*	*Who are the key personnel that the work has an impact or effect upon?*	*What and where are the sources of information, and what type of information is required?*	*What are the best methods for capturing the information needed and from the personnel identified?*	*What and how is the process of the evaluation being captured, reflected upon and used to inform ongoing activities?*	*What and how will the evaluation be recognised and/or measured in terms of successful outcomes, and for whom?*
Improved Delivery of: • practice education; • programme; • service; • others Understand delivery mechanisms to become more efficient and/or cost effective Verification/clarification of aspired and lived values (i.e. what we say we are doing matches what is being done) Exploration of complex processes for future strategic planning and knowledge advancement	Service users/Clients (where who and how to engage clients in meaningful engagement) Staff/employees Specific professional groups Management/Board members Funders/Commissioners Local Communities Populations Policy makers – national and international Evaluation team External scrutiny panel Supervisory relationships and mentorship potential Power sharing is transparent and expectations made clear of participants roles and responsibilities	Macro layer: • Economic evaluation • Strategic visioning Meso layer: • Unit/team plans • Values clarification • Vision statements • Philosophy of care delivery Micro layer: • Narratives • Audit • Survey data • Creative artefacts	• Participant observation • Questionnaires/surveys/interviews • Documentation review • Observing: clients/customers • Observing: staff/employees • Conducting focus groups • Action learning sets • Critical reflexion cycles • Project group meetings • External review/scrutiny • Panels • Baseline data • Time series repeat measures • Audit data (existing measures) • Comparison analysis • Narrative analysis/storytelling • Creative data gathering (artefacts, blogs, video, arts, etc.) • Resources required to achieve evaluation • Costing/funding the evaluation	Action-orientated activity cycles Critical reflexion Broad stakeholder inclusion Exposing strengths and weaknesses of product/service Co-construction with stakeholders of priority actions Exploring convergence and/or divergence of perspectives Greater clarification of processes to achieve goals	Greater understanding and clarification of impact of product(s), programmes, services, or specific interventions on stakeholders Report writing – representation is achieved Educational materials arising from new knowledge/understanding Planning how best to disseminate findings to stakeholder groups Variety of outcome measures identified suitable to original purpose and audiences/stakeholders

CONCLUSION

Within this chapter, we have shown how our understanding and use of evaluation within practice development has become increasingly sophisticated in line with the necessity to capture the complexity, implications and outcomes of practice in its multi-faceted forms. We have outlined how evaluation is a central component of global health care, at a time when attention is focused towards measuring value for money, product purpose and sustainable safe and effective health care delivery.

Further work is needed to amalgamate international data sets based on those emerging in practice development projects (being delivered locally, nationally and internationally), so as to create a data pool that provides substantial evidence of the impact and outcomes of practice development. There is increasing evidence of how practice development is able to penetrate and positively influence workplace cultures. A transformational practice development approach provides both how to apply and enable practice led innovation concurrent with producing evidence to further inform successful and sustainable transformational change. We reiterate that evaluation can provide a critical creative method for the ongoing generation of new knowledge that can contribute to the evidence base for improved health care experience that in turn promotes human flourishing for all participants, from all angles, perspectives and in any practice context.

What is becoming increasingly significant is the utility of outcomes in clarifying how practice development influences sustainable change. Manley et al. (2011) identifies the importance of demonstrating outcomes and impact when demonstrating evidence of the effectiveness of practice development approaches. Within the current context, there is a significant risk that enforced measures and means of evaluating clinical practice will result in ignoring the 'hidden treasures' of practice expertise (Manley et al., 2005) that contributes to new insights and critically informed actions, as a process of PRAXIS innovation. Further discussion of the outcomes of practice development is provided in Chapter 10.

REFERENCES

Bateman, W.L. (1824–1903) Famous inspirational quotes. http://www.quoteworld.org/quotes/1051 (Accessed 24 April 2012).

Black, A.D., Car, J., Pagliari, C., Anandan, C. & Cresswell, K., et al. (2011) The impact of eHealth on the quality and safety of health care: a systematic overview. *PLoS Medicine*, **8** (1), e1000387.

Benatar, S. & Brock, G. (2011) *Global Health and Global Health Ethics*. Cambridge University Press, Cambridge.

Bryce, A., Butler, C., Gnich, W., Sheehy, C. & Tappin, D.M. (2009) CATCH: development of a home-based midwifery intervention to support young pregnant smokers to quit. *Midwifery*, **25**, 473–482.

Carr, S., Lhussier, M., Wilcockson, J., Robson, L., Warwick, J., Ransom, P. & Quinn, I. (2008) Roles, relationships, perils and values: development of a pathway between practice development and evaluation research. *Quality in Primary Care*, **16** (1), 157–164.

Central Nursing Advisory Committee (CNAC). Research & Development (R&D) Subgroup (2012) *Understanding practice development in the context of R&D*. Paper produced by T. McCance, Northern Ireland.

Chenoweth, L. & Kilstoff, K. (1998). Facilitating positive changes in community dementia management through participatory action research. *International Journal of Nursing Practice*, **4**, 175–188.

Chin, H. & Hamer, S. (2006) Enabling practice development: evaluation of a pilot programme to effect integrated and organise approaches to practice development. *Practice Development in Health Care*, **5** (3), 126–144.

Coster, S., Redfern, S., Wilson-Barnet, J., Evans, A., Peccei, R. & Guest, D. (2006) Impact of the role of nurse, midwife and health visitor consultant. *Journal of Advanced Nursing*, **55** (3), 352–363.

Davidson, P., Digiacomo, M., Zecchin, R., Clarke, M., Paul, G., Lamb, K. & Daly, J. (2008) A cardiac rehabilitation program to improve psychosocial outcomes of women with heart disease. *Journal of Women's Health*, **17**, 123–134.

Dewar, D., Mackay, R., Smith, S., Pullin, S. & Toucher, R. (2009) Use of emotional touch points as a method of tapping into the experience of receiving compassionate care in a hospital setting. *Journal of Research in Nursing*, **15** (1), 29–41.

Gates, D., Gillespie, G., Smith, C., Rode, J., Kowalenko, T., Smith, B. & Arbor, A. (2011) Using action research to plan a violence prevention program for emergency departments. *Journal of Emergency Nursing*, **37**, 32–39.

Guba, E.G. & Lincoln, Y.S. (1989) *Fourth Generation Evaluation*. Sage Publications, Newbury Park, CA.

Hardy, S. & Park, A. (1997) Supervision and professional practice. In: *Stuart and Sundeen's Mental Health Nursing. Principles and Practice* (eds B. Thomas, S. Hardy & P. Cutting), Chapter 10. Mosby, Edingburgh.

Hardy, S.E., Titchen, A., Manley, K. & McCormack, B. (2009) *Revealing Practice Expertise through Practitioner Inquiry*. Blackwell Science, Oxford.

Hardy, S., Wilson, V., Brown, B. & Crisp, J. (2012) A "Praxis" evaluation framework: a tool for all seasons? *International Journal of Practice Development*, **1** (2), 2.

Hawes, S. (2009) 'Take the lead'. Strengthening the nursing/midwifery unit manager role across NSW. Report Phase One: August 2008. NSW Department of Health, Sydney.

Kemmis, S. & McTaggart (1998) *The Action Research Planner*, 3rd edn. Deakin University Press, Geelong.

Kirkpatrick, D.L. (1994) *Evaluating Training Programs*. Berrett-Koehler Publishers, Inc., San Francisco, CA.

Kushner, S. (2000) *Personalizing Evaluation*. Sage Publications, London.

Macfarlane, F., Greenhalgh, T., Humphrey, C., Hughes, J., Butler, C. & Pawson, R. (2011) A new workforce in the making? A case study of strategic human resource management in a whole-system change effort in healthcare. *Journal of Health Organization and Management*, **25** (1), 55–72.

Manley, K., Hardy, S., Titchen, A., Garbett, R. & McCormack, B. (2005) Changing patients' worlds through nursing practice expertise. Exploring nursing practice expertise through emancipatory action research and fourth generation evaluation. A Royal College of Nursing Research Report 1998–2004. RCN, London.

Manley, K. & Titchen, A. (2012) Being and becoming a consultant nurse: towards greater effectiveness through a programme of support. RCN, London. http://www.rcn.org.uk/__data/assets/pdf_file/0005/444299/003574.pdf (Accessed 28 September 2012).

Manley, K., Crisp, J. & Moss, C. (2011) Advancing the practice development outcome agenda within multiple contexts. *International Practice development Journal*, **1** (1), 4–11.

McCormack, B., Henderson, E., Wilson, V. & Wright, J. (2009) Making practice visible: the workplace cultural critical analysis tool (WCCAT). *Practice Development in Health Care*, **8** (1), 28–43.

McGill, I. & Beaty, L. (2001) *Action Learning. A Guide for Professional Management and Educational Development*, 2nd edn. Kogan Page Ltd., London.

Owen, J.M. & Rogers, P.J. (1999) *Program Evaluation – Forms and Approaches*. Sage Publications, London.

Pawson, R. & Tilley, S. (1997) *Realistic Evaluation*. Sage Publications, London.

Porter, S. & O'Halloran, P. (2012) The use and limitations of Realistic Evaluation as a tool for evidence based practice: a critical realistic perspective. *Nursing Inquiry*, **19** (1), 18–28.

Pross, E.A. (2010) Promoting excellence in nursing education (PENE): Pross evaluation model. *Nurse Education Today*, **30** (6), 557–561.

Quinn-Patton, M. (1997) *Utilisation – Focused Evaluation*, 4th edn. Sage Publications, London.

Reason, P. & Bradbury, H. (2006) *Handbook of Action Research*. Sage Publications, London.

Reifsnider, E., Hargraves, M., Williams, K.J., Cooks, J. & Hall, V. (2010) Shaking and rattling developing a child obesity prevention program using a faith-based community approach. *Family and Community Health*, **33**, 144–151.

Research and Development (R&D) Office (1999) *Research for Health and Wellbeing*. R&D Office, Northern Ireland.

Reynolds, C.J. & Wyatt, J.C. (2011) Open source, open standards and health care information systems. *Journal of Medical Internet Research*, **13** (1), e24.

Roulin, M.J., Hurst, S. & Spirig, R. (2007) Diaries written for ICU patients. *Qualitative Health Research*, **17**, 893–901.

Simons, H. (1996) The paradox of case study. *Cambridge Journal of Education*, **26** (2), 225–240.

Slater, P. (2006) *The Development and Testing of the Nursing Context Index*. Unpublished PhD thesis, Ulster University.

Soh, K.L., Davidson, P.M., Leslie, G., DiGiacomo, M., Rolley, J., Soh, K.G. & Rahman, A.B. (2011) Factors to drive clinical practice improvement in a Malaysian intensive care unit: assessment of organisational readiness using a mixed method approach. *International Journal of Multiple Research Approaches*, **5** (1), 104–121.

Stake, R.E. (1994) Case studies. In: *Handbook of Qualitative Research* (eds N. Denzin & Y. Lincoln), CA Publications, Newbury Park, CA.

Stufflebeam, D.L., Madaus, G.F. & Kellaghan, T. (2000) *Evaluation Models: Viewpoints on Educational and Human Services Evaluation*. 2nd edn. Kluwer Academic Publishers, Boston, MA.

Titchen A. (2000) *Professional Craft Knowledge in Patient-Centred Nursing and the Facilitation of its Development*. PhD thesis. Ashdale Press, Oxford.

Tolson, D. (1998) Practice innovation: a methodological maze. *Journal of Advanced Nursing*, **30** (2), 381–390.

Warfield, C. & Manley, K. (1990) Developing a new philosophy in the NDU. *Nursing Standard*, **4** (41), 27–30.

Whitehead, D., Keast, J., Montgomery, V. & Hayman, S. (2004) A preventative health education programme for osteoporosis. *Journal of Advanced Nursing*, **47** (1), 15–24.

Wilson, V. (2005) Developing a vision for teamwork. *Practice Development in Healthcare*, **4** (1), 40–48.

Wilson, V.J., Ho, A. & Walsh, R. (2007) Participatory action research and action learning: changing clinical practice in nursing handover and communication. *Journal of Children's and Young People's Nursing*, **1** (2), 85–92.

Wilson, V., Hardy, S. & Brown, B. (2008) An exploration of practice development evaluation: unearthing praxis. In: *Practice Development in Nursing: International Perspectives* (eds K. Manley, B. McCormack, &V. Wilson). Blackwell Publishing Ltd., Oxford.

Wilson, V.J. (2011) Evaluation of a practice development programme: the emergence of the teamwork, learning and change model'. *International Practice Development Journal*, **1** (1), 1–15.

FURTHER READING

House, E.R & Howe K.R. (1999) *Values in Evaluation and Social Research*. Sage Publication, London.

Ovretveit, J. (1998) *Evaluating Health Interventions*. Open University Press, Buckingham.

Patton, M.Q. (2008) *Utilization-Focused Evaluation*, 4th edn. Sage Publications, Beverly Hills, CA.

Shufflebeau, D.L. & Shinkfield, A.J. (2007) *Evaluation Theory, Models and Applications*. Jossey-Bass, San Francisco, CA.

Stringer, E.T. (2007) *Action Research: A Handbook for Practitioners 3e*. Sage Publications, Newbury Park, CA.

Winter, R. (1989) *Learning From Experience. Principles and Practice in Action Research*. Falmer Press, Lewes.

Approaches to evaluation. Checklists and other international resources. http://gsociology.icaap.org/methods/approaches.html (Accessed 29 February 2012).

Collaborative Action Research Network (CARN). The CARN is committed to supporting and improving the quality of professional practice, through systematic, critical, creative inquiry into the goals, processes and contexts of professional work. http://www.esri.mmu.ac.uk/carnnew/ (Accessed 29 February 2012).

NMAHP Practice Development Centre (March, 2010) Guidance for evaluation of training, education and development programmes for Nurses, Midwives, AHPs and their support workers. http://www.lanpdc.scot.nhs.uk/PracticeandLearning/PoliciesGuidelines/Policies%20and%20Guidelines/Guidance%20for%20Development%20of%20Training,%20Education%20and%20Dev%20Programmes%20for%20NMAHPs.pdf (Accessed 25 September 2012).

New South Wales. Essentials of care programmes. http://www.health.nsw.gov.au/nursing/projects/eoc.asp (Accessed 29 February 2012).

10 Outcome Evaluation in the Development of Person-Centred Practice

Brendan McCormack[1],Tanya McCance[1,2] and Jill Maben[3]

[1]University of Ulster, Newtownabbey, UK
[2]Belfast Health and Social Caret Trust, Belfast, UK
[3]King's College London, London, UK

INTRODUCTION

This chapter explores the evaluation of outcomes arising from the development of person-centred practice and person-centred cultures. The focus of the chapter will be on articulating the different meanings and dimensions of person-centred practice and identifying what outcomes can be evaluated, as well as approaches to evaluating these outcomes. We show how the complexity of the term (person-centredness) and its multidimensionality makes it difficult to clearly articulate outcomes that can be evaluated. In addition, the different stakeholder agendas and perspectives, each of which comes with particular expectations of outcomes means that evaluation frameworks need to be able to 'hold' these different (and sometimes competing) agendas in healthy suspension.

In the context of the practice development journey introduced in Chapter 2, this chapter transcends each stage of the journey. Knowing that the ultimate purpose of practice development is the development of person-centred cultures, with an integral part of such a culture being the delivery of safe and effective person-centred care, gives a clear direction for outcome evaluation. However, it is essential that at the beginning of the journey, practice developers consider how progress towards achieving the ultimate purpose will be evaluated as well as the particular outcomes pertaining to the delivery of person-centred care. The evaluation of processes used to enable change as well as outcomes arising from particular developments is important considerations throughout the whole journey. This issue was introduced in Chapter 1 and illustrated in the *'the framework for holding on to the whole practice development journey'* (Chapter 1, Figure 1.3). In particular, 'ongoing and integrated action, evaluation, learning, planning and celebration' are interwoven components of the framework.

In this chapter, we provide an overview of person-centred practice and its key characteristics. We then identify the challenges associated with evaluating outcomes in practice development activities with a particular focus on person-centred outcomes. We explore the need for an evaluation framework that takes account both of the complexity of practice development itself and the concepts embedded in person-centred practice. An evaluation framework is proposed and examples of the framework in use are offered. The examples offered are drawn from the work of experienced practice developers, because if you are new to practice development and person-centred practice, then it is important that you connect

Practice Development in Nursing and Healthcare, Second Edition. Edited by Brendan McCormack, Kim Manley and Angie Titchen.
© 2013 John Wiley & Sons, Ltd. Published 2013 by John Wiley & Sons, Ltd.

with experienced practitioners who are familiar with practice development processes and evaluation methods. Finally, a case study that integrates the different components of the framework is provided in order to illustrate ways in which evaluation can be embedded in an organisational approach to practice development.

PERSON-CENTREDNESS AND PERSON-CENTRED PRACTICE: BEING CLEAR ABOUT THE DEVELOPMENT FOCUS

Person-centred practice has become a key focus of international policy and strategy in health care. Since the 1990s when health care reform became an international movement, the development of services that are respectful of persons has become a significant concern. Whilst to many commentators, the fact that the 'person' needs to be made so explicit represents a failure of health systems and an admission that professionals have lost their way in terms of knowing what matters to service users and in ensuring that patients and their families are held central. To others, it is no surprise that person-centredness has become such a prominent issue, given the shift in philosophy underpinning health care delivery – from one that was primarily focused on the hospital, acting as a place of safety, cure and healing, to the development of whole-system models of health care delivery with a dominant 'business and management' culture (Maben et al., 2010). Whilst the central ethos of care, treatment and cure has not disappeared, a significant shift has occurred in the way these values are needed to operate within a business philosophy, with profit, loss, efficiency and effectiveness becoming key interests.

The management agenda of achieving efficiency, increased throughput, increasing demands for evidence and information and customer orientation all within a focus on cost-effectiveness have brought nursing work into line objectively, rationally and authoritatively with outcomes that have been pre-determined to be desirable, indicative of success and which demonstrate quality of care (Rankin & Campbell, 2006). Rankin and Campbell argue that the new public management approach to managing health care, now evident in many countries, means that nurses are caught up in standardised organisational practices that sometimes disregard their own beliefs about good nursing care. The pressure to achieve standardised efficiencies competes with nurses getting to know the individual needs of patients. The dominant discourse of efficiency overwhelms nurses' abilities to draw upon knowledge of patients as whole people (Rankin & Campbell, 2006). Indicative of this managerial discourse is the consistent message given to nurses, which is that the objectified knowledge of patient surveys, audits and other measures of the top-down targets embedded in managerialism, supercede their own judgement and expert decision-making. As a result, Maben (2008) argues that many nurses, therefore, question their ability to give good care under the new systems. Others have argued that the irony of this approach is that the very objectified methods considered by managers to benefit service-user experience fail to do so and, in addition, increase cynicism and decrease commitment among staff (Kivimäki et al., 2000; Chadwick et al., 2004; Ronson, 2011)

In contemporary, health service systems, the concepts of equality, partnership, power, collegiality and holism are usually subsumed under the umbrella concept of 'person-focused services' with a particular emphasis on removing barriers to making choices about treatment options and people are encouraged to make choices about their own treatment with as much help as they need. There is increasingly more openness about service provision, continuous changes in public expectation and more access to effectiveness information. However, despite these developments, the number of reported incidents of insensitive, thoughtless and undignified care continues to increase (CQC, 2011; Patients Association, 2011; NHS Confederation, the Local Government Association and Age UK, 2012)

The current focus on 'patient experience' represents some attempt to redress that balance and ensure that it is given equal priority (DHSSPS, 2008). Increasingly, patients' experiences are of central importance to health care systems worldwide, where it is common to judge the quality of care not only by measures of clinical quality and safety such as mortality rates but also by gathering the views of patients receiving care. The rationale for doing so is that a better understanding of patient experience is believed to have a positive influence on health care by delivering services that patients, their families and carers need (Shaller, 2007; Goodrich & Cornwell, 2008). Evidence suggests that insights into patient experience can potentially improve patient's satisfaction with their care and clinical outcomes (Stevenson et al., 2004; Shaller, 2007). Furthermore, shared decision-making between patients and health providers may lead to improved patient knowledge, more realistic perceptions of the potential benefits and harms as well as a greater ability to reach decisions that reflect patient values and preferences (Stevenson et al., 2004; Goodrich & Cornwell, 2008).

From a professional perspective, there is a desire to reaffirm the importance of the fundamentals of care, emphasised by the Royal College of Nursing report, which highlights the challenges for nurses and midwives in providing sensitive and dignified care (RCN, 2008). There has been an increasing emphasis on improving the service user experience (DHSSPS, 2008), where the focus is explicitly on the promotion of 'person-centred standards' across the health and social care sector. However, the drive within the health service to demonstrate effectiveness and efficiency through performance management processes has never been greater. This has resulted in a range of quality and clinical indicators that pay little attention to how patients, clients and their families experience care (Davies & Nolan, 2006; DHSSPS, 2008). Whilst nurses have a significant contribution to make in determining the patient experience, a review of the evidence reveals a greater emphasis on areas of nursing and midwifery practice that can be quantified (e.g. pressure ulcer incidence, rates of health care associated infection and incidence of falls), and indeed that reflect on occurrence of negative incidences, with a dearth in indicators that measure the impact of nursing and midwifery care with a person-centred orientation (Griffiths et al., 2008).

Whilst the meaning of the term 'person-centredness' is open to debate and indeed there has been some 'kick-back' to the use of the term at all (e.g. Nolan et al., 2004), the values that underpin person-centred practice are synonymous with international movements that focus on humanising the health care experience. Principles such as autonomy, citizenship, dignity and respect (that also underpin principles of person-centred practice) are central to patient experience and ways of working that focus on meeting the needs of people.

Developing models of practice that enable person-centred principles to be realised across all services is a key issue in health care developments. Most notably is the influence of the 'Institute for Health care Improvement (IHI)' in the United States. The transformation of health and social care services is a focus of many western governments and many of the innovation frameworks and tools have emanated from the IHI. The focus of much of the work is on the development of person-centred practice mainly through the transformation of health care systems, structures and the redesign of clinical services. The terminology relating to person-centredness, whilst the subject of less intense debate, has also been discussed in the literature. Person-centred, patient-centred, client-centred and individualised cares are examples of terms often used interchangeably to express the idea of person-centredness

(Slater, 2006; Leplege et al., 2007). Several analyses have been conducted in an attempt to define the core attributes of person-centredness, although this activity is only a relatively recent development in the contemporary literature (McCormack, 2004; Slater, 2006; Leplege et al., 2007). The later definition of person-centredness adapted from McCormack et al. (2010) identifies the essential characteristics of person-centredness whilst also highlighting the importance of the development of culture to support person-centredness:

> *Person-centeredness is an approach to practice established through the formation and fostering of healthful[1] relationships between all care providers, older people and others significant to them in their lives. It is underpinned by values of respect for persons, individual right to self-determination, mutual respect and understanding. It is enabled by cultures of empowerment that foster continuous approaches to practice development.*

Drawing on this definition we suggest that five key principles need to be in place if a service is considered to be person-centred and so when thinking about an evaluation framework for practice development activities, it is important to be clear about these principles:

1. The meeting of needs through caring processes
2. The existence of nurturing relationships
3. The promotion of social belonging
4. The creation of meaningful spaces and places
5. The promotion of human flourishing

Caring processes

McCormack and McCance (2010), in the development of their framework, identify a range of activities that operationalise person-centredness within the nurse–patient relationship. These activities include working with patient's beliefs and values, engagement, having sympathetic presence, sharing decision-making and providing holistic care. Working with patients' beliefs and values reinforces one of the fundamental principles of person-centred practice, which places importance on developing a clear picture of what the patient values about his/her life and how he/she makes sense of what is happening from their individual perspective, psychosocial context and social role. This is closely linked to shared decision-making, which focuses on how patients and others significant to them are supported to be involved in decisions made about their care and treatment. Facilitating authentic involvement of patients in the decision-making process requires the health professional to engage in a process of negotiation that takes account of individual values, experiences, concerns and future aspirations. Engagement that supports this way of working reflects the connectedness of the practitioner with a patient and others significant to them, determined by knowledge of the person, clarity of beliefs and values, knowledge of self and professional expertise. This, in turn, is linked to having sympathetic presence, which highlights engagement that recognises the uniqueness and value of the individual by appropriately responding to cues that maximise

---

[1] We use the term 'healthful' here to describe the multifaceted nature of the kinds of relationships that patients/residents/families/communities have with care providers, including therapeutic, social, loving, functional, meaningful, superficial and nurturing relationships (for example). The word healthful also embraces a broad perspective of health that focuses on individual achievement in daily living, as captured by Seedhouse (2001).

coping resources through the recognition of what is important in their life. Finally, providing holistic care describes the provision of treatment and care that pays attention to the whole person through the integration of physiological, psychological, socio-cultural, developmental and spiritual dimensions. All the care processes described in this section are interlinked and complimentary, and whilst on the surface, they appear fundamental to any care experience, their effective delivery can be challenging, reflecting the interplay between the expertise of the health professional and the care environment (McCormack & McCance, 2010).

Nurturing relationships

Nolan and colleagues have introduced the concept of relationship-centred care, arguing for a move away from what they perceive as a focus on meeting individual needs, to focusing on interactions among all parties involved in care whose needs should be taken account of if good care is to result (Nolan et al., 2004). To suggest that person-centredness does not consider the importance of relationships represents a fundamental misunderstanding of the concept of 'person'. Being in relation emphasises the importance of relationships and the interpersonal processes that enable the development of relationships that have a healthful benefit. Whilst the importance of relationships in person-centred practice can never be disputed, 'relationship' is only one component of personhood. In person-centred practice, the relationship between care workers, service users and their families is paramount and it has been argued that sustaining a relationship that is nurturing requires valuing of self, moral integrity, reflective ability, knowing of self and others and flexibility derived from reflection on values and their place in the relationship (Nolan, 2001; Nolan et al., 2001; Dewing, 2002; McCormack, 2003; Packer, 2003; Titchen & McGinley, 2003; Dewar, 2011). Relationships are also reflected in one of seven attributes of person-centredness identified by Slater's (2006) concept analysis – evidence of a therapeutic relationship between person and health care provider. Slater (2006) describes this as a partnership between the person and carer that ensures the person's own decisions are valued, in a relationship that is based on mutual trust, is non-judgemental and does not focus on the balance of power.

Social belonging

The philosopher Merleau-Ponty (1989) considers persons to be interconnected with their social world, creating and recreating meaning through their being in the world. Irrespective of the care setting or the focus of care, staff and patients bring with them their own unique values and beliefs to the care situation. These values shape each of our 'being in the world', including the groups with which we belong, the communities we are part of, the social engagements we commit to and the decisions we make. Knowing what a patient values most about the way they live their life is hugely important to enabling a continued sense of social belonging. No matter how 'short-term' the health care experience is for a person, the experience has the potential to create a disconnect between the person and their sense of 'self'. How a person copes in terms of crisis, knowing their need for support, identifying the connections and relationships that are important to them are key considerations in maintaining social belonging. However, being attentive to these aspects of the patient experience is only possible if we are aware of how our own values influence our decisions and actions. As already highlighted, the need for shared values and a practice culture that facilitates discussion of values, particularly when they are in danger of being compromised/are compromised is a key consideration. Being supported in understanding how our values, decisions and actions are inter-related enables the potential for a more honest relationship between a practitioner, patient and families and goes some way towards creating a negotiated approach to care decision-making.

Meaningful spaces and places

Few studies have been undertaken to assess the impact of physical spaces on patients' experiences. Dementia care mapping has been well developed in dementia care (Kitwood & Bredin, 1992; Brooker, 2005), and it has a particular focus on the 'milieu of care' and how this impacts on the care experience. Paying attention to 'place' in care relationships is important. In the United States, a number of developments are promoted that focus on the environment of care in residential settings for older people. These include *The Eden Alternative* with a focus on the integration of inside and outside spaces and the creation of spontaneity in a home-like setting by infusing the nursing homes with plants, animals, and children (http://www.edenalt.org/). *The Culture Change Movement* emphasises the de-medicalisation of the care environment in nursing homes and the creation of 'ordinary home' type facilities (http://www.pioneernetwork.net/). Many of these ideas have influenced the development of person-centred services for older people in other countries. Other movements such as The Planetree Project (http://planetree.org/), the Kings Fund healing environment programme (Lowson et al., 2006) and the Hospice Friendly Hospitals Programme in the Republic of Ireland (http://www.hospicefriendlyhospitals.net/) have all emphasised the redesign of hospital services towards ones that promote healing and care at all stages of the life course.

Andrews (2003) argues that the concept of 'place' and its impact on care experiences is poorly understood in nursing. From the perspective of residential services for older people, it is increasingly acknowledged that 'place' has significant meaning. How older people are helped to create a sense of place in a nursing home, for example, is critical to their ability to transition from the loss of what may often have been their lifelong home to a new 'sense of home'. Creating meaningful places ensures that there is respect for the values that the person holds and that these values shape their interaction with the care environment and on the relationships that are formed. Within this context, systems of decision-making, staff relationships, organisational systems, power differentials and the potential of the organisation to tolerate innovative practices and risk taking are all important factors in the creation of places that are person-centred.

Human flourishing

In their development of 'critical creativity' as a methodology for transformational practice development, McCormack and Titchen (2006) identified human flourishing as a means and the end of transformative practice development. What is meant here is that the engagement with critical and creative approaches enables aspects of the human spirit to be energised, resulting in the release of potential for seeing new opportunities for growth and development that may not have been seen before. So the creative approaches release energy for self-exploration and the potential for transformation, and if these are embraced, then patients, families and staff can experience a sense of flourishing (Titchen et al., 2011). In this context, human flourishing is described by McCormack and Titchen as being a whole human being ourselves and promoting others being as whole human being. For human flourishing to exist in a care setting, care environments need to enable a variety of approaches to learning, particularly active learning (Dewing, 2008b), need systems and processes in place that enable staff to release energy for creative practice through creative thinking and problem-solving, and promote creative practices.

However, as we have highlighted earlier, the increase in managerial techniques and discourses do not help create flourishing human environments for staff or patients (Maben, 2008; Maben et al., 2010). Cost containment and rationalisation have a detrimental impact on nurses' ability to deliver care and practice in a person-centred way. The art of caring does not fit easily into a managerial discourse, where caring may be invisible, marginalised and subordinated (Maben, 2008). Rankin and Campbell (2006) examined the effects of the health care reforms in Canada on nurses abilities to care and concluded that 'Hospitals are being restructured to accomplish goals that are not traditionally those of nurses, and the standpoint of nurses in the activities of caring is being subordinated' (p. 165). There is now much evidence to suggest that what matters to staff in caring environments is being able to deliver high quality care, with a supportive manager, where staff are treated with respect, trusted and listened to and where a friendly working and caring environment is positively encouraged. Staff also need to feel valued by other staff. Maben (2008) argues that the work environment is key to human flourishing and to both good staff and patient experience and outcomes:

> *Many nursing scholars have identified optimal environments for nurses to work in and for patients to receive good care. These are not mutually exclusive – far from it, they are one and the same. To be able to care, a nurse or indeed any person needs to feel well supported and cared about – to feel valued and to have adequate resources to do the job well. So often in an acute health care environment this is compromised or does not exist (p. 337).*

Work in Magnet hospitals in the United States also suggests that staff flourish in areas where there is the opportunity to work with others who are clinically competent and where concern for the patient is paramount, where there are good nurse–physician relationships and communication, nurse autonomy and accountability, supportive nurse managers, control over nursing practice and the practice environment, support for education, and adequate nurse staffing (Mallidou et al., 2011). Where these factors are not present or not enough of them are present in practice environments there is growing evidence that nurses are prevented from practising how they would wish to – forcing them to make compromises in how they care for others.

So far, in this chapter, we have explored the concept of person-centredness and identified a range of issues that need to be considered when developing person-centred practice. However, being committed to developing person-centred practice is one thing, whilst identifying outcomes arising from these developments is yet another! So we now turn to the issue of outcome evaluation in person-centred practice and explore a range of considerations when considering the identification and evaluation of outcomes.

OUTCOME EVALUATION IN PERSON-CENTRED PRACTICE: THE STATE OF THE ART

Practice development has as its ultimate outcome, the development of person-centred practice cultures. The evaluation of outcomes arising from the development of person-centred cultures is still in the early stages of development. Descriptive accounts of person-centred practice leave little doubt that it does impact on patients/families experience of care services and practitioners' experiences of practice. However, there is a need to develop creative strategies for evaluating the complex processes that underpin person-centredness in practice as described earlier.

Determining outcomes arising from practice development, in general, is a significant challenge. As practice development methodologies have evolved and matured, tried and tested linear models of outcome evaluation do not capture the complexity of the processes involved and how these processes relate and interact in the achievement of person-centred outcomes. In addition, for many people engaged in practice development, it is often difficult to determine a 'beginning and end' to the work undertaken, and so, pre- and post-intervention outcome evaluation models are compromised. Further, many practice developers start their work with a commitment and passion for changing an aspect of practice, and it is only through the process of development that they discover they are engaged in significant changes that need to be evaluated in order to be retained and sustained. Not all practice developers have the necessary skills for undertaking evaluations that are outcome orientated.

In their review of the evidence underpinning practice development and particularly the outcomes arising from practice development activities, McCormack et al. (2006, p. 118) identified a range of outcomes identified in the literature and that can be grouped into five themes:

1. Improved collaborative and interpersonal relationships
2. More use of evidence in practice
3. Improved workplace culture
4. The development of learning cultures
5. The implementation of person-orientated caring practices

McCormack et al. highlighted a range of challenges associated with evaluating practice development outcomes, including the use of multiple change processes in bringing about small changes, a lack of connection between practice development processes and the predicted/anticipated outcomes, a lack of creativity in the development of evaluation frameworks, a lack of skill in designing evaluation frameworks, and a failure to recognise practice development as a complex intervention, and thus the need for evaluation frameworks to reflect this complexity. If we accept that practice development reflects a complex intervention, then we cannot rely on simplistic linear and input–output models of evaluation. Most emancipatory practice development activities involve, for example, a series of behavioural, attitudinal and/or contextual changes, and therefore, evaluation frameworks need to be able to 'hold' these different components, as well as be capable of linking the different and often small changes to the staged outcomes along the way. A linear model of evaluation is not appropriate in this context, but instead a series of different evaluations may be necessary in order to capture the complexity and determine the range of possible outcomes.

A recent review of aspects of nursing linked to patient outcome from the UK 'National Nursing Research Unit' (Griffiths et al., 2008) highlighted the complexity of measuring outcomes in patient care. The authors highlighted 'failure to rescue' and health care associated infection as nurse sensitive outcomes, but falls and pressure sores were less sensitive. They also highlight that positive contributions of nursing to outcomes such as well-being or recovery are less well addressed in nursing outcome frameworks. However, Griffiths et al. (2008) highlight those aspects of care that patients most value, including:

- a holistic approach to physical, mental and emotional needs, patient-centred and continuous care;
- efficiency and effectiveness combined with humanity and compassion;
- professional, high-quality evidence-based practice;
- safe, effective and prompt nursing interventions;
- patient empowerment, support and advocacy;
- seamless care through effective teamwork with other professions.

These aspects of patient care feature less strongly in nursing outcomes frameworks but yet are consistent with the principles and values underpinning person-centred practice. In an attempt to address this gap in the evaluation of nursing effectiveness, McCance et al. (2011) conducted a study using consensus methodology to identify key performance indicators (KPIs) relevant for nursing/midwifery practice in the current policy context. The findings from this study identified a different but complimentary set of indicators for nursing/midwifery, which include:

1. consistent delivery of nursing/midwifery care against identified need;
2. patient's confidence in the knowledge and skills of the nurse/midwife;
3. patient's sense of safety whilst under the care of the nurse/midwife;
4. patient involvement in decisions made about their nursing/midwifery care;
5. time spent by nurses and midwives with the patient;
6. respect from the nurse/midwife for patient's preference and choice;
7. nurse/midwife's support for patients to care for themselves, where appropriate;
8. nurse/midwife's understanding of what is important to the patient.

These indicators are strategically aligned to work on the patient experience and are reflective of the fundamentals of nursing and midwifery practice, with the focus on person-centred care. As a consequence, measurement of the KPIs requires an alternative approach that challenges traditional ideas regarding the nature of evidence.

Maben (2008) has argued that, while critically important, much of what matters to staff and patients in terms of person-centred care and practice is largely invisible to others and indeed to audit and measurement:

> *Part of the problem certainly lies in the difficulty of measuring many of the core caring skills, and it is important that these aspects of nurses' work should not become add-ons or marginalized because they are not readily counted (p. 336).*

As Einstein said 'everything that counts cannot necessarily be counted'. Whilst the work of Griffiths et al. (2008) and McCance et al. (2011) resonates with much of the desires of practice developers in terms of demonstrating outcomes such as increased efficiency and effectiveness set within a framework of humanity and compassion, capturing these complex relationships is challenging. Manley et al. (2011a) considered practice development outcomes in the context of global health reform agendas and argue that the outcomes agenda needs consensus around parameters of practice development interventions, process outcomes and the major health outcomes that drive practice development work. Practice development has as an explicit outcome, 'the development of evidence-informed and person-centred workplaces' (ref) and as such outcome evaluation needs to reflect both these agendas.

The literature on the translation of research evidence into practice, knowledge utilisation and knowledge translation is growing, and the science of knowledge translation is becoming increasingly sophisticated. Numerous publications since the 1990s have demonstrated that determining the existence of an evidence-informed practice culture is predicated by a number of factors including staffing levels and years of experience, availability of information and data, the ability to interpret information and data, the nature of the organisational support infrastructure, team relationships, leadership practices and team effectiveness . . . to name but a few (Kitson et al., 2008). In the field of knowledge translation, there continues to be a dominance of the use of experimental or quasi-experimental approaches to evaluation, with some evidence of the use of mixed-methods beginning to emerge. The increased recognition in the field of knowledge translation has led to increased demand for evaluation methodologies that can take account of contextual factors, for example, in outcome measurement that would previously be reported as the 'black box' of knowledge translation, that is the unknown factor. Taking account of context in evaluation creates opportunities for the development of methodologies that are theory informed and reflective of the realities of practice.

However, whilst practice development as a methodology has contributed to the broadening of the knowledge translation agenda and greater recognition of the importance of context, a key challenge as it further grows and develops is that of retaining its primary focus of working with clinical teams to bring about sustained changes in the workplace in order to make them more evidence-informed and person-centred. A key distinguishing feature between practice development and other methodologies is that it is led by practitioners and practice teams with a commitment to working for person-centred care and better patient outcomes (Manley et al., 2011a). Thus, creating a balance is important between the development of evaluation frameworks that are integral to the work of practitioners, are owned by them and are context specific with the dominance of organisational desires to achieve outcomes in major health care agendas. This is not to suggest that these are mutually exclusive agendas, but the challenges of balancing power relationships, ownership of data, staff and service user empowerment, with macro health care agendas, are not to be underestimated. Manley et al. (2011a) suggest that there is a need for practice developers to balance the need for different forms of data by different key stakeholders with the need to be strategic in a health-outcomes orientated challenging global health care environment.

Evaluation has often focused on the development of instruments that evaluate the existence of person-centredness or not, and/or the evaluation of key parts of person-centredness (Slater & McCormack, 2007; McCance et al., 2008; Edvardsson & Innes, 2010). Whilst these studies are important in terms of the development of instruments that may have broad applicability in practice, they are limited in their capacity to unearth the complex interpersonal relationships and contextual factors that enable or hinder effective person-centred practices.

As discussed earlier, evidence from research such as magnet hospitals and models of nursing practice shows that changing an organisation's culture has an impact on the issues concerning nurses' working life. The bulk of this evidence draws a causal link between organisational culture change and working environment factors such as retention of staff, job satisfaction and job stress. A number of authors have identified the need for a unified approach to workforce planning that takes account of organisational culture issues that impact on nursing job satisfaction, stress, commitment and nurse retention (e.g. Newman et al., 2001; Spence-Laschinger, 2009; Sheingold et al., 2012). The Institute of Medicine in the United States reiterated the importance of organisational culture as an aspect of improving nurses working environment and proposed guidelines for hospitals based on research conducted into 'magnet hospitals' where it identified a number of traits such as professional autonomy and practice control as key in keeping nurses working. The report authors concluded that:

> Quality problems (nurse retention and patient satisfaction levels) occur typically not because of a failure of goodwill, knowledge, effort, or resources devoted to health care, but because of fundamental shortcomings in the way care is organised (2001: 25).

Person-centred practice involves the reorganisation of the context of care to promote continuity of care amongst other things. The context of care offers the greatest source of facilitation (or hindrance) to the development of a person-centred ethos in the nurse's workplace (Manley et al., 2011b).

Whilst the values and principles of person-centred practice are increasingly espoused in policy and strategy, its evaluation and particularly outcome evaluation is poorly developed. Debates persist about the meaning of underpinning concepts, the appropriateness of models and their implementation, whilst at the same time, approaches to outcome evaluation receive less attention. Some of this lack of attention is due to the limitations of existing methodologies to capture the complexity of person-centred practice in its entirety and thus it is easier to evaluate sub-elements.

A framework for outcome evaluation: paying attention to processes and outcomes

Drawing upon the person-centred theoretical framework of McCormack and McCance (2010), we suggest that there are four outcomes that could be achieved from the development of a person-centred culture. NB: These outcomes apply to staff, patients, residents, families:

1. Satisfaction with care
2. Involvement with care
3. Feeling of well-being
4. Creating a therapeutic culture

From the perspective of evaluating person-centredness, we specifically focus on 'experience of good care' as the particular aspect of satisfaction that we are concerned with. Patient experience is a critical part of the evaluation of effectiveness in health care internationally and it is commonplace for 'patient experience' to be an explicit part of management roles and audit/evaluation methods. However, we argue that the experience of good care is not an exclusive measure applied to patients only. For staff the experience of delivering good care and the positive feedback that can follow is a key factor in creating a culture that is motivational and respectful of staff and promotes human flourishing. These are important considerations in the literature that focuses on effective environments of care, staff satisfaction, staff retention and positive workplace cultures (Manley et al., 2011b).

Story 10.1: What can a practice developer do to evaluate if service users are more satisfied with care?

Felicity is an experienced manager of a vascular surgical ward. She adopts a transformational leadership approach and incorporates principles of emancipatory practice development into her work. In September 2010, Felicity reviewed all the complaint letters that had been received about her service, and whilst there were not many, she identified a dominant theme of inconsistent patient-care decisions – in particular she identified that complainants reported, for example, poor management of pain with different nurses giving patients and families different reasons why analgesia could or could not be administered, with the result that pain was poorly managed. Felicity instigated a local evaluation of their team effectiveness using observations of practice (ward rounds, case reviews, handovers and patient/family consultations) and a review of care plans (particularly focusing on who completed care plans, how they were reviewed and the evidence upon which changes to plans of care were made – in this, she was particularly interested to see how the 'patient's voice' was captured). As a result of the observation work, Felicity identified an inconsistent approach to decision-making, thus adding strength to her theming of the complaints. This was also reflected in the care plans and their review; that is, different inputs from different nurses and changes to plans made without explicit rationale/evidence for these changes. She also identified a complete absence of the patient's voice in care reviews.

Felicity established a practice development project that focused on achieving more consistency in care planning and delivery. She set up a multi-disciplinary group and a comprehensive action plan based on the evidence from the complaints and her evaluation. Over 8 months, the team changed a number of their team processes to achieve greater consistency. They undertook peer-reflection to learn how to make the rationale for care decisions more explicit and supported each other in doing that. A template for capturing the patient and family voice in care review meetings and in care plan reviews was also introduced.

Whilst Donna and the multi-disciplinary team undertook process evaluations of each change (reflective notes, meeting notes, ad hoc observations and discussions for example), follow-up evaluation in September 2011 using patient/family stories of their care experiences, observations of practice and discussions with staff showed that the majority of people were satisfied with how the system worked, that most patients and families had a good care experience and that their respective voices were 'heard' in the new system. There were still a few 'gremlins' in the system and the ongoing action plan and multi-disciplinary group continued to work on these.

Feeling involved is a key part of contemporary health care strategy and policy and there is an explicit expectation that patients will be active participants in their own care. Examples such as 'the expert patient initiative' are predicated on this assumption and that they work in partnership with health care professionals. Models of care that are focused on working in partnership with patients and families have the explicit aim of trying to enhance the experience of being involved in care. Evaluating the extent to which people feel involved is also a key focus of person-centred outcome evaluation. In addition from a staff perspective, being involved and 'engaged' is a key focus of many models of care that aim to ensure that care decisions are made by nurses working directly with patients and is a key indicator in developments such as the Magnet Hospitals. Robinson et al. (2004) suggest an engaged employee experiences a blend of job satisfaction, organisational commitment, job involvement and feelings of empowerment. It is a concept that is greater than the sum of its parts. Employee engagement is a much contested concept, but there is a good body of evidence to suggest that if employees are engaged and committed it will increase productivity and performance and engagement with users (see, e.g., Macleod & Clarke, 2011). Focusing on increasing individuals' perceptions of their involvement with and their value to the organisation will increase engagement levels, contributing to increased retention and performance. Increasing the levels at which staff feel valued can be achieved through:

- managers listening to employees;
- employees having the opportunity to develop their jobs;
- good suggestions being acted upon;
- employees feeling able to voice their opinions;
- senior managers showing employees that they value them;
- employers showing concern about employees' health and well-being;
- employees being involved in decision-making.

(Robinson et al., 2004)

Story 10.2: What can a practice developer do to evaluate if team members feel involved in care?

Jean is the manager of a nursing home. She has had feedback from some of the registered nurses that the care assistants do not do what they are asked to do and that some residents have complained about their attitude. The registered nurses feel that they have no authority over the care assistants and they just seem to 'do their own thing'.

Jean was aware that there seemed to be poor relationships between the care assistants and registered nurses from how she observed them interacting. The most recent quality monitoring visit from the inspection and regulation authority had suggested that registered nurses were weak in their leadership of care and so Jean was beginning to see that there was an issue that needed to be addressed.

Jean convened a meeting with the care assistants that she framed using a Claims, Concerns and Issues (CCI) exercise[2]. The key issue emerging from this was that the care assistants did not feel involved in care decisions. In exploring this issue, they identified their non-participation in handovers, lack of continuous assignment to residents,

---

[2] Claims, Concerns and Issues (CCIs) is derived from 4th Generation Evaluation (Guba & Lincoln, 1989) and its purpose is to enable a democratic approach to the 'voices' that are heard in the evaluation of a programme/team etc. Fourth generation evaluation, a constructivist approach, makes repeated use of CCIs when working with stakeholder groups. *Claims* are favourable assertions about the topic and its implementation. *Concerns* are any unfavourable assertions about the topic and its implementation. *Issues* are questions that reflect what any 'reasonable person' might ask about the topic and its implementation, and usually emerge from claims and concerns.

a feeling of not being appreciated by the registered nurses and a lack of interest among the registered nurses of the care assistants' knowledge about particular residents. Jean instigated observations of practice by training a volunteer registered nurse and care assistant in the method and together they observed practice over three different shifts. The observations of practice highlighted how the issues raised in the CCI exercise with the care assistants manifested themselves in practice. The registered nurse also could see this and realised that there was a problem with their ways of working. Together they fed-back their observations to the whole team and there was a sense of relief among the team that the issues had been 'exposed'.

The team worked together to develop an action plan that included team-building work, involvement of care assistants in handovers, consistent assignment with residents, participation in care planning and role clarification activities. In addition, the registered nurses were provided with leadership development. Each development was evaluated using simple audit techniques as it progressed and the action plan was altered accordingly. Follow-up CCI sessions with all staff demonstrated that a very different team had emerged. The sense of involvement in care by the care assistants was particularly noticeable and feedback from residents and families also was really positive. Jean coordinated writing the work up as evidence for the next inspection visit and as evidence of their commitment to continuous improvement.

Having a feeling of well-being underpins the aims of many caring theories, rehabilitation models and care practices. McCance (2003), for example, clearly articulated how positive care experiences engendered feelings of well-being among patients and is indicative of the patient being valued. Studies of well-being have focused on 'subjective well-being' (e.g., Davern et al., 2007) – a theory derived from positive psychology that focuses on how people make cognitive and affective evaluations of their lives. It aims to understand how people set goals in their lives, adapt throughout their lives and the influence of culture on well-being. It is argued that an individual's happiness is predicated on their sense of well-being derived from these evaluations of their lives. Practice cultures have a significant impact on patient well-being, and whilst patient outcome studies tend to focus on well-being in the context of alleviation of symptoms and effective management of ill-health, assessment of subjective well-being has also an important role to play in the evaluation of care effectiveness. As shown earlier, the culture of a care setting is increasingly understood as a key determinant in how patients experience care and ultimately their sense of well-being. Positive feelings of safety, security and being valued as a person are critical components of an effective care environment and again ultimately on patients' sense of well-being.

Similarly, nurses need to feel valued for their work and well-being at work is also considered a key aspect of outcome evaluation in person-centred nursing (Maben et al., 2012). A review of the health and well-being of staff in the NHS (Boorman, 2009a) identified that over 80% of staff surveyed felt that their health and well-being impacts upon patient care, and virtually none disagreed. The review found that NHS organisations that prioritise staff health and well-being perform better; they have improved patient satisfaction (up to 10% better), stronger quality scores and better outcomes for patients (half Methicillin-resistant *Staphylococcus aureus* rates), as well as higher levels of staff retention and lower rates of sickness absence. The review encouraged a long held belief that there is a 'clear link between staff health and well-being and standards of care'. Brown and McCormack (2011) highlighted the importance of workplaces being 'psychologically safe' in order for safe and effective evidence-informed practice to happen and, in particular, for effective collaborative teamwork to happen. This finding has been confirmed by other literature that suggests that certain management practices can contribute to stress and mental health problems among staff, including reported high levels of bullying and harassment, a deep-seated culture of long working hours and a lack of managerial interest in, and support for, staff concerns about their health and well-being (Firth Cozens, 1990; Edwards & Burnard, 2003; Cox et al., 2009). Attention to job design or organisation in many health care organisations requires more attention be paid to developing jobs into 'good jobs' with meaningful work that help staff to feel valued (Boorman, 2009a: 12).

Story 10.3: What can a practice developer do to evaluate patient and staff well-being?

Margaret has been working as a practice development facilitator in the orthopaedic out-patients department of the hospital. The department has been involved in the 'releasing time to care' project that the hospital is taking part in, and it has made significant improvements towards the aim of nursing staff spending more time with patients rather than on administrative work. Margaret integrated the methods promoted in the releasing time to care framework with emancipatory practice development facilitation processes. Overall, she identified that this resulted in a greater potential to sustain the changes made as the team felt real ownership for the changes. Whilst staff were pleased with the progress they had made with changing practices and ways of working, they felt like they were 'pawns' at the hands of management and were mistrusting of the overall agenda for the changes and the continuous non-replacement of staff. It was clear that the staff experienced high levels of job demands and stress in the department and this did not seem to get any less. Margaret was also conscious that some of the evaluation work she had undertaken with patients attending the department revealed that they often felt that they spent a lot of time 'hanging around' the department waiting to be seen by the relevant clinician, even though significant changes had been made to waiting times. Therefore, in addition to the use of an emancipatory approach, Margaret created 'communicative spaces' where staff spent time together regularly expressing emotions and feelings about their work and how this impacted on their sense of well-being. Margaret facilitated open, honest and partici-pative discussion and together the team reached consensus on how to move forward. The team engaged the Psychologist in the hospital and connected with the Point of Care pro-gramme at the King's Fund to establish and facilitate 'Schwartz rounds'[3] which offered staff opportunities for compassionate dialogue about their experiences of delivering care-its challenges, frustrations and rewards and time for the multi-disciplinary team to dis-cuss the thoughts and feelings these experiences evoke for them. The team also continued

---

[3] Schwartz rounds have been brought to the UK by the King's Fund Point of Care programme from Boston Massachusetts where they originated. The rounds take place in 195 sites in the USA and currently 7 in the UK with expansion planned. The rounds (usually 1 hour each month) provide space for 'renewal' by practition-ers and recognition, re-inforcement and support from colleagues and managers. http://www.kingsfund.org.uk/current_projects/point_of_care/schwartz_center_rounds/index.html

with the communicative spaces over the following year as well as seeking continuous feedback from patients. The team contracted with a researcher from the local university to have two training sessions in how to analyse narratives. Together they adopted a narrative analysis approach to analyse the discussions and feedback and were able to demonstrate a significant shift in how team members talked about their work and how patients felt about their time in the department. Together they concluded that the well-being of team members and patients had improved. They communicated their experience and findings to the Head of Research and Development in the organisation and the team developed a proposal to undertake an outcomes focused evaluation of the approaches implemented.

Creating a Therapeutic Culture has been discussed earlier as a key factor in the delivery of person-centred nursing and the extent to which the environment supports and maintains person-centred principles has been shown to be critical to person-centred practice. To recap, the essence of a therapeutic culture is one where staff are supported and enabled to deliver therapeutic care and which consequently enhances retention and job satisfaction. It is known that the majority of health care staff are (at least initially) motivated by ideals of altruism and making a difference to people's lives (Becker & Geer, 1958; Maben et al., 2007), but these ideals can be eroded over time by less than therapeutic working environments (Maben et al., 2006, 2007). In Maben et al.'s study, nurses at the end of their pre-qualifying education were very clear that they wanted to give high quality, patient-centred, holistic and evidence-based care with care being 'centred around needs of the patient'. However, over 20 of these nurses went onto describe the ways in which their ideals and values of person-centred practice were undermined, undervalued and did not count in ways that other more task-orientated aspects of their work did. The organisational constraints identified included increased turnover and throughput of patients – the intensification and routinisation of nursing work (Maben et al., 2006) – and also incorporated work overload and time pressures as a result of staff shortages or poor skill mix. This, in turn, created routinised and task-orientated care giving, which was seen to militate against a whole person approach to caring. The majority experienced frustration and some level of 'burn out' as a consequence of their ideals and values being thwarted.

Thus, a therapeutic culture is crucial to helping staff to maintain their ideals of care. McCormack and McCance (2010) identified the attributes of a therapeutic culture as being one that:

- empowers practitioners;
- promotes autonomy;
- fosters a sense of accountability;
- enables reflection in and on practice;
- has systems and processes in place for evidence use;
- provides patient-centred care, which includes:
  - working with Patient's Beliefs and Values;
  - providing for physical needs;
  - sharing decision-making;
  - having sympathetic presence;
  - engagement.

> **Story 10.4: What can a practice developer do to evaluate the extent to which a therapeutic culture exists in a care setting?**
>
> Barbara is a practice development coordinator for the 'person-centred care programme' in a large acute care facility. The facility has 25 inpatient units, a large outpatients department and a variety of tertiary services as well as a regional critical care service. Barbara's role involves working with clinical teams to continuously improve the effectiveness of care delivery and patient experiences of care. In order to do this work, Barbara has developed a programme incorporating a package of tools and processes that she uses collaboratively with clinical teams to help them evaluate how person-centred their culture is and to inform ongoing practice developments. The evaluation programme is implemented on an 18-month cycle with each ward and department. Staff in each clinical unit have been trained in the use of each of the tools and processes and so the evaluation process and outcomes are owned by the staff teams and so their commitment to the programme is high. Each year, Barbara does an overarching analysis of the findings from the individual unit evaluations, the action plans developed and progress with developing person-centred cultures. She maps the data against the person-centred practice framework of McCormack and McCance (2010), which is the theoretical framework underpinning the programme of work in the Trust. She uses these findings to report to the Trust Board about developments in person-centred care and to make the case for particular resources to support the programme. In addition, the results are used to inform the commissioning of education programmes from the local Higher Education Institutions as well as the in-house facilitated work-based learning programme. The learning from the programme is being used by other organisations as a model of good practice and has gained support from the Regional Board to be disseminated to other facilities.

PUTTING IT ALL TOGETHER: DEMONSTRATING THE ACHIEVEMENT OF THE ULTIMATE PURPOSE

So far in this chapter we have explored the challenges associated with evaluating outcomes in practice development work and in particular those associated with evaluating the outcomes associated with person-centred practice. We have argued that more traditional linear/input–output models of evaluation are inappropriate for evaluating person-centred practice developments due to the complexity of the work involved. We have suggested that four outcome themes can be used to evaluate the development of person-centred practice in health care organisations:

1. Satisfaction with care
2. Involvement with care
3. Feeling of well-being
4. Creating a therapeutic culture

However, we have treated these as separate areas of evaluation when clearly they connect and overlap with each other. So, in this section of the chapter, we present a case study that integrates the whole framework and shows how an evaluation framework can be used to demonstrate progress towards achieving the ultimate purpose of practice development, that is the creation of a person-centred culture. We hope that by considering this case study, it will identify ways in which you could establish your own evaluation framework for evaluating progress with your person-centred practice development activity. However, it is important to remember that achieving a person-centred culture is never an end-point as it is always a work in progress! So the evaluation framework you develop needs to take account of the need for ongoing evaluation and commitment to it as a process rather than an outcome. The following case study illustrates how one organisation has developed and implemented a comprehensive evaluation framework dealing with all aspects of person-centred practice.

Story 10.5: Developing an evaluation framework to assess progress within person-centred practice development programme

The Belfast Trust is one of five health and social care providers within Northern Ireland, which employs approximately 20 000 staff, of which almost 6800 are nurses and midwives. The organisation provides services for 340 000 people in Belfast and regional services for the population of Northern Ireland, with services organised through directorates that span acute and community sectors. The delivery of person-centred care was one of the priorities identified within the Trust's Nursing and Midwifery Strategy, and in response to this, the Research and Practice Development Team set out to develop and implement a practice development programme that would be delivered across the specialities and within different settings. A pilot programme was initiated involving 10 sites, the overarching aim of which was to enable nursing teams to explore the concept of person-centredness within their own clinical setting, in order to improve care delivery. The programme was underpinned by the Person-centred Nursing Framework (McCormack and McCance, 2010) and integral to it were the four outcome themes already discussed in this chapter. A range of evaluation methods were repeatedly used to establish impact, which not only included claims, concerns and issues undertaken globally at Project Team meetings but also used with individual participating sites, qualitative interviews using focus groups with programme participants and facilitators, and patient stories from service users cared for in each of the participating sites. There were also process evaluation methods (e.g. participant feedback on workshops and reflective accounts) in place to generate data and increase understanding of approaches to engagement and the learning journey experienced by programme participants. Figure 10.1 maps the measures used within the programme evaluation to the four outcomes expected from person-centred practice and illustrates a comprehensive approach to evaluation of practice development activities (McCance et al., 2011).

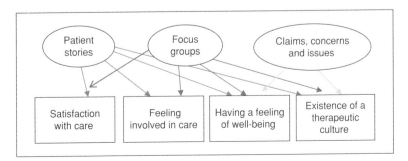

Fig. 10.1   Outcome measures linked to expected person-centred outcomes.

CONCLUSIONS

In this chapter, we have explored how we can evaluate outcomes arising from the development of person-centred practices. Whilst emancipatory and transformational practice development methodologies have as their focus, the development of person-centred cultures, evaluating outcomes from this work continues to be a challenge. We have identified many of these challenges, and we argue that to evaluate person-centred outcomes there is a need to be guided by a theoretical framework. In that way, particular and specific outcomes can be identified and systematically evaluated. This we would argue is a more effective approach to evaluation than trying to evaluate person-centredness as a global measure of quality. The evaluation of person-centred outcomes requires the use of multiple methods of data collection and analysis and so whilst there are various evaluation instruments available, these do not provide a comprehensive evaluation of person-centredness. Therefore, as practice developers, we need to be cognisant of the focus of our activities and have an 'open-mind' to the most appropriate evaluation methods.

When thinking about evaluating the development of person-centred practices in your organisation, you might like to consider questions such as these:

1. What is the specific purpose of the practice development activity?
2. What theoretical perspective is driving our person-centred practice developments?
3. What are the key components of that theory?
4. What activities are we engaging in that implement particular components of the theory into practice?
5. What information are we collecting as part of our development work that could 'double up' as evaluation data?
6. What help do we need with evaluating the processes and outcomes from our work?

REFERENCES

Andrews, G. (2003) Locating a geography of nursing: space, place and the progress of geographical thought, *Nursing Philosophy*, **4** (3), 231–248.

Becker, H.S. & Geer B. (1958) The fate of idealism in medical school. *Journal of Health and Social Behavior*, **23**(1), 50–56.

Boorman, S. (2009a) NHS Health and Wellbeing Review. Department of Health.

Brooker, D. (2005) Dementia care mapping: a review of the Research Literature. *Gerontologist*, **1** (1), 11–18.

Brown, D. & McCormack, B. (2011) Developing the practice context to enable more effective pain management with older people: an action research approach. *Implementation Science*, **6** (9), 1–14.

Care Quality Commission (CQC) (2011) *Dignity and Nutrition Inspection Programme: National Overview*. Newcastle upon Tyne, England.

Chadwick, C., Hunter, L. & Walston, S. (2004) Effects of downsizing practices on the performance of hospitals. *Strategic Management Journal*, **25**, 405–27.

Cox, T., Karanika-Murray, M., Griffiths, A., Wong, Y. & Hardy, C. (2009) *Developing the Management Standards Approach within the Context of Common Health Problems in the Workplace: A Delphi Study*. Health and Safety Executive, Research Report RR687, Her Majesty's Stationery Office, Norwich. http://www.hse.gov.uk/research/rrpdf/rr687.pdf (Accessed 10 April 2012).

Davern, M.T., Cummins, R.A. & Stokes, M.A. (2007) Subjective wellbeing as an affective-cognitive construct. *Journal of Happiness Studies*, **8**, 429–449.

Davies, S. & Nolan, M. (2006) 'Making it better': self-perceived roles of family caregivers of older people living in care homes: a qualitative study. *International Journal of Nursing Studies*, **43** (3), 281–291.

Department of Health and Social service and Public Safety (DHSSPS) (2008) *Improving the Patient and Client Experience*. DHSSPS, Belfast.

Dewar, B. (2011) *Caring about Caring: An Appreciative Inquiry about Compassionate Relationship-Centred Care*. Unpublished Doctoral Thesis, Napier University, Edinburgh.

Dewing, J. (2002) From ritual to relationship: a person-centred approach to consent in qualitative research with older people who have a dementia, *Dementia*, **1** (2), 157–171.

Dewing, J. (2008b) Becoming and being active learners and creating active learning workplaces: the value of active learning. Chapter 15. In: *International Practice Development in Nursing and Healthcare* (eds K. Manley, B. McCormack & V. Wilson), pp. 273–294. Blackwells, Oxford.

Edvardsson, D. & Innes, A. (2010) Measuring person-centered care: a critical comparative review of published tools, *The Gerontologist*, **50** (6), 834–846.

Edwards, D. & Burnard, P.A. (2003) A systematic review of stress and stress management interventions for mental health nurses. *Journal of Advanced Nursing*, **42** (2), 169–200.

Firth-Cozens, J. (1990) Sources of stress in women junior house officers. *British Medical Journal*, **301**, 89–91.

Goodrich, J. & Cornwell, J. Seeing the Person in the Patient Review Paper: The Kings Fund 2008.

Griffiths, P. Jones, S. Maben, J. & Murrells, T. (2008) *State of the Art Metrics for Nursing: A Rapid Appraisal*. King's College, London.

Guba, E.G. & Lincoln, Y.S. (1989) *Fourth Generation Evaluation*. Thousand Oaks, CA, Sage.

Kitson, A.L., Rycroft-Malone, J., Harvey, G., McCormack, B., Seers, K. & Titchen, A. (2008) Evaluating the successful implementation of evidence into practice using the PARIHS framework: theoretical and practical challenges. *Implementation Science*, **3**, 1. http://www.implementationscience.com/content/3/1/1 (Accessed 10 October 2012).

Kitwood, T. & Bredin, K. (1992) A new approach to the evaluation of dementia care. *Journal of Advances in Health and Nursing Care*, **1** (5), 41–60.

Kivimäki, M., Vahtera, J., Pentti, J. & Ferrie, J. (2000) Factors underlying the effect of organisational downsizing on health of employees: longitudinal cohort study. *British Medical Journal*, **320**, 971.

Leplege, A., Gzil, F., Cammelli, M., Lefeve, C., Pachoud, B. & Ville, I. (2007). Person-centredness: Concepetual and historical perspectives. *Disability and Rehabilitation*, **29** (20–21), 1555–1565.

Lowson, K., Beale, S., Kelly, J. & Hadfield, M. (2006) *Evaluation of Enhancing the Healing Environment Programme*, Final Report for the Department of Health (NHS Estates), York Health Economics Consortium, University of York, York, England.

Maben, J. (2008) The art of caring: invisible and subordinated? a response to Juliet Corbin: 'is caring a lost art in nursing?' *International Journal of Nursing Studies*, **45**, 335–338.

Maben, J., Peccei, R., Adams, M., Robert, G., Richardson, A. & Murrells, T. (2012) *Patients' Experiences of Care and the Influence of Staff Motivation, Affect and Wellbeing*. Final report. NIHR Service Delivery and Organisation Programme.

Maben, J., Cornwell, J. & Sweeney, K. (2010) In praise of compassion in nursing. Guest editorial. Special edition. *Journal of Research in Nursing*, **15** (1), 9–13. doi: 10.1177/1744987109353689

Maben, J., Latter, S. & Macleod-Clark, J. (2006) The theory-practice gap: impact of professional-bureaucratic work conflict on newly-qualified nurses. *Journal of Advanced Nursing*, **55** (4), 465–467.

Maben, J., Latter, S. & Macleod-Clark, J. (2007) The challenges of maintaining ideals and standards in professional practice: evidence from a longitudinal qualitative study. *Nursing Inquiry*, **14** (2), 99–113.

Macleod, D. & Clarke, N. (2011) *Engaging for Success: enhancing performance through employee engagement – report to government*. UK Government Department for Business, Innovation and Skills. http://www.bis.gov.uk/files/file52215.pdf (Accessed 10 April 2012).

Mallidou, A.A., Cummings, G., Estabrooks, C. & Giovanetti, P.B. (2011) Nurse specialty subcultures and patient outcomes in acute care hospitals: a multiple-group structural equation modelling. *International Journal of Nursing Studies*, **48** (1), 81–93.

Manley, K., Crisp, J. & Moss, C. (2011a) Advancing the practice development outcomes agenda within multiple contexts. *International Practice Development Journal*, **1** (1), 1–6, Article 4. http://www.fons.org/library/journal/volume1-issue1/article4 (Accessed 10 October 2012).

Manley, K., Sanders, K., Cardiff, S. & Webster, J. (2011b) Effective workplace culture: the attributes, enabling factors and consequences of a new concept. *International Practice Development Journal*, **1** (2), 1–29.

Article 1. http://www.fons.org/Resources/Documents/Journal/Vol1No2/IPDJ_0102_01.pdf (Accessed 10 October 2012).

McCance, T.V. (2003) Caring in nursing practice: the development of a conceptual framework. *Research and Theory for Nursing Practice: An International Journal*, **17** (2), 101–116.

McCance, T., Telford, L., Wilson, J., MacLeod, O. & Dowd, A. (2011) Identifying key performance indicators for nursing and midwifery care using a consensus approach. *Journal of Clinical Nursing*, **21** (7-8), 1145–1154.

McCance, T., Slater, P. & McCormack, B. (2008) Using the caring dimensions inventory (CDI) as an indicator of person-centred nursing. *Journal of Clinical Nursing*, **18**, 409–417.

McCormack, B. & McCance, T. (2010) *Person-centred Nursing: Theory, Models and Methods*. Blackwell Publishing Ltd., Oxford.

McCormack, B. & Titchen, A. (2006) Critical creativity: melding, exploding, blending. *Educational Action Research*, **14** (2), 239–266.

McCormack, B., Dewing, J., Breslin, L., Tobin, C., Manning, M., Coyne-Nevin, A., Kennedy, K. & Peelo-Kilroe, L. (2010) *The Implementation of a Model of Person-Centred Practice in Older Person Settings. Final Report*, Office of the Nursing Services Director, Health Services Executive, Dublin, Ireland.

McCormack, B., Dewar, B., Wright, J., Garbett, R., Harvey, G. & Ballantine, K. (2006) A Realist Synthesis of Evidence Relating to Practice Development: Final Report to NHS Education For Scotland and NHS Quality Improvement Scotland http://www.healthcareimprovementscotland.org/previous_resources/policy_and_strategy/a_realist_synthesis_of_evidenc.aspx (Accessed 10 October 2012).

McCormack, B. (2004) Person-centredness in gerontological nursing: an overview of the literature. *Journal of Clinical Nursing*, **13** (3A), 31–38.

McCormack, B. (2003) A conceptual framework for person-centred practice with older people. *International Journal of Nursing Practice*, **9**, 202–209.

Merleau-Ponty, M. (1989) *Phenomenology of Perception* (translation by C. Smith with revisions by F. Williams & D. Gurriere). Routledge, London.

Newman, K., Maylor, U. & Chansarkar, B. (2001) The nurse retention, quality of care and patient satisfaction chain. *International Journal of Health Care Quality Assurance*, **14** (2), 57–68.

NHS Confederation, the Local Government Association and Age UK (2012) *Delivering Dignity. A Reform Plan for the Care of Older People by the Commission on Improving Dignity in Care for Older People*. NHS Confederation, London.

Nolan, M. (2001) Successful ageing: keeping the 'person' in person-centred care. *British Journal of Nursing*, **10** (7), 450–454.

Nolan, M., Davies, S., Brown, J., Keady, J. & Nolan, J. (2004) Beyond 'person-centred' care: a new vision for gerontological nursing. *International Journal of Older People Nursing (in association with the Journal of Clinical Nursing)*, **13** (3a), 45–53.

Nolan, M., Davies, S. & Grant, G. (2001). *Working with Older People and their Families: Key Issues in Policy and Practice*. Open University Press, Buckingham.

Packer, T. (2003) Turning rhetoric into reality: person-centred approaches for community mental health nursing. In: *Community Mental Health Nursing and Dementia Care* (eds J. Keady, C. Clarke & T. Adams), pp: 104–119. Open University Press, Maidenhead.

Patients Association (2011) *We Have Been Listening, Have You Been Learning?*. Patients Association. Middlesex, England.

Rankin, J.M. & Campbell, M.L. (2006) *Managing to Nurse: Inside Canada's Health Care Reform*. University of Toronto Press, Toronto, ON.

Robinson, D., Perryman, S. & Hayday, S. (2004) *The Drivers of Employee Engagement*. Institute for Employment Studies, Brighton.

Ronson, J. (2011) *The Psychopath Test: A Journey Through the Madness Industry*. Picador, London.

Royal College of Nursing (2008) *Defending Dignity: Challenges and Opportunities for Nursing*. Royal College of Nursing, London.

Seedhouse, D. (2001) *Health: The Foundations for Achievement*. John Wiley & Sons, Chichester.

Shaller, D. Patient-centred care: what does it take? Picker Institute and the Commonwealth Fund 2007.

Sheingold, B.H., Hofmeyer, A. & Woolcock, M. (2012) Measuring the nursing work environment: can a social capital framework add value?. *World Medical & Health Policy*, **4** (1), 1. Article 3.

Slater, L. (2006) Person-centredness: a concept analysis. *Contemporary Nurse*, **23**, 135–144.

Slater, P. & McCormack, B. (2007) An exploration of the factor structure of the Nursing Work Index. *Worldviews on Evidence-Based Nursing*, **4** (1), 30–39.

Stevenson, F., Cox, K., Britten, N. & Dundar, Y. (2004). A systematic review of the research on communication between patients and health care professionals about medicines: the consequences for concordance. *Health Expectations*, **7**, 235–245.

Titchen, A., McCormack, B., Wilson, V. & Solman, A. (2011) Human flourishing through body, creative imagination and reflection. *International Practice Development Journal*, Article 1. http://www.fons.org/library/journal/volume1-issue1 (Accessed 10 October 2012)

Titchen, A. & McGinley, M. (2003) Facilitating practitioner research through critical companionship. *NTResearch*, **8** (2), 115–131.

11 Practice Development as Radical Gardening: Enabling Creativity and Innovation

Angie Titchen[1] and Ann McMahon[2]

[1]Fontys University of Applied Sciences, Eindhoven, The Netherlands
[2]Royal College of Nursing, London, UK

Ann: (Entering the gates of Regent's Park in London) Practice development as radical gardening! What do you mean by that Angie?

Angie: I use the term radical gardening as a metaphor for doing practice development in workplaces where it is difficult to find space to plan, implement, reflect on and evaluate the development. It's all about re-framing the mindset that it's impossible to do practice development, as described in this book, given the current pressures we are all facing in health care. Radical gardening symbolizes, for me, thinking out of the box, being imaginative and doing things differently. In other words, being creative and innovative! The idea of radical gardening comes from people in different parts of the world, including the United Kingdom, growing their own food in urban areas or where land is disappearing or flooding due the effects of global warming. So volunteers use any space they can find – roof tops, walls, school grounds, roundabouts, derelict land or railway station platforms (see Figures 11.1 and 11.2)! And everyone in the community can forage for free (http://www.incredible-edible-todmorden.co.uk/).

Ann: What an amazing idea! In terms of our chapter on creativity and innovation, I can see how your metaphor could work. It's like the radical garden is the innovation, say the development of a nurse-led clinic and creativity is the growth process and its nurture to enable the innovation to happen.

Angie: Yes. it's not that we are literally encouraging readers to develop actual gardens in their workplaces! (As we turn a corner in the park) I don't believe it. Look, there is a vegetable garden! Right in the middle of London! And it's a community allotment garden!

INTRODUCTION

Creativity is concerned with bringing something into existence. It requires being able to create and be inventive and imaginative in thought, as well as involving routine skill and thinking. So creativity uses both left (rational) and right (creative) sides of the brain. These capacities have been shown to be key features of expertise, whether it is in clinical nursing (see Hardy et al., 2009), practice development or research (see Higgs et al., 2007). Innovation, on the other hand, is the new thing or novelty that is being brought in. It can be introduced creatively that is where creativity and innovation are linked, but it can also be brought in using

Practice Development in Nursing and Healthcare, Second Edition. Edited by Brendan McCormack, Kim Manley and Angie Titchen.
© 2013 John Wiley & Sons, Ltd. Published 2013 by John Wiley & Sons, Ltd.

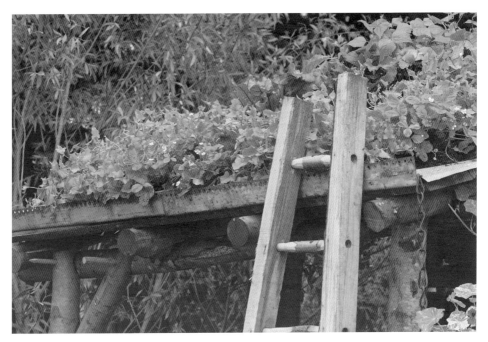

Fig. 11.1 Thinking out of the box when the waters rise (Photo reproduced by permission of The Royal Horticultural Society).

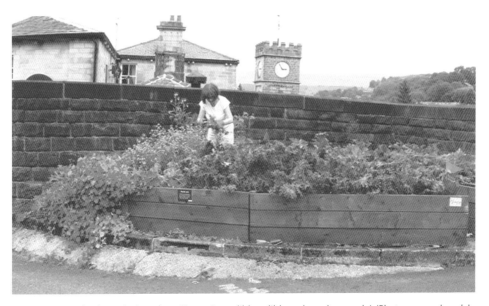

Fig. 11.2 Radical gardening. http://www.incredible-edible-todmorden.co.uk/ (Photos reproduced by kind permission of Incredible Edible Todmorden).

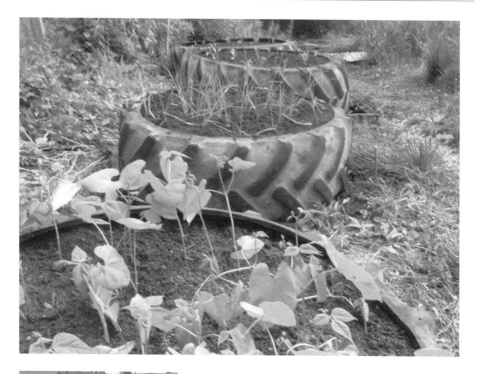

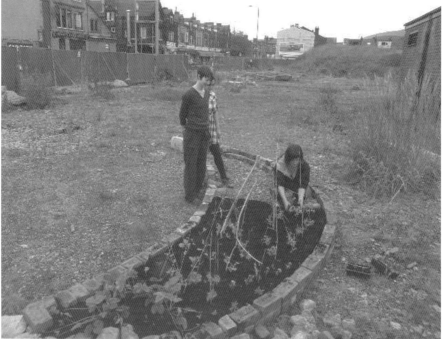

Fig. 11.2 (Continued)

unimaginative or non-inventive processes that may hinder the planning, implementation or evaluation of the innovation.

The purpose of the chapter is to begin to answer questions, in the context of practice development, about the nature of creativity and innovation and their connections. We do this creatively by drawing on our experiences of our dialogue as we walked together in Regent's Park. By posing questions, we invite you to dialogue between your own thoughts and values and ours. We hope to stimulate more questions than answers for you. And we model how creative imagination and thought can be facilitated through critical-creative dialogue.

Angie is an experienced practice developer and action-orientated researcher. She explores the use of creative imagination and expression with nurses and health professionals in many fields of practice. She has written and researched extensively about this work (e.g. Higgs & Titchen, 2001; Titchen & Horsfall, 2011). With Brendan McCormack, Annette Solman, Val Wilson and others within the International Practice Development Collaborative (IPDC) and beyond, she is creating a new worldview called critical creativity and philosophical, theoretical and methodological frameworks to underpin it within practice development (see Chapter 3; McCormack & Titchen, 2006; Henderson, 2009; Titchen & McCormack, 2010; Titchen et al., 2011). In this chapter, Angie sets out the contextual and values background for being a practice developer working within this new worldview. Vignettes with fictional characters are drawn on the basis of her own and others' real experiences of practice development. The vignettes show how groups of stakeholders work with the values of critical creativity and how they use creative processes during the elements of the practice development journey (see Figure 1.1). The vignettes illustrate how novice practice developers can contribute to creating person-centred cultures in their workplace where everyone can flourish.

Ann continues by setting out what innovation means in the context of her innovation work at the Royal College of Nursing (RCN) in the United Kingdom. Ann has worked as a clinical nurse and in research and development for approximately 30 years. She has been committed to improving patient care through the generation of new knowledge (research) and the development of health policy and nursing practice, informed by the best available research evidence, throughout her career (McMahon & Darby, 1993; Kitson et al., 1997; McMahon, 1998; Scott et al., 1999). In 2008, Ann completed her doctoral studies where she critically examined the conditions in which innovation in health care may flourish (McMahon, 2008). As professional research policy adviser at the RCN, Ann has worked with RCN members to lobby for investment to build nursing research capacity and capability, the development of sustainable clinical academic careers in nursing and investment into the research priorities of nursing practice. She is a founding member of the Academy of Nursing, Midwifery and Health Visiting Research and currently edits the *Journal of Research in Nursing*.

Next, we pull together principles for creativity and innovation in practice development and weave our conclusions for novice practice developers. We round off by setting out some resources and a glossary of possibly unfamiliar words.

CRITICAL CREATIVITY AND THE PRACTICE DEVELOPMENT JOURNEY

Ann: (Walking down the long straight path from the gate) Angie, given that practice developers talk a lot about clarifying and making values and assumptions explicit at the beginning of a practice development project, what are they in terms of creativity?

Angie: Good question. Many of us practice developers frame creativity in the philosophical ideas and frameworks of critical social science. The key value held by critical social scientists is social justice for all. So, this is the ultimate purpose of any changes that a group of people in a particular context aim to bring about. The values underpinning the change processes include democracy, collaboration, inclusion and participation amongst others. It is assumed that social justice will be achieved if there is a focus on the enlightenment, empowerment and emancipation of all stakeholders involved in the change. Change is brought about by communicative action (Habermas, 1972). Communicative action involves creating spaces where stakeholders can communicate with each other through dialogue, discussion, agreeing and disagreeing whether something is valid or not until a mutual decision on cooperative action is reached.

Ann: This sounds like emancipatory practice development (see Chapter 3) to me . . . (Angie nods). So what about creativity if you are striving to become an emancipatory practice developer?

Angie: Well, creativity for such practice developers is bound up not only with communicative action but also with communicative rationality. Big words, but let's break it down. We are all familiar with rationality or rational thinking. It involves us using our heads – our mental or cognitive processes. An example is reflexivity (something that practice developers promote) that is a term that means us having self-knowledge and a conscious awareness of the impact of ourselves when we are interacting with others. Now communicative rationality not only involves a person being reflexive but also includes being open to communication with others through dialogue and differing arguments and searching for new meanings together. The idea is that new understandings to inform action come from questioning and challenging historical, cultural, social and political assumptions that usually go unquestioned because they are so taken for granted. For example, a group of stakeholders may assume that practice development is not possible in their workplace because they do not have enough time or staff to do it, let alone get through the everyday work. If they don't challenge this assumption about lack of time themselves, they will never become 'radical gardeners' who find creative ways to grow vegetables and flowers in busy, crowded urban environments or, in other words, make space to do practice development that enables everyone to flourish.

So creativity or bringing something into existence is facilitated by searching together for understanding, learning from each other and different arguments and critiquing the status quo. And the first search might be for odd little corners of time and space that can be used for talking and listening to each other about what, for example, they could let go of to make time for change. The effectiveness of these radical gardens and little corners can be increased by helping each other to reflect in structured ways in say, 15 minute reflection spaces.

Ann: So, if emancipatory practice developers use cognitive, rational ways of knowing, coming to know and talking, how is this different in critical creativity?

Angie: Another good question! The short answer is . . . but let me go back a bit first. Practice developers who frame their work in the critical creativity worldview also hold these values and assumptions, but they add human flourishing to social justice as the ultimate purpose of practice development. By human flourishing they mean maximising people's achievement of their potential for growth and development as they go through the turbulence of a change experience as well as everyone flourishing when the desired changes have been achieved.

In this worldview, creativity emerges within critical-creative spaces and little corners that we create for self and/or others. In these spaces, critical consciousness or knowing with the mind is blended with non-rational creative imagination and the knowing of our heart, body (includes gut feelings and intuition) and soul. These non-rational ways not only help us to grasp the meaning of the whole of something but also reveal meanings and things that are hidden inside ourselves or in the external context. When these meanings and things are blended with what we know with our heads, we can get a much deeper understanding of the whole and its parts. Working with non-rational ways of knowing helps the inclusion of stakeholders who may not know about the theory of person-centred cultures, that is, head knowledge, for example, but they can know it with their hearts and body if they are helped to express it. So, if patients, families and domestic staff, for instance, can be helped to understand what a person-centred culture is through what their bodies, heart and soul know, they can contribute to creating a vision for such a culture and take a part in genuinely person-centred action to achieve it.

However, what we know in the heart, body and soul can be difficult to talk about and this is where the use of creative arts media like painting, metaphor, writing a poem or making a sound or gesture can be useful. Practice developers create the conditions for the blending of these creative expressions with communicative rationality and communicative action.

So the short answer to your question is that practice developers working within critical creativity create conditions that enable embodied, imaginative and symbolic meaning to be brought into the cognitive critique of a context, situation or event!

Ann: I find what you say about ways of knowing really interesting. It seems to me that people's values are likely to influence their ways of knowing that, in turn, will shape the practice development journey and people's response to it! Some people will resist heart, body and soul knowing and stay with the more comfortable with head knowing, whilst others might feel more adventurous or willing to move out of their comfort zone and work with creative expression that brings heart, body and soul knowing to the surface.

Angie: Yes, you are absolutely right. Many people are very wary of using creative arts media in any context let alone at work, usually because they have been socialised to think that it is too 'touchy-feely', and therefore, not to be messed with or they feel it is silly, trivial and a waste of time or that they have been told, usually at school, that they are not creative or artistic. I find that many people are afraid of exposing their artwork to others and being criticised, so it is really important for facilitators to ensure that everyone understands that their expression is not going to be judged or interpreted by anyone as if it were a work of Art. Rather, it is a means of expression for that person to help them put words to things they know but cannot say.

Ann: Yes, and I can see that the role of the facilitator is really important here. So tell me, how do you define creativity in this worldview of yours?

Angie: Well, in the work I have been doing with Brendan (McCormack & Titchen, 2006) (in which we have been studying our own practice development work), we have set out a new theory of the creativity in the context of taking what Brian Fay (1987) calls, 'transformative action'. So Brendan and I propose that creativity is:

the blending and weaving of art forms and reflexivity (critical consciousness) located in the critical paradigm. Blending and weaving occur through professional artistry in order to achieve the ultimate outcome of human flourishing. Thus this theory has critical, moral and sacred dimensions.

These theoretical statements summarise a lot of what I have just been saying, but I think it is important now to show our readers how this kind of creativity is facilitated in practice development contexts particularly those that are full of choking brambles, weeds and unfavourable or toxic conditions for transformative action. In such conditions, flourishing for all is supported through contemporary facilitation strategies that connect with beauty and nature and blend ancient wisdom, creative traditions and the active learning that is described in Chapter 8.

Radical gardeners: vignettes of critical creativity

Health care organisations and workplaces often say that their purpose is to deliver effective, safe and person-centred care. However, the reality for patients (and staff) is that they often do not deliver it (see Patient Opinion, 2011). Doing practice development has always been very challenging. This is often because organisations and workplaces do not pay attention to creating democratic structures and collaborative, inclusive and participative ways of working. Nor do they put energy into creating workplace cultures that support person-centred practice and transformation. It seems that other beliefs and values, especially around costs and top-down change strategies carry more weight in decisions about how energy and resources are to be used. However, despite such challenges, research and project reports (e.g. Binnie & Titchen, 1999; McCormack et al., 2008; Wilson & Walsh, 2008) have demonstrated that practice development in health care has effectively brought about changes in structures, team working, leadership and workplace cultures that have resulted in improved patients' and staff experience. To do this, as if radical gardeners in urban environments, practice developers have had to be creative in finding spaces and time in the busy working day to engage stakeholders collaboratively within the elements of the practice development journey (see Figure 1.1). In addition, practice developers working within critical creativity often use creative arts approaches to speed up and deepen this engagement (see Figure 11.3). Three vignettes here introduce how this can happen in practice.

Although the vignettes are fictional, they are based on practice development research and experience, notably, through the IPDC schools and research (e.g. McCormack & Titchen, 2006; Titchen et al., 2011) and the work of others (e.g. Coats, 2001; Titchen & Horsfall, 2011; Wilson & Walsh, 2008; McCormack et al., 2010). Various health care settings have been chosen to help you identify with what is going on, but remember, the principles for using creative arts approach for the communicative action and rationality can be used in any context or setting.

Vignette 1: Knowing and demonstrating values and beliefs: bringing radical gardeners together

A group of six nurses, including four staff nurses, a clinical nurse specialist and the ward leader in a cardiac unit, have undertaken an audit of intravenous cannulation on their ward. They identify that the rate of phlebitis resulting from cannulation is unacceptably high. They decide that their group will carry out a year-long project to introduce clinical guidelines to the ward team to reduce phlebitis through a series of teaching sessions for the nurses. They will then monitor the implementation of the guidelines. The group repeat the audit a year later and find that the rate of phlebitis has dropped dramatically! The unit and hospital are delighted. The work is done and so the group disband. At the end of the following year,

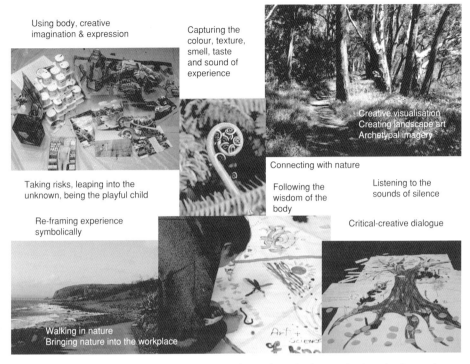

Fig. 11.3   Principles for using creative arts approaches to bring body, creative imagination and expression into communicative action and rationality (Photos 2 (middle) and 4 (lower left) by Brendan McCormack and the rest by Angie Titchen).

however, another audit is carried out and the phlebitis rates are almost back to where they were before the guidelines were introduced.

The group re-assemble and discuss what might have contributed to this situation. In other words, they engage in communicative rationality. They recognise now that they had been using a technical approach to practice development. They have identified that this approach assumes that it is sufficient just to provide people with sound research evidence for a particular change and then training in the new practice and that that will be sufficient. Unfortunately, it rarely is and so it was for them. They conclude that because there is no agreed vision for care on the ward, perhaps members of the team are pulling in different directions according to what they value most. They also recognise that by not engaging staff stakeholders in the project, no-one has taken responsibility for continuing to use and monitor the guidelines, once the group disbanded. They think that this is an effect of the kind of culture that prevails in the unit and that this culture is not supporting person-centred care and enabling all staff members to take responsibility for the quality of patient care. If they are going to transform that culture then all stakeholders, including patients and families, need to work together in a coordinated way for each person to make their values explicit, so that a shared vision can be created from the points of connection between their values. They agree that they should become a visioning group for this purpose.

Some group members have heard about using creative arts approaches to help people to talk about things that are held in their hearts and bodies and embedded in what they do. They think that values are embodied and embedded like that and so are really difficult to talk

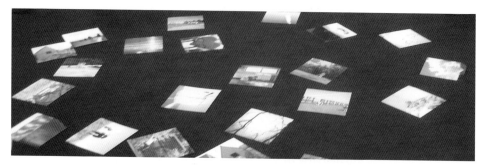

Fig. 11.4 Using picture cards for expressing values (Photo by Angie Titchen).

about. They discuss the pros and cons of using picture cards (see Figure 11.4) as a simple way of bringing people's values to the surface, so that they can share them. Some people think they are a good idea, but others disagree arguing that people will dismiss using picture cards considering them childish or ridiculous. After listening and valuing all view points, the group agree that, despite there being some reservations about people feeling comfortable with using them, they will take the risk. They decide to invite people to use them at the next unit meeting.

The cards go down a storm. People say they are fun to use and that they could talk more easily about their values and what really matters to them when they had an image in front of them. They also say that they learned things about each other that they did not know before, even about people who they had been working with for years. Other people in the unit who were not at the meeting start asking group members if they can join in.

At the next group meeting, this evaluation of the use of the cards leads to an agreement to use them with others at events that are happening anyway in the unit, like shift handover, coffee break or meeting with relatives. They will use them not only to get to know each others' values but also to start building person-centred relationships in the unit and to prepare for a visioning exercise that will involve the whole unit. Each group member commits to introducing the cards whenever they can.

Vignette 2: Developing a shared vision: creating a shared expression of the radical garden of the future

The visioning group is made up of seven volunteers (two patients, a physiotherapist, two staff nurses, the ward leader and one relative, Mrs Jones). Mrs Jones has made the poster (Figure 11.5) and bought the creative arts materials with money donated by the hospital's League of Friends. All staff who work and visit the ward and patients and their visitors are invited to make a wish and tie it on the tree. Although there is a lot of curiosity about what is going on, messages are slow to start. But when ward staff start encouraging everyone to spend a few minutes making a wish and begin doing it themselves, the momentum grows. People often stop at the tree and look at the wishes. And that gets conversations going.

Three weeks later the tree is groaning with the weight of the 'fruit'. The visioning group begin their 30-minute meeting in the dining space. Ellen Jones is facilitating and she invites group members to gather round the tree and then using all their body senses, to take in the laden tree as a whole. She suggests that when people feel ready they could move around the tree to look at each offering individually. When everyone has done this, Ellen invites them to begin to share, not how they make sense of it all at this point, but what they actually see, feel and imagine. One of the group members who has been a patient on the ward several

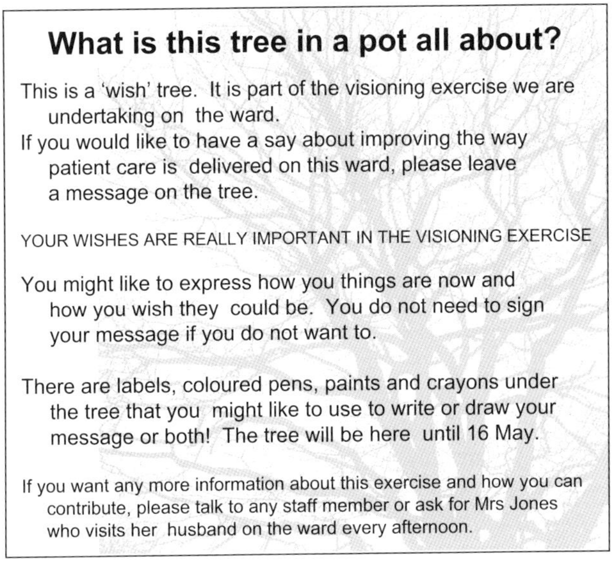

What is this tree in a pot all about?

This is a 'wish' tree. It is part of the visioning exercise we are
undertaking on the ward.
If you would like to have a say about improving the way
patient care is delivered on this ward, please leave
a message on the tree.

YOUR WISHES ARE REALLY IMPORTANT IN THE VISIONING EXERCISE

You might like to express how you things are now and
how you wish they could be. You do not need to sign
your message if you do not want to.

There are labels, coloured pens, paints and crayons under
the tree that you might like to use to write or draw your
message or both! The tree will be here until 16 May.

If you want any more information about this exercise and how you can
contribute, please talk to any staff member or ask for Mrs Jones
who visits her husband on the ward every afternoon.

Fig. 11.5   Poster placed by the visioning group in the dining area of a ward caring for older people.

times this year starts off and says, 'I see a lot more colour and positive energy in the way people would like the ward to be in comparison with their experience of the ward now'. One of the staff nurses who has agreed to record what people say, writes up 'more colour and positive energy in the future' on a flipchart . . . When people have finished sharing, the fruits are harvested and set out on a dining table and people sit down.

The group now begin a critical-creative dialogue about the key things that are coming up and points of connection between the images, meanings and words. When they reach agreement, they write them down on sticky notes and put them on the table. Then they cluster the sticky notes into themes and give each theme a name. Themes like 'trust', 'respect', 'active listening' and 'not being rushed' emerge. It is nearly time for the meeting to end, so actions are agreed. The staff nurse who has been recording the themes on the flipchart offers to prepare a presentation of the themes for the ward notice board. One of the patients suggests that each theme should be presented with some of the messages that support it, so that people can see where the themes come from. Everyone but the ward leader thinks this is a good idea. She has some reservations about this, but is eventually convinced by the others that it will show particularly patients and families that they have been listened to. It is agreed that the presentation will invite patients, staff and visitors to look at the themes and leave a message (in a box attached to the notice board) about whether they can feel their values and voice somewhere in the themes. What people say will help to establish the trustworthiness of the analysis the group has done. Later, the visioning group will take agreements and disagreements into account as they develop vision statements from the themes. After further checking by as many stakeholders as possible (in a series of 15-minute spaces in the dining area), the final statements will set the new direction the ward will take.

Questions for you:

- Why do you think this visioning group took so much trouble to ensure that everyone got a chance to contribute to the vision statements?

- How did you feel as you read the two vignettes and looked at the imagery? Why did you feel like this?
- What are your thoughts about this use of the body, nature and creative imagination and expression as an addition to just talking about a vision for the future?
- Why do you think the ward leader had initial reservations? Does this say anything to you about the current culture on the ward?

Vignette 3: Integrated evaluation, learning, planning, action, evaluation…

Service users and staff in a unit providing complex continuing care and rehabilitation have agreed a vision for a person-centred culture. The vision is set out in their own words from their own values. They feel as though they own the vision, rather than it being someone else's or their organisation's alone. This makes them feel committed to it. Some stakeholders think that the vision is already a reality, but others have become more aware during the visioning activity that the unit has a long way to go in creating a culture that will genuinely support learning and inquiry into, for example, service users' experiences of care and working in teams that include staff and service users. Such a team has been set up to act as a practice development coordinating group.

Group members attended an IPDC school recently that was hosted by their organisation and paid for by a trust fund that supports improved services in the group their organisation is part of. Like many others who have attended practice development schools, they experienced practice development (and learning about it) as a journey. The journey is premised on the idea of never-ending and integrated cycles of evaluation, learning, planning and acting. Each new cycle begins to look at the impact of the actions and to see if they achieved what they set out to do. And if not, what new learning, inquiry and planning of action might be required. They know that the first step for them now is to evaluate more deeply where they are starting from. Whilst the visioning activity has given them a beginning sense of what is working well and what is not, they need to gather evaluation evidence to understand why. This evidence will enable them to devise an overall practice development plan based on the vision.

At the school, group members were introduced to a number of tools to collect empirical, quantifiable evidence and they experienced the power of gathering qualitative evaluation evidence using all the body senses and creative imagination. This kind of evidence is usually unconscious or so obvious that it goes unnoticed; just as we go about our lives without seeing the air we breathe. It is evidence known by the body, heart and soul. It is very different from, but complementary to, evidence held in the head. This latter kind of evidence can be accessed in more traditional ways like questionnaires, interviews and conversations. In addition to evidence that can be quantified, they decide to collect both kinds of qualitative evidence by taking reflective walks followed by creative expression and then critical creative dialogue.

The coordinating group put out a call for volunteers to gather this evidence and six staff and service users come forward. They meet with Nadia who is a nurse and a member of the coordinating group for 1 hour in the late afternoon when the unit is quieter. Nadia has set up a circle of chairs in room off one of the wards in the unit. There is a table at one side where she has placed some paper, tin foil, crepe paper, paints, pastels and magazines and other materials she has retrieved from her recycling box at home.

Once people have settled, she explains that the purpose of the activity today is to gather evidence about the current culture in the unit and the culture within their teams. She invites them to introduce themselves and how they are feeling today – as if they were a garden! What kind of garden would they be; what colours and smells and so on. They have fun doing that and there is a lot of laughter. Then Nadia suggests that they close their eyes for a moment

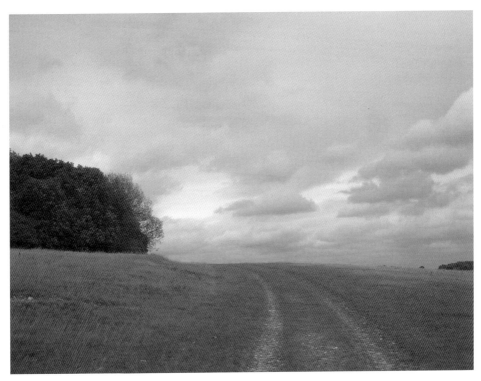

Fig. 11.6 Image symbolising inner openness and space that can be facilitated for reflective walks in busy workplaces or grounds.

and bring their focus back to themselves and to their breath. After a moment of silence, she asks them to stand up with their eyes closed and move slowly forward into the circle with their arms outstretched. The first person they bump into will be their partner for a walk! When the pairs have found themselves, she demonstrates a shadow-hands activity where the partners mirror each other's movement in silence. Partner's place their hands close together, palm to palm, but they do not touch. Leading and following the movement is shared by both but the change from being leader or follower is imperceptible; it is not indicated by word, gesture or facial expression. Eye contact is maintained throughout. The imperceptible shift from leading to following and vice versa comes through being attuned to the other's body. When Nadia signals, the pairs talk briefly about this experience. The buzz and energy in the room is extraordinary. Although the activity is simple and quick, some people experience an unexpectedly deep connection with the other person. Others are amazed at the magical attunement their bodies possess of which they were previously unaware:

> Now Nadia explains that each pair will go on a reflective walk (see Figure 11.6) together and that each will take with them a pen and piece of A4 paper folded into four. They might choose to walk within the unit or in the grounds outside or both. 'You have 20 minutes' she says. 'The first 10 minutes is to be spent walking in silence (see Figure 11.6). Pause for a moment or two before you set off to take a few deep breaths and let go whatever thoughts are in your mind. You can do this 'letting go' by really looking around you, as if you had never seen these surroundings and things before. As you walk, notice what you really notice, what captures your attention, what you feel and write these things down (a word, phrase or image) or sketch them roughly. Even pick them up and bring them back with you if it is appropriate. There doesn't have to be any

reason at all for what you notice. The important thing is that these particular things just happen to attract or repel you. And it is this noticing that often reveals what we have previously been unaware of. In the second 10 minutes share what you noticed and help each other to search for meaning. Perhaps you might see parallels for your experiences or meanings in the physical environment that surrounds you.

When you come back into this room, come in silence and express what you have noticed and the meanings that have emerged for you during the walk using any of these creative materials and or the things you have brought back with you – either on your own or in your pair.

. . . The group have presented their creative expressions of reflections and insights that emerged for them during the walk. One pair chose to walk around the ward where they work. They were completely stunned by the amount of noise there with all the beeps of machinery, bells constantly ringing, staff shouting at each other down the corridor, loud chatter coming from the ward office where a meeting was in place with the door open and the banging of equipment in the kitchen. Having entered the ward as if it was strange and in a completely different way from their usual, unconscious going about their business, they began to appreciate at a deep level what it might be like to be a service user staying in this ward . . . This insight was transformational, a turning point, in terms of staff and service users committing to work together to create a person-centred culture.

Although this vignette is fictional, it is based on the experiences of a practice development school in Canada where Brendan and Angie were facilitators. You might like to read an article by Haynes and Janes (2011) to hear what really happened after such an experience!!! You can access it online for free.

Questions for you:

- Why didn't Nadia just send people straight off on their reflective walk? Was she wasting time with the introductions, breathing and the shadow-hands partner activity?
- Why was silence used in this evidence gathering activity?
- Could you use such walks for other purposes in the practice development journey?
- What have you learned so far from the real walk that we (Ann and Angie) had in Regent's Park when we were preparing to write this chapter?
- Do you think that you might become a radical gardener working with others in your setting?
- Can you see communicative action and rationality playing out in any of these three vignettes?

INNOVATION

Back in Regent's Park . . .

Angie: Ann, what does innovation mean to you within the context of your current role at the RCN?

Ann: Thank you Angie for asking that question and asking me to answer 'within the context of my role at the RCN' because I think it can be particularly challenging to talk about innovation without understanding the context in which innovation is being talked about! The reason I think that is because in my experience and from my research, innovation can mean many things to different people. It can, therefore, be quite hard to pin it down! It is almost like a visually impaired person walking into this beautiful garden and asking you 'what does a flowering plant look like?' When you look around and see the huge range of flowers we can see here in this garden and then if you think about all of the flowers in all the gardens all over the world, you can begin to imagine the scale of the challenge, to answer what at first may seem like a simple straightforward question!

Angie: OK Ann, but there are certain common features of a flower that I might describe such as sepals, petals, stamens and pistils, not to mention colour and smell.

Ann: Yes for sure. But think about the debates over 'what is a weed?' Remember that natural border filled with glorious wild flowers, dancing gracefully in the gentle breeze that we have just walked past and which we both thought were truly magnificent? And yet we acknowledged that some people perceive wild flowers as nothing but weeds, the gardener's enemy, to be attacked with chemicals and destroyed. My point here is that there are multiple meanings of innovation and whilst definitions may have some common features, what actually constitutes an innovation is often highly contested!

Angie: I see what you are saying. So what would you say are the common features of innovation?

Ann: I think there are two key fundamental features of innovation. The first is some sense of novelty and the second is about change. Therefore, innovation is generally understood to be the introduction of something new. You immediately get into hot water though, Angie, when you talk about 'new'. What does 'new' mean? Innovation is often linked to creativity and this is where the sense of newness can come from. However you'll have heard the biblical reference that 'there is nothing new under the sun'. So understanding what we mean by new can be tricky!

If you introduced a flower into the United Kingdom that is traditionally grown in the Mediterranean, for example, and you are able to create the conditions where that flower flourished, then I would describe that as an innovation. It is not a new flower but it is growing successfully in a different place. The skill of the garden innovator I would recognise as having the ability to create and sustain the right conditions for the flower to grow. For this reason, I see innovation very much as context specific.

I think this is a really important point and I passionately would like all nurses to share this understanding of innovation because nursing does have something of a reputation of 'eating its own'. For example, when nurses write up and publish in a nursing journal, for example, a new initiative they have been involved in, I have heard other nurses scoffing at the article by saying: 'That's not new, we've being doing that on my ward for the last 6 months!' And I think, well that's great for the patients in your care. But if you do not tell other nurses about it then how will other, equally deserving patients reap the benefits of your creativity and innovation? In many cases, however, nurses do not recognise their own creativity and do not consider that the changes that they make in their practice may be regarded as innovative. Equally, I do not think nurses necessarily think about the potential 'scalability' of their innovations.

It is for this very reason, at the RCN, that we see innovation as being context specific. We are not necessarily looking for something that is 'brand new' because in reality that may be something of the holy grail! Our take on innovation is that there are creative and innovative nurses up and down the country introducing new products and services into the context in which they are working. And we want to hear about it because we can play a key role in helping to spread innovation across the profession.

The second key feature of innovation is that it is about change. Innovation is not just about an idea or a proposal, it is about what is done with the idea. I would argue that for an idea to be innovative it has to be tested out and there has to be some evidence that it works.

The RCN's focus on innovation is currently within the context of a campaign to mobilise members of the college to share their experiences. It is absolutely about creating a vehicle for members who may not necessarily actively engage in the work of the RCN to get involved. In the current economic climate, health services are required to reduce costs. The RCN recognises that austerity measures are required, however, it wants to make sure that decisions made to save money are good for patients and good for nurses. By capitalising on the power of the internet, the campaign, therefore, encourages and enables RCN members to report on cuts that are being made where they work and the impact this is having on nursing and patient care. It enables RCN members to highlight where they see waste in the system, that if addressed could save significant amounts of money. And thirdly the campaign invites its members to report on nursing solutions or innovations in practice that, as stated earlier, the RCN can help to actively promote.

(We arrive at huge ornamental gates and enter into a formal rose garden.)

So Angie, in our walk together today, we have visited the community garden here in Regent's Park. It was a wonderful and inspiring example of what can be achieved when a group of people, often unknown to one another at the start, come together with a common purpose. The produce grown so successfully in that garden was not only of great beauty, it could feed the community gardeners and perhaps their friends and families too. The potential that can be realised when like-minded people are connected and can collaborate can be incredibly productive and beneficial.

Angie: You are right Ann, and this can happen both politically as well as practically. Just as we see the potential that modern information and communication technologies have to mobilise like-minded people in organizations like Avaaz (meaning 'voice') (see http://www.avaaz.org/en/). Such organisations bring together citizens around the world to campaign, for instance, for social justice, environmental issues and the end of poverty.

Ann: Exactly. The RCN campaign seeks to connect the reality of nursing on the front line with its political activities as a professional organisation and trade union. So in order to encourage nurses to share their innovations we decided to offer an RCN innovation award at the end of 2010. This posed us with a challenge. How do you discriminate when you have more than 300 submissions, which innovations should be long listed and then shortlisted for such an award? As in all the things that we do, this was about being clear about our purpose. Did we want a wild flower garden like the one we saw earlier with potentially endless biodiversity or did we need a much more structured and regimental rose garden like the one we are sitting in now?

We were looking at nurse-led innovations within the context of our campaign that, in turn, was operating within the context of the political and economic climate that called for 'austerity measures'. As well as demonstrating that nurses on the front line were the solution to the current crisis, we recognised that we had a key role to play in supporting the spread of innovation. This clarity of purpose helped us define meaningful criteria against which we could assess the submissions that we received. The process of selection is often described as a funnelling process. You start with 300 and you end up with 3. Our top three (Bell, 2011) were selected on the strength of their evidence of impact and effectiveness and because of their potential scalability.

Angie: What do you mean by scalability?

Ann: Good question Angie. This links back to my earlier point about the importance of telling your story. If you have brought about an innovation in the area where you work that has demonstrated making a real difference, you need to ask yourself – *could other patients/service users benefit from what we are doing here if the nurses working with them adopted or adapted our innovation and changed their practice too?* If the answer to this question is yes, whether that is with a similar client group or a different client group, then your innovation is scalable. Arguably, the more scalable an innovation, the greater its potential impact.

In Northern Ireland, Marina Lupari had developed and implemented a new model of community nursing for managing long-term conditions. Her innovative nurse-led service working with high-risk older people in their own homes led to a reduction in unplanned admissions to hospital. Focusing on people with serious respiratory problems, heart failure and diabetes, 16 full-time district nurses were appointed and given additional training on the identification and management of risk factors associated with these conditions. Patients at risk were, therefore, quickly identified and supported to manage their symptoms themselves. Through a controlled trial, Marina demonstrated that together these nurses and patients not only improved their health but also reduced hospital admissions by more than 59% and saved their local health services more than £400,000 in 9 months!

In Bradford, Carol Gill had introduced an early warning system to prevent older people in care homes from getting pressures sores. Carol reduced the number and severity of pressure ulcers through an innovative health care assistant (HCA) early reporting and recording system. A district nurse who had been a HCA herself, Carol set about reducing the incidence of pressure sores by enabling HCAs working in the care homes to recognise the early warning signs and to escalate concerns to a registered nurse before problems became intractable. The HCAs empowered themselves through a training and development programme that Carol designed and delivered herself after negotiating with her employer. In addition, Carol developed and introduced a traffic-light system that identified HCAs' role and responsibility in identifying and escalating concerns. The human cost of a pressure sore is immeasurable. The cost of this largely preventable condition is £2.4 billion per annum to the NHS in England. Carol and her colleagues reduced the incidence of pressure sores by 25% in 12 months. The human and financial benefits that could be realised through the adoption of this innovation across the country are enormous!

In Wakefield, Sheila Hayward and her colleagues Leanne Cook and Karen Jordan had improved the health of substance misusers. Their innovation aimed to meet the health care needs of clients who were working to overcome drug dependency. These are clients with relatively chaotic lives and who do not routinely access mainstream primary care services. The team operate both a drop in and an outreach service. The service had grown and developed over 3 years and, at the time of the award nomination, provided health services including dentistry, sexual health, nutrition and family planning in venues as varied as cafes, pubs, clubs and prisons. The team was also helping clients address the side effects of intravenous drug misuse, namely, venous ulceration and deep vein thrombosis. Clients who presented in accident and emergency with venous ulcers were proactively followed up by the team to ensure they received active and ongoing wound care treatment until their ulcers healed. The strong focus on keeping these clients healthy not only benefits the individual clients but also benefits society as a whole. And it impacts on the service up-stream by preventing avoidable hospital admissions.

Ann: Upon reflection Angie, I think the case studies of innovation, shortlisted by the RCN Frontline First innovation award judging panel, were metaphorically drawn from and beautifully represent the wild flower border we both enjoyed so much rather then the somewhat regimental rose gardens that equally gave us so much pleasure. For me, these case studies reflect the diversity of nursing innovation and the care and compassion that is the hallmark of nursing practice. My fear that the application of a funnelling process could constrain our celebration of the 'biodiversity' that is nursing was, thankfully, unfounded.

After an online vote, Marina's was identified as the winning innovation and since the award was made she has been an ambassador for nursing innovation and the RCN in key forums both in the United Kingdom and in Europe.

(A butterfly lands on Angie's hand...)

Angie: Ah, how amazing that a butterfly (an ancient symbol for transformation) appears at the end of your story! For me, in this moment, the butterfly symbolises the incredible potential for transformation that this campaign could bring about!! On another note, I would call Marina, Carol, Sheila and her colleagues practice developers as well as garden innovators. I wonder whether they see themselves that way and whether they intentionally worked to transform the culture and conditions to enable the success of their innovations!

Questions for you:

- What strikes you about this conversation about innovation and the RCN campaign?
- If you wanted to bring in a particular innovation that was relevant to your own practice setting, what might be worthwhile considering in order to promote its success?
- What more do you think you could do to celebrate and raise the profile of nursing innovation where you work?

PRINCIPLES FOR CREATIVITY AND INNOVATION IN PRACTICE DEVELOPMENT

As we walked in Regent's Park, we agreed that the following principles were equally relevant to improving practice whether the focus is on creating person-centred cultures or bringing in a particular innovation or both. They are based on the premise that creating such cultures and engaging with stakeholders will enable the achievement of desired innovations. If you want to work particularly within critical creativity, then principle 4b is relevant. All the other principles are relevant to emancipatory practice development and innovation:

1. All stakeholders have the potential to be innovative and creative.
2. This potential can be developed by the individual alone or with others and enhanced by a skilled person-centred facilitator of learning in and from practice.
3. Such a facilitator is likely to have engaged in deep personal and professional development to achieve the level of skill required.

4. The facilitator is like a gardener enabling people to grow and flourish and who:
   (a) creates conditions that enable risk-taking but provides safety nets if and when necessary when people deal with ambiguity and uncertainty and flow through the turbulence of transformational change, that is by creating silent, reflective and reflexive spaces in busy, noisy workplaces; embodying or modelling being creative and innovative in everyday work and nurturing understanding and growth;
   (b) creates spaces in everyday work and environments for artistic and cognitive critique through using all aspects of self, that is body, heart, mind and soul, through an interplay of art forms and rational thinking:
       (i) spaces are seen as having boundaries, form, colour, texture, fragrance, sounds, movement, stillness;
       (ii) helps people to be playful, curious, questioning, challenging of assumptions;
       (iii) enables people to respect each others' creative expressions and critical views/judgments and, if requested by the creator to give feedback, to take care not to interpret the creator's experience/judgment, but to own "what I see/hear, feel and imagine about the other's expression/view/judgment.
5. Privileging different ways of knowing shapes creativity and innovation and people's responses to them.
6. Putting the familiar into different contexts enables transferability of knowledge and ideas. It also reveals the unexpected that can enchant or delight.
7. There is freedom to use the same space and natural resources differently to bring about different effects, for example, entering the workplace as a space we have never been in before in order to notice and bring the taken-for-granted to consciousness; or using the work space as a reflective space by re-framing it metaphorically.
8. Creativity and innovations that are unassuming and yet alluring are cost-effective.
9. Creativity and innovation speak for themselves – their secrets can be shown or pointed out and then enhanced by snippets of information. These snippets beckon rather than overwhelm.
10. Symbols of transformation bring joy and amazement, so achievements, large and small, are celebrated along the way with wonderment and sensitivity.

HERE-NOW AND BEYOND

In this chapter, we have shared what we know in mind, body, heart and soul about enhancing creativity and innovation in the workplace and in a professional body. We have walked our talk by sharing with you our experiences of a real walk in Regent's Park. This walk and the metaphor of radical gardening inspired our own creativity and innovation in writing this chapter, as well as helping us to understand each other's meanings in relation to creativity and innovation. The metaphor helped us to show the connection between them by symbolising the innovation as the garden and the practice developer or innovator as the gardener who creates the conditions for people and the innovation to flourish. This idea is fundamental to critical creativity that sees human flourishing as both the ends and means of transformational practice development. This may contrast with mainstream where flourishing is seen as end and not as means.

This contrast shows up the politics of working in development environments and perhaps it can be seen in the different foci of the critical creativity vignettes and the descriptions of the shortlisted innovations within the RCN campaign. The former are concerned with process and process outcomes along the practice development journey, whilst the latter focus on the innovation outcome. Also relating to the political dimension, the vignettes differ from the innovation descriptions in that they are concerned with creative imagination and expression in combination with communicative action and rationality. Perhaps the way the innovators worked with their stakeholders is more similar to what happens in the mainstream where creative arts approaches are rarely used. Is this because people tend to shy away from the use of creative imagination and expression (for a variety of reasons some of which are presented in this chapter); sometimes to the point of a visceral aversion to an alien form or counter-culture?

Given this political dimension, if you want to experiment with using creative imagination and expression in your workplace, it is important to be aware that their introduction needs to be carefully facilitated. People often need to help to overcome resistance to or fear of this way of working. If you are a novice practice developer, we do not want to put you off trying. This way of working is definitely within your reach. We urge you to find someone, for example, a buddy, colleague or your manager, who can en-courage you by offering you support and feedback as you develop your facilitation or use of creative approaches. The creative approaches in this chapter are usually well received and are suitable for newcomers to facilitation. There are also resources below to help you. Remember not to feel too downhearted if you find that some people resist finding new spaces and trying new ways; even the most skilled facilitators experience this situation. You will probably find that once people have experienced the power of bringing the whole of themselves to development work, they are more open to using such approaches again and introducing them to others.

We wish well on your journeys!

RESOURCES

Creativity

If you are a beginner wanting to explore your own creativity, then the resource, 'Opening Doors' (Coats et al., 2006) is recommended. If you decide that you want to learn more about the practical ideas behind using these approaches, then we recommend a chapter by Titchen and Horsfall (2011). Although this chapter is about research spaces, the ideas are also relevant to practice development. The articles by McCormack and Titchen (2006), Titchen and McCormack (2010) and Titchen et al. (2011) will give you more in-depth theoretical and methodological background if you want to explore these in the future.

Innovation

http://www.rcn.org.uk/development/researchanddevelopment/innovation
http://www.fons.org/

GLOSSARY

Communicative action: Stakeholders communicating with each other in a variety of spaces that promote dialogue, discussion, agreeing and disagreeing until a mutual decision on cooperative action is reached.

Communicative rationality: Being open and cognitively self-aware when communicating with others (through dialogue and posing different arguments) in the shared search for new meanings.

Creativity: Bringing some thing into existence.

Critical creativity: A world view for transformational practice development, education, research and practice that values bringing both sides of our brains into our work, that is, through blending of creative imagination and expression, ancient wisdom and rationality.

Innovation: Some thing, not necessarily new or novel, that is introduced into a different context and demonstrated to be effective.

Reflexivity: Self-knowledge and awareness of the impact of self on others.

REFERENCES

Bell, K. (2011) Fresh ideas from the frontline. RCN Bulletin, 12th January, pp. 6–7.

Binnie, A. & Titchen, A. (1999) *Freedom to Practise: The Development of Patient-Centred Nursing.* Butterworth Heinemann, Oxford.

Coats, E. (2001) Weaving the body, the creative unconscious, imagination and the arts into practice development. In: *Professional Practice in Health, Education and the Creative Arts* (eds J. Higgs & A. Titchen), pp. 251–263. Blackwell Science, Oxford.

Coats, E., Dewing, J. & Titchen, A. (2006) *Opening Doors on Creativity: Resources to Awaken Creative Working.* A learning resource, Royal College of Nursing, London. http://www.rcn.org.uk/__data/assets/pdf_file/0020/64514/opening_doors.pdf (Accessed 26 September 2012).

Fay, B. (1987) *Critical Social Science.* Polity Press, Cambridge.

Habermas, J. (1972) *Knowledge and Human Interests* (translator J.J. Shapiro). Heinemann, London.

Hardy, S., Titchen, A., Manley, K. & McCormack, B. (2009) *Revealing Nursing Expertise through Practitioner Inquiry.* Wiley-Blackwell, Oxford.

Haynes, J. & Janes, N. (2011) Visioning with service users: tensions and opportunities for a new facilitator. *International Practice Development Journal*, **1** (1), 8. http://www.fons.org/library/journal.aspx (Accessed 26 September 2012).

Henderson, L. (2009) Critical creativity in the development of clinical nurse specialists' practice. In: *Revealing Nursing Expertise through Practitioner Inquiry* (eds S. Hardy, A. Titchen, B. McCormack & K. Manley), pp. 194–215. Wiley-Blackwell, Oxford.

Higgs, J. & Titchen, A. (eds) (2001) *Professional Practice in Health, Education and the Creative Arts.* Blackwell Science, Oxford.

Higgs, J., Titchen, A., Horsfall, D. & Armstrong, H. (2007) *Being Critical & Creative in Qualitative Research.* Hampden Press, Sydney.

Horsfall, D. & Titchen, A. (2009) Disrupting edges – opening spaces: pursuing democracy and human flourishing through creative methodologies. *International Journal of Social Research Methodology*, **12** (2), 147–160.

Kitson, A., McMahon, A., Rafferty, A.M. & Scott, E. (1997) On developing an agenda to influence policy in health-care research for effective nursing: A description of a national R&D priority-setting exercise. *NT Research*, **2** (5), 323–334.

McCormack, B. & Titchen, A. (2006) Critical creativity: melding, exploding, blending. *Educational Action Research: an International Journal*, **14** (2), 239–266.

McCormack, B., McCance, T., Slater, P. F., McCormick J., McArdle C. & Dewing J. (2008) Person-centred outcomes and cultural change. In: *International Practice Development in Nursing and Healthcare* (eds K. Manley, B. McCormack & V. Wilson), pp. 189–214. Blackwell Publishing Ltd., Oxford.

McCormack, B., Dewing, J., Breslin, L., Tobin, C., Manning, M., Coyne-Nevin, A. & Kennedy, K. (2010) The implementation of a model of person-centred practice. In: *Older Person Settings*. Final Report, Health Service Executive, Republic of Ireland, Office of the Nursing & Midwifery Services Director, Republic of Ireland & University of Ulster. Northern Ireland.

McMahon, A. (2008) *The politics of innovation: a critical analysis of the conditions in which innovations in health care may flourish*. PhD thesis, The University of Salford.

McMahon, A. & Darby, M.-A. (1993) *Research and Development: Nurse Led, Unit Wide*. International Council of Nurses, Madrid.

McMahon, A. (1998) Developing practice through research. In: *Research and Development in Clinical Nursing Practice* (eds B. Roe & C. Webb), pp. 219–246. Whurr Publishers Ltd., London.

Patient Opinion (2011) In their words: what patients think about our NHS. www.patientopinion.org.uk/resources/POreport2011.pdf (Accessed 25 March 2011).

Scott, E., McMahon, A., Kitson, A. & Rafferty, A. M. (1999) A national initiative to set priorities for R&D in nursing, midwifery and health visiting: investigating the method. *NT Research*, **4** (4), 283–290.

Titchen, A. & McCormack, B. (2010) Dancing with Stones: Critical creativity as methodology for human flourishing. *Educational Action Research: An International Journal*, **18** (4), 531–554.

Titchen, A. & Horsfall, D. (2011) Embodying creative imagination and expression in qualitative research. In: *Creating Spaces for Qualitative Researching . . . Living Research* (eds J. Higgs, A. Titchen, D. Horsfall & D. Bridges). The Netherlands: Sense, Rotterdam.

Titchen, A., McCormack, B., Wilson, V. & Solman, A. (2011) Human flourishing through body, creative imagination and reflection. *International Practice Development Journal*, **1** (1), 1. http://www.fons.org/library/journal.aspx (Accessed 26 September 2012).

Wilson, V. & Walsh, R. (2008) Changing the culture and context of practice: Evaluating the journey towards family-centred care. In: *International Practice Development in Nursing and Healthcare* (eds K. Manley, B. McCormack & V. Wilson), pp. 215–240. Blackwell Publishing Ltd., Oxford.

12 Building Capacity for Transformation through Practice Development: Two Case Studies in NHS Trusts, England

Jan Dewing[1], Jill Down[2] and IrenaAnna Frei[3]

[1]East Sussex Healthcare NHS Trust & Canterbury Christ Church University, Canterbury, UK
[2]Cambridge University Hospitals NHS Foundation Trust, Cambridge, UK
[3]University Hospital Basel, Basel, Switzerland

INTRODUCTION

There is some published evidence on how practice development manages to establish a strategic foothold within an organisation. There is less evidence on how it can be embedded and sustained in large organisations over time. The aim of this chapter is to offer an insight into practice development work within two NHS Trusts. We begin with Jill updating on the practice development work undertaken at Cambridge University Hospitals (CUH) NHS Foundation Trust 2000–2005, previously Addenbrooke's NHS Trust, to see how it has been able to maintain a presence within this organisation. The main section of this chapter is about an innovative practice development partnership between an NHS Trust in East Sussex (East Sussex Healthcare NHS Trust (ESHT)) and The England Centre for Practice Development at Canterbury Christchurch University in Kent. The partnership has led to a collaborative strategic approach to practice development within nursing and midwifery, committed to developing flourishing people and places (Gaffney, 2011; Seligman, 2011). At the heart of this work lies a creative new joint professorial position driving forwards practice development. One of the authors (Jan) presents an overview of how this work is being achieved in the Trust during organisational redesign and ongoing complexities and also includes examples of some of the current work. Finally, the chapter concludes with an external perspective from IrenaAnna offering a short critique of the preceding sections.

BACKGROUND: THE NATIONAL CONTEXT

Clearly, practitioners will both be influenced by and need to influence and make a significant contribution to national and even international health care policy. All countries have national frameworks with major outcomes. Amongst these are often aims or outcomes related to preventing avoidable harm, providing safer environments and safer care, preventing premature deaths and enhancing quality of life for people with specific illnesses and conditions. Further, more action is needed to facilitate sustainable clinical academic career pathways and further develop research skills (DH, 2010c, p. 7).

There appears to be an increasing demand for health care, spiralling costs and complexity about health care organisation and delivery alongside ever-greater social and professional complexities (Ham, 2012). For example, there are a plethora of new roles (or old roles

Practice Development in Nursing and Healthcare, Second Edition. Edited by Brendan McCormack, Kim Manley and Angie Titchen.
© 2013 John Wiley & Sons, Ltd. Published 2013 by John Wiley & Sons, Ltd.

rebranded); reduced lengths of stay in hospital; expanding roles for health care assistants; and increased specialist, advanced and consultant roles (National Nursing Research Unit, 2008). Government policies, it seems, can be perceived as, on the one hand supportive, such as Essence of Care (DH, 2010a) and on the other, undermining, for instance, targets and extreme economic efficiencies (Baillie et al., 2008, p. 6). Within this there is a consequent practice agenda. For example, the report on nursing and midwifery in England, Front Line Care (DH, 2010b) sets out three overarching sets of challenges for nursing and midwifery:

1. Fewer human and financial resources.
2. Changing health needs, both with supply and demand.
3. Sustainable changes to practice and ways of working.

Fiscal and economic downturns, as hard as they are, offer a time of opportunity to begin the longer term work needed to achieve sustainable change. The Point of Care programme (2009) recommends action is needed at four levels to create sustainable change in health services: (1) the individual staff member; (2) the team, unit or department; (3) the institution as a whole, directed by the board and executive team; and (4) the wider health care system. This is complementary with what practice development has been arguing for many years (e.g. Webster & Dewing, 2007; McCormack et al., 2008, p. 21, 2010).

Practitioners will have to work in new ways and sometimes in new roles in response to service users' needs and in response to the wider business and political agendas. This will probably mean looking at what can be done differently at micro, meso and macros levels. To clarify the micro level concerns, the day-to-day aspects of practice of individual practitioners and clinical teams; the meso, the ward or departmental level; and the macro, the organisational level. These shifts in the philosophy and practice within service delivery will provide important opportunities to increase practitioner impact and strengthening of connections between high-quality care, cost effectiveness and staff and practice development. The Front Line Care report (DH, 2010b, p. 34) clearly advocates local empowerment for the creation of local solutions and states that supporting innovation and creating positive practice environments needs the right leadership and support (Solman & Fitzgerald, 2008, p. 262). Strong leadership at all levels is needed, with those in senior management positions accountable for championing quality in their organisations, from the point of care to the board. Those already in leadership positions will need to support, encourage and challenge staff and inspire and nurture the next generation (DH, 2010b, p. 34). The shift from working in isolated pockets at the micro and meso levels, to developing and delivering practice development in a coordinated way across an organisation is complex and challenging, as we now go onto describe.

PART 1: CAMBRIDGE: FROM CONCEPTION TO DELIVERY AND 7 YEARS ON (JILL)

Back in 2000, a small group of practice development facilitators (PDFs), a patient, audit staff and allied health practitioners worked with an external practice developer/facilitator on an ambitious action research project across CUH NHS Foundation Trust. The project had research ethics committee approval and aimed to refocus their work to develop and implement: a practice development vision, an implementation strategy and an evaluation plan. The starting point of the work was to develop a shared vision with key stakeholders, which would form the central tenet for all the work:

To work in partnership with patients ensuring they are the focus of effective care.

This led to five key areas of work believed to be necessary to achieve the vision:

1. Patient focus: increasing patient involvement in care/services provision.
2. Culture: developing a work-based learning culture.
3. Facilitation skills development: individuals and teams taking responsibility for quality.
4. Evidence-based care: developing, implementing and evaluation of evidence-based practice.
5. Continuous evaluation of care and services.

(Down, 2004, p. 275)

The work had executive backing and was purposefully aligned to deliver the Trust nursing and midwifery strategy, Trust objectives and national policies. However, it is important to note that the practice development strategy was managed separately and in addition to the other strategies because the organisation was complex, large and with multiple agendas and multiple reporting mechanisms.

The practice development project was 'new territory' as it involved very different ways of working for those leading it and a determination to move from a technical approach to project work to an emancipatory style, where the focus is on changing the culture and context of care using a systematic approach with skilled facilitation, using methods that enable teams to learn about and take ownership of changing their culture and practice.

During the early years, there were no written or experiential protocols for undertaking the work and it was very time-consuming to be learning about what we needed to do, how we were to do this and then to actually get on and do the practice development. Tension was created as the PDFs came under increasing pressure to complete the work, and other staff considered it a rather indulgent piece of work when there was a pressure in clinical areas to provide care to patients. However, as a result of this emancipatory approach, the Trust now has in place processes and tools to describe and measure care. It also has a number of staff skilled in facilitation who are now in influential leadership roles.

On reflection of the original work, greater exploration of the organisational culture and the organisation's readiness for the work would have provided some useful information to assist in the preparation and delivery of the project. As the project began, the work was primarily led by PDFs, which resulted in it being perceived as 'their work'. This was, in effect, a barrier to other staff, particularly ward leaders, becoming engaged in the work. As the project neared completion, most PDF's roles in the Trust were cut; a situation reflected across many other organisations at that time. At the same time, authors of a report recommended the need to de-emphasise the PDF role and for organisations to review the variety of roles needed to operationalise practice development methods and develop an infrastructure to enable senior staff to coordinate this work (McCormack& McCance, 2006, p. 7).

The loss of practice development roles was a concern at the time. This period of change and uncertainty proved difficult for the group and the individuals working in it. There was a general sense of loss and grief associated with the rather abrupt ending to an incomplete project and the personal fears of role change or redeployment. Mixed with this was a sense of rejoicing and liberation in the recognition that they had developed new ways of working and

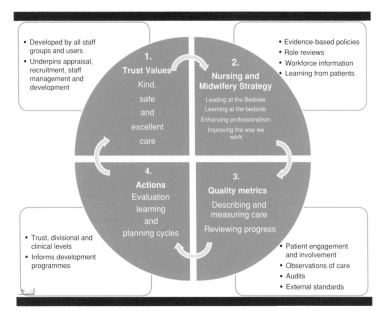

Fig. 12.1   Cambridge University Hospital (CUH) framework for integrating measurement, evaluation and care improvement.

skills development that resulted in personal flourishing and a new confidence in their ability to understand and work in changing cultures. Several of the group gained promotion in the organisation and external to it enabling them to influence the work in different ways and with different groups of stakeholders, using their refined facilitation skills and knowledge of tools to measure and improve practice. Thus, it provided a real opportunity to address some of the concerns highlighted about lack of ownership.

Along with a change in senior leadership and the creation of matron and divisional nurse leaders in the Trust, new opportunities for involving and engaging staff provided clear reporting structures that would influence and shape future practice development work. In particular, the collaborative development of Trust values, a new nursing and midwifery strategy and the development of care quality metrics, all formed a sound framework on which to base future work, particularly as they were all developed by the workforce, patients and users using some of the practice development methods and processes and practice development facilitation skills. A strong patient engagement and involvement strategy was also realised.

Seven years on, the Trust has a more sophisticated and integrated framework for the ongoing measurement, evaluation and improvement of care at Trust, divisional and team levels that encompass several of the original project objectives. It is a shared framework that is a real focus for staff and is now embedded in the everyday working of the Trust (see Figure 12.1).

Sustainability

The original practice development project has pervaded many current areas of work across the Trust with some of the original objectives being sustained more successfully than others.

A patient focus: increasing patient involvement in care/services provision

This area of work has improved and developed considerably with increasing patient involvement since the project:

- Focus groups are regularly facilitated to inform and develop general areas of care and policy such as dignity, nutrition, and more specific areas of care – dementia, management of falls prevention and care of people with learning disabilities whilst in CUH. These are always productive and enjoyed by staff and patients alike, whilst also providing tangible outcomes such as changes to patient documentation and recruitment of volunteers to assist at patient mealtimes. They also provide an opportunity for experienced facilitators to work with and develop the skills of those less experienced.
- Clinical staff interview patients in clinical areas and outpatients weekly for their views on several issues including noise levels, assistance with eating, awareness of their plan of care, the attitude of the staff and their responsiveness to their needs. These areas were all highlighted in the original project by patients as important to them. The feedback is triangulated with weekly care quality audits and additional patient surveys.
- Patient representatives assist clinical staff by working with them to undertake observations of care in clinical areas. Most recently, by observing mealtimes.

Culture: developing a work-based learning culture

Work in this area remains stable:

- The use of observations to understand and learn about the culture of the workplace has been really valued. They are used extensively by the Trust to engage staff and to provide a catalyst for change in the workplace either by: undertaking them across all clinical areas to obtain topic-specific information at micro, meso and macro levels; or providing additional information for an area that has had specific issues, such as an increase in infections or a rise in falls by observing the workplace.
- Reconfiguration of wards and ensuring maximum patient contact time by staff has been positive in assisting the development of work-based learning opportunities, with particular success in dementia training and care of patients with mental and physical health issues. We have learnt that 20-minute sessions in the workplace have had a tangible positive impact.
- Recognition of the project work has provided an opportunity for the Trust to be involved in the development and critique of, and its participation in, the observational component of a national dementia audit.

Facilitation skills development: individuals and teams taking responsibility for quality

This area has a less structured approach now than during the project due to the constraints in releasing staff for regular action learning and development. We now focus this area of work on the large numbers of registered mentors. This has had a direct impact in clinical areas and the development of work-based learning cultures:

- Coaching and coach training for all staff has been developed since the project and is integral to any leadership training.

- Training is provided to ensure that the staff have the skills to facilitate the weekly interviewing of patient in an exploratory way (thus building on the work of the original project).

Evidence-based care: developing, implementing and evaluating evidence-based practice

There is now a structured approach to staff collecting weekly care quality metrics from clinical areas in relation to policy and patient needs. This involves reviewing areas of care including the completion of documentation, pain management, nutritional assessments and management of tissue viability. These data are triangulated with feedback from the patient interviews and workforce information. Dedicated staff now analyse and produce reports monthly, which are available electronically for all staff to access and use. This is a major improvement since the project when clinical staff were collecting, analysing and reporting on the evidence they had collected across the Trust, resulting in delayed review of evidence and thus action planning.

Continuous evaluation of care and services

This work has continued to develop and improve into a much more sophisticated and robust process and is an example of how national directives, regulatory bodies and performance management relating to financial incentives have provided an added impetus for development. Clear processes for the collection, review, reporting and action planning at Trust, divisional and clinical levels are in place, together with regular benchmarking internally between departments and more widely sharing the problems and identifying solutions with other organisations. It has become part of the everyday practice led by strong clinical leaders.

Summary

It is clear from the work at CUH that progress has been made since completion of the project. Some systems and processes still need to be in place to work towards delivering clearly articulated and shared Trust vision and objectives. In addition, the work needs to be iterative and responsive to changes in the context of care. This work is the domain of all teams and individuals. Practice development principles and processes have made an important contribution in determining how outcomes are achieved. On the basis of our experience, I (Jill) would argue that these principles and processes need to be integral, and not additional to, any Trust's strategic planning.

PART 2: THE EAST SUSSEX HEALTHCARE NHS TRUST AND CANTERBURY CHRISTCHURCH EXPERIENCE

In this next section, I (Jan) aim to explore how practice development has begun to get a foothold within one large NHS Trust on the south coast of England. In this case study, the following inter-related activities are described:

- Strategic leadership.
- Influencing at different levels and boundaries.

- Multiple start points.
- Dynamic critical questioning and strategic incrementalisation.
- Voicing positive future and new certainties.
- Stakeholder experiences and false consciousness.
- Diagnostics and evaluation.
- Building and maintaining direction, connections and momentum.

Note: There are more activities in the process of embedding practice development than shown above. This chapter is simply focusing on the ones above.

The organisational context: strategic leadership

The preparation for a strategic approach to practice development began in 2008, when two influential nurse leaders, the Deputy Director of Nursing in a Community Trust and Head of the Nursing Department at Canterbury Christchurch University met and began discussing how to do things differently. This has been likened by both as 'two worlds colliding' (Jackson & Webster, 2012). Although both leaders had strong values and beliefs about practice development and shared a similar vision, at that point in time, others did not place a high value on practice development and it was absent in strategy, policy, principles and in everyday talk and action. Therefore, strategic leadership and building relationships were a first step in this context.

Both organisations were undergoing significant change with redesign and senior management changes. Although turbulent, it was felt important to seize an opportunity to influence, moving the respective organisations from being focused on one path: 'the way we've always done it' (Bate & Robert, 2007) to being open to investing in new ways of working that could offer different benefits within the new organisation. From this initial collision, a partnership was established that aimed to:

> *develop a transformative partnership that demonstrates excellence in academic and professional practice thereby enriching the individuals, teams, organisations and communities we serve.*
> *(Jackson & Webster, 2012)*

Influencing at different levels and boundaries

The next set of activities was about influencing for a new vision. Both recognised that the priority was to secure influential support for a new partnership at the earliest opportunity at a senior level within the two respective organisations. This plus some financial planning enabled the creation of a joint clinical professorial post in person-centred research and practice development. This signalled a change of direction, as such a post is highly unusual, if not unique. The post provides evidence of the visible and integrated approach to strategic leadership and steers in both organisations. Some of the challenges in setting up this post and the early competing agendas have been described elsewhere (Jackson & Webster, 2012). Just as the post was beginning to achieve outcomes and demonstrate some impact in key services, another organisational redesign took place. In March 2011, the local acute and community NHS Trusts were dissolved and a new joint Trust, ESHT was created. A relatively seamless transfer, at least on paper, was achieved, although for practice development it was once again a time of uncertainty as practice development did not have a formal 'place' in the acute Trust.

The immediate challenges were the following:

- Having the purposes, principles and methods of practice development recognised and understood.
- Finding a place for it in the new organisation along with senior leadership support.
- A massively enlarged organisation and workforce to work with and no additional resource to begin with.
- Engaging staff who have moved into the new organisation, as well as staff new to practice development.
- Beginning during a period of instability about organisational, nursing and midwifery strategies.
- Ongoing redesign in senior clinical and support posts.

The new organisation brought into the existing partnership another key player in the shape of the Director of Nursing. An unknown entity to begin with, the director had previous experience of practice development and was highly supportive with a strong vision for the future. She had an understanding, combined with an appreciation, of how practice development could contribute, plus she could vision the benefits of a more direct partnership with academia in the longer term.

Multiple starting points

It is tempting to think that the priority was to establish a practice development strategy and that elements of practice development strategy for a whole organisation would consist of linear steps approached sequentially, which should include:

- reaching consensus on shared vision;
- agreeing on purpose, aims and objectives;
- developing a plan for achieving the objectives;
- marshalling and allocating the resources required to implement the plan;
- monitoring and evaluation.

And yes, it would be very convenient if creating a practice development strategy was done in this way, with the bigger picture requirements dealt with first and then the smaller operational needs addressed. However, the reality in ESHT was that there are already in existence multiple, complex large and small strategies, policies and agendas at play, as in any large organisation, and of course, patients and families were already receiving services and care. The organisation brought with it history and baggage and varying areas and levels of effectiveness. In addition, resources, as is the way in the NHS, are seldom available at the time of need and the complexity of practice agendas meant that there was often a multi-layered and inter-dependent picture. Thus, all the elements of the strategy would be inter-dependent and must be situated within current workplace and corporate cultures (Johnson et al., 2008). Working out where practice development should sit in the organisation was challenging, given that the historic organisational structure encouraged 'silo' working. The solution was not to make practice development fit somewhere, but to focus on the methods and processes incorporating matrix working by:

- capturing opportunities for moments of moment (Dewing et al., 2009): starting with small pilot projects and working with practitioners, leaders and managers who demonstrated potential;
- bringing added value to existing work streams and projects;
- bringing in other sources of evidence and more effective processes to add rigour to local work;
- role-modelling effective facilitation and leadership;
- creating positive futures and visions;
- talent identification;
- building up a learning culture through critical connections and critical mass (Kolb, 1984, p. 3).

Dynamic critical questioning and strategic incrementalisation

The initial task in our strategy development was probably seen as the compilation and dissemination of a mission statement, or in practice development terms, a vision statement generated from shared values and beliefs. As has been argued before, in the 'real world', there is no one single task or starting point. In the ESH Trust case, this was further compounded because of organisational instability, the ongoing redesign and a large number of senior management and leadership posts being rebranded and appointed to. Therefore, the context did not lend itself to the typical initiation activities. Instead, multiple activities took place at micro, macro and meso levels as opportunities emerged and as they could be created. For example, there were already in existence stated core values and beliefs about the purpose of nursing and midwifery from both previous organisations, so these were used as a basis to show how practice development could bring added value to strategic work. An initial simple framework illustrated this (Figure 12.2).

Small pilot projects were created to illustrate potential. And with a view to the longer term, an integrative dynamic method was used for strategy development. This method included drawing on current realities around the organisation both about where practice patterns, especially patient experience, were at and what the possibilities were, from small micro level practice development projects (or those with practice development potential) already in place along with a dynamic critical questioning process; similar to the one described by de Wit and Meyer (2008). These authors offer a perspective known as strategic incrementalisation that involves creating a dynamic relationship between questions about aims and objectives, the planning for implementation and the available resources. Interestingly, Moncrieff (1999) discusses strategy dynamics whereby strategy is partially deliberate and partially unplanned. And Wheatley (1999, p. 38) further describes how strategies should be 'just in time'. The planned and unplanned or even chaotic elements constituted our emergent strategy in the short term. In turn, this enabled us to be highly attuned to the emergence of opportunities and threats in the environment and also to 'strategies in action' or the *ad hoc* actions by many people from all parts of the newly forming organisation, who were creating new meaning and new realities around them. The practice developer, because of their understanding of practical knowledge and contexts and their expertise, can capture this evidence and potentiality in a

Nursing and midwifery values are:
working together;
delivering the right outcomes;
highly educated and developed workforce;
creating the conditions that enable
empowerment for practitioners; and
innovation.

Practice development aims to:
transform care and services so that they are person-centred,
safer and more effective;
ensure that the best evidence and research informs everyday
practice; and
enable people to flourish and create good places to work.

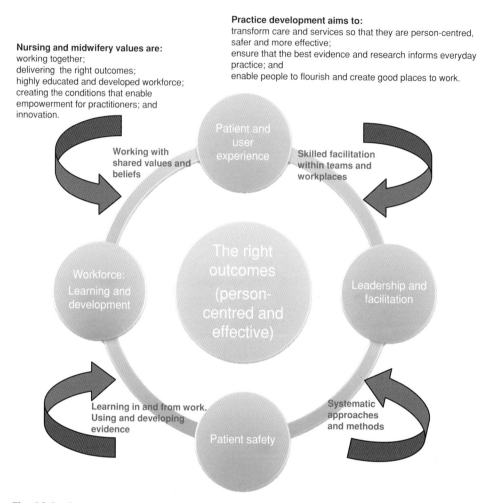

Fig. 12.2   Practice development: adding value to nursing and midwifery.

way that many conventional strategy developers miss. This of course meant that our initial planned strategy did change quite radically in the first few months. Although messy in the early phases, the key benefits of this method are that it led to a more effective strategy. In particular, one that is more:

- suitable for others or fit for purpose;
- feasible, in that it can be made to work by others;
- acceptable, in that others will want to make it work in their place of work.

(Johnson & Scholes, 2000, p. 8).

On reflection, the sequential strategic incrementalisation approach is probably beneficial for practice development, as it is much more 'real' as it enables the dynamic evolution of strategy rather than a forced conception and delivery on paper within a very tight timescale. As many point out, strategy development should be a repetitive learning cycle not a linear progression towards a (single) clearly defined and final destination. This approach accommodates complexity and even chaos reasonably well. The method requires the practice developer to have enough experience to see the connections between smaller and larger aspects of the strategy, between practice and policy, as well as to adapt practice development models, and yet remain consistent to its core principles, especially around patient and user experience. In other words, to contemplate and plan for influencing within webs of connections that seem to be everywhere in the organisation, whether or not they are effective. Inadequate understanding of larger scale organisational agendas and how these tend to play out must be a key concern for many practice developers when 'upgrading' their work and moving into macro or larger scale strategy development.

Example: the nursing and midwifery documentation project

This 2-year project was a 'must do' for the Trust for compliance reasons. It provided an opportunity to (1) demonstrate practice development principles, methods and processes; (2) develop the facilitation skills of a cohort of practitioners and (3) introduce peer review and enhance governance connections across the Trust. This is in addition to improving evidence of personalised and evidence-based patient care.

A participatory action research approach, with ten foci, was used with practitioners being the main stakeholder groups.

Achievements in year 1 include the following:

- Increased awareness about the contribution of documentation to personalised, safer and effective patient care.
- Improved documentation as measured by various evaluation methods.
- Increased and informed compliance in using the Trust-wide integrated patient document and in developing integrated care pathways.
- Focus on 'patient choice and voice' in daily documentation and on evidencing work around consent and mental capacity.
- Drop in work place session to support and encourage real time discussion about documentation of patient care.
- Quick response email query and help service.
- Move away from the small-scale 'hidden' *ad hoc* alterations to documentation to a more open and transparent process.
- Enhanced governance by practitioners including peer review. Increased awareness about the contribution that individuals and teams can make.
- A regular Trust documentation newsletter and various workplace learning resources.

Voicing positive future and new certainties

Transformational leaders (Kouzes & Posner, 2007, p. 130) and effective, enabling facilitators (Shaw et al., 2008, p. 152) must voice beliefs in a positive future and create certainties, especially when turbulence is a feature; although, it serves little purpose to provide certainties where they do not exist. Not promising the undeliverable is important. What matters for the purposes of our strategy development is having a clear view – based on the best available evidence and on defensible assumptions from acquired professional expertise – of what it seems possible to accomplish within the constraints of a given set of circumstances. Using the best available evidence is often a major omission in how many strategies are developed. We recognise that as the situation changes, some opportunities for pursuing objectives will disappear and others arise. Some implementation approaches will become impossible, while others, previously impossible or unimagined, will become viable.

Our strategy needed to start work with stakeholders early on, including working with their perceptions and expectations. Being 'out and about' and engaging with different stakeholders, from a shared exploratory stance, is important as this helps with knowing what the realities of different stakeholders are. However, for the practice developer, there is the challenge of false consciousness to be addressed. False consciousness can be thought of as self-misunderstandings (Fay, 1996, p. 128). This can be an individual state or a 'whole group state' where members are stuck within limited and inadequate schemes of meaning and ultimately, argues Fay, they are unable to perceive that they are stuck by their own thinking. Morgan (1997, p. 4) conceives of this as psychic imprisonment. People who have become so encultured that they are unable to see any other way of being and working, and find it very hard if not impossible to conceive and perceive any other realities (Brown & McCormack, 2009). Thus, as a practice developer, I need to accept this position as a starting point but not, myself, become constrained from seeing and voicing a more positive future (Wheatley, 2007, p. 13).

Diagnostics and evaluation

Diagnostics and then ongoing evaluation work, including culture scanning, is being undertaken to establish current patterns and practices and to estimate the degree of false consciousness that exists. Scanning can help ascertain the orientation and focus of the organisation. For us, this particularly is true in regard to:

- person-centred moments (compliance only focused organisation);
- person-centred patterns (compliance and quality improvement focused organisation);
- person-centred culture (compliance, quality improvement and innovation focused organisation).

All of the above mean that we need to focus more on the relationships with their patterns of critical connections rather than on the 'things' to be achieved. I perceive each relationship as a bundle of potentiality to bring into a network of connections. For the practice developer, the essence of being 'strategic' probably lies in the capacity for emotionally intelligent gardening (Titchen, 2011), rather than being able to write and direct detailed strategic plans or simply being a project manager. Strategic thinking is about interpreting, and continuously reinterpreting, the desired direction alongside the possibilities presented by shifting circumstances. However, this alone is insufficient, and strategic doing and being must also be achieved.

Direction: building and maintaining direction, connections and momentum

Although a sense of direction is important, it can also stifle creativity, especially if it is rigidly enforced. In a complex world, coordinated fluidity becomes more important than a finely tuned strategy on paper. When a strategy becomes too internalised into an already existing corporate culture, it can lead to 'groupthink' with no space to think outside of the box or to be creative; in itself, another form of collective false consciousness. People can become inward looking and focus on building up ever more complex structures and processes rather than simplifying matters. This is another argument for having a more process-orientated approach to strategy development. Strategy development should not be an analytical exercise undertaken by the few – but instead, it needs to be creative and involve the majority. By this, I do not mean simply holding awareness or information sessions about strategy once it is planned. It is the building of connections that is vital (Wheatley, 1999, p. 127). Connections, especially rich connections, according to Donde et al. (2000), transmit information and enable the creation of meaning among people working in sub-cultures across the organisation. In the longer term, this mechanism will enable the establishment of systems with an improved capacity for learning (Dewing, 2009). After 1 year, the sense of momentum and of a culture change beginning has just started being noticed and commented on by some practitioners and clinical leaders in nursing.

Learning opportunities to experience the connection and early experiences to feel the contribution that practice development can make

- Local team and ward projects on a variety of topics or needs.
- Piloting opportunities.
- Master classes for senior nursing and midwifery leaders and managers in the Trust.
- Practice development workshops, which bring in external people via The England Centre for Practice Development working in practice development and related fields.
- Master classes on key topics: for example essential care rounds, observation of practice, patient's stories and clinical supervision.
- Building a culture of facilitation – focus in year 1–2 is on clinical supervision.
- Participating in practice development open spaces (associate practice development team membership).
- University staff setting up practice development roles with clinical wards/departments.
- Writing and presenting.

As our practice development strategy comes to life, there are many concerns and issues that can be addressed because of apparent complexity within the organisation. To add to this, many people seem to absorb this as chaos and start to replicate it, which needlessly adds to its potency and lifespan. Chaos theory (Wheatley, 1999, p. 117) deals with turbulent systems that rapidly become disordered. Nevertheless, complexity is not quite so unpredictable. It involves multiple agents interacting in such a way that a glimpse of patterning may appear, however unconnected it may seem. Chaos is a part of order in systems and can also indicate a time and space for a new ordering to emerge. Practice development can thrive in complexity and can begin work in chaos or where there are spaces of discontinuity. Drucker (1969), of course, used the phrase 'Age of Discontinuity' to describe the way change forces disruptions into the continuity of our lives. He identifies four broad sources of discontinuity: (1) new technologies, (2) globalisation, (3) cultural pluralism and (4) knowledge capital. This work was later expanded on by Handy (1998), and Toffler (1970) also added to this, describing the trend for accelerating of change. Therefore, we cannot assume that trends that exist today will continue into the future. Further, all strategy has a limited lifespan and will decay (Hamel, 2002) to make way for something else. Practice development at a strategic level needs to be multi-faceted (Melton et al., 2011) and yet relatively simple to survive in complex cultures.

In the short term, it feels like being part of a web or constellation (Proctor-Thomson, 2008) where complexity is escalating, and where many of the existing enterprises are not equipped

Table 12.1 The five disciplines of a learning organisation.

Personal responsibility, self-reliance and mastery
We accept that we are the masters of our own destiny. We make decisions and live with the consequences of them. When a problem needs to be fixed, or an opportunity exploited, we take the initiative to learn the required skills to get it done.

Mental models
We need to explore our personal mental models (e.g. values and beliefs) to understand the subtle effect they have on our behaviour.

Shared vision
The vision of where we want to be in the future is discussed and communicated to all. It provides guidance and energy for the journey ahead.

Team learning
We learn together in teams. This involves a shift to 'a spirit of enquiry'.

We look at the whole rather than the parts.
This is what Senge (1990) calls the 'fifth discipline'. It is the glue that integrates the other four into a coherent strategy.

to cope with this complexity. Because of this, being creative in the workplace and making use of the learning that comes from being creative is becoming the single most important survival competency in the health care workforce. Tied into this is the ability to be resilient. As we move towards becoming more simplified and effective, we will become more of a learning organisation. Revans (1983) famously pointed out that in a learning organisation, the rates of learning must be faster than or equal to the rate of change in an organisation. Then Senge (1990) popularised the notion of the learning organisation, with the underlying theory that an organisation's capability is strongly influenced by its ability to gather, analyse and use information. Much of that information or knowledge capital lies within the potentiality and connections of the workforce itself. Senge argues that an organisation needs to be structured in such a way that it enables people to continuously expand their capacity for learning and to be productive, to have new patterns of thinking, to be an active part of collective aspirations that are encouraged, and that people in the organisation can see the 'whole picture' together (see Table 12.1). Practice developers, such as I, in ESHT are working out the most effective ways of making a major contribution to creating learning that is necessary for driving forward an effective culture and that will ultimately enable flourishing.

These five disciplines are all captured in the values, principles and methods of practice development. To help build that strategic discipline, our longer term vision is to have a closer formalised partnership with a local education and research provider institution. Work has also begun on this aspect of our strategy.

PARTNERSHIP WITH CANTERBURY CHRISTCHURCH UNIVERSITY

Having a more formal relationship with the university based around shared values and needs makes sense on a number of fronts. It brings added value to the academic context and can refocus the ultimate purpose of learning and teaching. Boyer (1990) has advanced four forms of scholarship: (1) discovery, (2) integration, (3) application and (4) teaching. Discovery (pp. 17–18) is generally what is understood as research committed to developing new knowledge. The scholarship of integration (pp. 18–19) is focused on developing perspectives on knowledge. It is '. . . serious, disciplined work that seeks to interpret, draw together, and bring new insight to bear on original research' (p. 19). This scholarship is represented by work at the boundaries of a discipline where it overlaps and connects with other disciplines. The scholarship of application (pp. 21–23) is often characterised as 'service', which is not currently given much reward (Thompson & Watson, 2008; Rolfe, 2011). Boyer argues that service activities must be connected to faculty specialty, must be serious, demanding and accountable, and flow out of the expertise in the specialty. It may be more collaborative to say that both service and faculty knowledge need to be connected. We are engaged in a collaborative endeavour to work out how to do this in ways that bring mutual learning and benefits. The development of both in the Trust and the faculty linked to practice development work in the Trust helps to develop scholarly capacity. Mutual learning and benefits also engage staff in influencing front line practice development work that is then brought back into the classroom to bring student experience more alive. Practice development work also enables academic staff to develop a different sort of credibility and impact in their support of learning in the practice environment that is so important in curricula that are 50% assessed in practice. This will become more important especially where our professional body expectations are that education creates future leaders capable of managing complexity at the point of registration. Practice development does not replace traditional forms of scholarship and research, rather it complements them and is vital in enabling educationalists to look more creatively at learning and at how practitioners make use of patient experience and other forms of evidence.

To summarise our engagement to date:

Constellationing
Beginning small, beginning quietly,
Multiple places, multiples of everything.
Nothing flows, disconnections abound,
Being in realities, still not seeing.
Everyone has a truth, the few have a true grasp,
The walking are asleep.
Being too late, missing in the fog,
Another opportunity goes passing by.
Chaos, unorganised movement,
Complexity with a dash of chaos.
Too much, it seems the same as before,
Repainting the landscape scene by scene.
Taking hold, taking shape.
Not too tight, steer a constant course.
Re-organising, unpicking 'business as usual',
Weathering the planned, working with the unplanned.
To do and be different, connect potentials,
No guarantee of permanency.

PART 3: A CRITIQUE

The complexity of large health care organisations presents a challenge to establish a successful practice development strategy. It is far from being an easy endeavour, as we can see in Jill and Jan's accounts. The journeys they have taken to build a Trust-wide practice development strategy are diverse. To achieve sustainable change within the constraints of an economically driven health service, frequent reorganisations on a small or even large scale, and changing health needs seems difficult at first sight. At second sight, the approaches taken prove that considerable success can be achieved.

As an outsider to the United Kingdom, I view policy papers on health care services provided genuinely at a national level as a strength. The Front Line Care report (DH, 2010b) supports a framework for practice development strategies and the recommendations offer direction for involvement of all levels of health care practices, professionals and patients. In this lie a driver and the power to successfully change health care practice and to reach the ultimate aim of person-centred health care (McCormack & McCance, 2010).

In the first case study of a practice development journey, Jill points at some important issues worthwhile to be taken into consideration for a Trust-wide strategy. Firstly and particularly important is that practice development is on the agenda of the Trust's executive board, hence an integral part of the institutional strategy. Secondly, time is often underestimated when planning a change process. Jill's account shows clearly that cultural change such as being responsive to service users' needs, cutback of resources, and building capacity takes time. Thirdly, pursuing a vision requires both flexibility as progress is made along the path of practice development and making use of influences of parallel processes and changes.

The initial intention of the practice development strategy was the engagement of all stakeholders within the organisation. However, having the PDF role got in the way of achieving that process outcome. The crisis caused by the cutting of that role and placing the PDFs in operational roles was an enabler in eventually achieving broader engagement and involvement of staff who continued the development work. This gives evidence of well-thought-out work supporting those people in becoming capable to organise and execute the courses of action needed to produce the given results (Bandura, 1997). The effect of this long-term journey is considerable. Above all, a refined framework illustrating the core issues of the practice development work is embedded in everyday practice. Everyone working in a large institution knows what that means. Moreover, it serves as a frame for evaluation and reporting improvements. There will hopefully be no end of the practice development journey in CUH and the challenge to navigate the boat through tidal waves will remain. However, they can draw on a broad experience and outcomes that will take practice development to the next level of maturity.

There are several common issues raised in the two accounts in this chapter that are important to a practice development strategy, for example, being flexible and working with what is happening anyway. However, in Jan's report there is one special aspect of networking: the partnership of ESHT with Canterbury Christchurch University. This is a real asset to practice development. To engage in an academic-service partnership challenges the traditional partnership of working alongside within highly structured organisations by requiring people to step out of their own silos. The driving forces for an academic-service partnership, as De Geest et al. (2010) describe them, are: the epidemiological and demographic imperative; the preparation and availability of the health care workforce; the new research imperative to demonstrate impact on outcomes; the patient safety and quality imperative; and the health care economic and policy imperative. A service and an academic organisation with a joint appointment of a clinical professor enables the pursuit of aims concerning the building of human capacity for innovations, investing in person-centred care and hence, improving service users' experience:

> *Each will need the courage to let go of prior behaviours that segregate resources and learn instead to embrace interdependence. This requires communication transparency, clarity of mutual goals, political vigilance as resources are shared, and clarifying policies (Warner & Burton, 2009, p. 333).*

This second more comprehensive case study also draws the readers' attention to the important role of leadership. The presence of strong leadership affects structural empowerment and can influence professional practice behaviours through self-efficacy (Manojlovich, 2005). Managers and practice developers are at the forefront in influencing policy. Thus, they are key players in shaping and developing a practice development strategy. Consequently, investment in leadership and facilitation development is also an investment in health care staff. In turn, this is of great value since practice development is only successful and sustainable if it is at the heart of everyone working in health care services.

SUMMARY

The immediate aim of practice development is to enhance patient experience, although this must be achieved through enhancing the work experience of health care staff. Even though competence is important, many senior leaders and managers still fail to value and nurture human knowledge capital and social networking. These factors are as important as the technical aspects in creating effective cultures and organisations. Practice development in the Trusts discussed here has been systematically working at enhancing social networking and learning. Ultimately, as practice developers, the purpose of practice development work is human flourishing (McCormack & Titchen, 2006; Gaffney, 2011; Seligman, 2011).

Would exactly the same method be used again in these organisations? Probably not, as the local context and events at any one time play a significant part in how practice development evolves. However, the guiding principles would be the same or similar: strategy needs to be both planned and fluid enough to allow for an element of the unplanned aiming to offer a complexity-realist perspective rather than an ultimate and fixed master plan; dynamism needs to be injected into strategic work, which can otherwise feel quite 'dry' and meaningless to many practitioners in their everyday work; and this work needs to be both visionary and realist. However, the real test of strategy, and therefore of how effective practice development will be, is not what is written but what is lived by health care staff through their practices and crucially what is experienced by patients and service users. Thus, in organisations that find it very difficult to break away from their emphasis on over-learned behaviours, practice developers strive to create enough of the best conditions that enable others to make different choices about how they work and learn how to do this:

> *One's philosophy is not best expressed in words; it is expressed in the choices one makes... and the choices we make are ultimately our responsibility. Eleanor Roosevelt (1884–1962)*

REFERENCES

Baillie, L., Gallagher, A. & Wainwright, P. (2008) *Defending Dignity: Opportunities and Challenges for Nursing*. Royal College of Nursing, London.

Bandura, A. (1997) *Self-efficacy: The Exercise of Control*. WH Freeman and Company, New York.

Bate, S.P. & Robert, G. (2007) *Bringing User Experience to Healthcare Improvement: The Concepts, Methods and Practices of Experience-Based Design*. Radcliffe Publishing, Oxford.

Boyer, E.L. (1990) *Scholarship Reconsidered: Priorities of the Professoriate, A Special Report*. The Carnegie Foundation for the Advancement of Teaching, Princeton, NJ.

Brown, D. & McCormack, B. (2009) Developing the practice context to enable more effective pain management with older people: an action research approach. *Implementation Science*, **6** (9). http:www.implementationscience.com/content/6/1/9 (Accessed 2 May 2011).

De Geest, S., Sullivan Mark, E. M., Rich, V., Spichiger, E., Schwendimann, R., Spirig, R. & Van Malderen, G. (2010) Developing a financial framework for academic service partnership: models of the United States and Europe. *Journal of Nursing Scholarship*, **42** (3), 295–304.

Department of Health (DH) (2010a) *The Essence of Care: Patient-Focused Benchmarking for Health Care Practitioners*. Department of Health, London. http://www.dh.gov.uk/en/Publicationsandstatistics/ Publications/PublicationsPolicyAndGuidance/DH_119969 (Accessed 3 March 2012).

Department of Health (DH) (2010b) Front-line care: the future of nursing and midwifery in England 2010. The Prime Minister's Commission on the Future of Nursing and Midwifery in England. Department of Health/The Stationery Office, London. http://cnm.independent.gov.uk (Accessed 22 November 2011).

Department of Health (DH) (2010c) *NHS Outcomes Framework*. Department of Health, London.

Dewing, J. (2009) Moments of movement: active learning and practice development. *Nurse Education in Practice*, **10** (1), 22–26.

Dewing, J., Titchen, A. & McCormack, B. (2009) Practice development and the potential for integrating transformational practice with research: A response to Editorial: Thompson, D.R., Watson, R., Quinn, T., Worrall-Carter, L., O'Connell, B. 2008. Practice development: what is it and why should we be doing it? *Nurse Education in Practice*, **8** (4), 221–222. *Nurse Education in Practice*, **9** (1), 1–4.

de Wit, B. & Meyer, R. (2008) *Strategy: Process, Content and Context*. Thomson Learning, London.

Donde, P., Ashmos, D.P., Duchon, D. & McDaniel, R.R. (2000) Organisational responses to complexity: the effect on organizational performance. *Journal of Organisational Change Management*, **13** (6) 577–594.

Down, J. (2004) From conception to delivery: a journey towards a trust-wide strategy to developing a culture of patient centredness. In: *Practice Development in Nursing* (eds B. McCormack, K. Manley & R. Garbett), pp. 207–287. Blackwell Publishing Ltd., Oxford.

Drucker, P. (1969) *The Age of Discontinuity*. Heinemann, London.

Fay, B. (1996) *Contemporary Philosophy of Social Science: A Multicultural Approach*. Blackwell Publishing Ltd., Oxford.

Gaffney, M. (2011) *Flourishing*. Penguin Ireland, Dublin.

Ham, C. (2012) Inertia rather than privatisation is the biggest threat facing the NHS. http://www.kingsfund.org.uk/blog/nhs_inertia.html (Accessed 4 March 2012).

Hamel, G. (2002) *Leading the Revolution*. Penguin Books, New York.

Handy, C. (1998) *Understanding Organisations*. Penguin Books, London.

Jackson, C. & Webster, A. (2012) Swimming against the tide; developing a flouirshing partnership for organisational transformation. *International Practice Development Journal*, **1** (2).

Johnson, G. & Scholes, K. (2000) *Exploring Public Sector Strategy*. FT Prentice Hall, London.

Johnson, G, Scholes, K & Whittington, R (2008) *Exploring Corporate Strategy*, 8th edn. FT Prentice Hall, Essex.

Kolb, D.A. (1984) *Experiential Learning: Experience as the Source of Learning and Development*. Prentice Hall, Upper Saddle River, NJ.

Kouzes, J.M. & Posner, B.Z. (2007) *The Leadership Cahllenge*, 4th edn. Jossey-Bass, San Francisco, CA.

Manojlovich, M. (2005) The effect of nursing leadership on hospital nurses' professional practice behaviors. *Journal of Nursing Administration*, **35** (7/8), 366–374.

McCormack, B., Dewar, B., Wright, J., Garbett, R., Harvey, G. & Ballantine, K. (2006) A Realist Synthesis of Evidence Relating to Practice Development: Final Report to NHS Education For Scotland and NHS Quality Improvement, Scotland. http://www.healthcareimprovementscotland.org/previous_resources/ archived/pd_-_evidence_synthisis.aspx (Accessed 4 November 2012).

McCormack, B., Dewing, J., Breslin, L., Coyne-Nevin, A., Kennedy, K., Manning, M., Peelo-Kilroe, L., Catherine Tobin, C. & Slater, P. (2010) Developing person-centred practice: nursing outcomes arising from changes to the care environment in residential settings for older people. *International Journal of Older People Nursing*, **5** (2), 93–107.

McCormack, B., Manley, K. & Walsh, K. (2008) Person-centred systems and processes. In: *International Practice Development in Nursing and Healthcare* (eds K. Manley, B. McCormack & V. Wilson), pp. 17–41. Blackwell Publishing Ltd., Oxford.

McCormack, B. & McCance, T. (2006) Development of a framework for person-centred nursing. *Journal of Advanced Nursing*, **56** (5), 1–8.

McCormack, B. & McCance, T. (2010) Person-centred processes. In: *Person-Centred Nursing: Theory and Practice*. Wiley-Blackwell, Oxford. doi: 10.1002/9781444390506.ch6.

McCormack, B. & Titchen, A. (2006) Critical creativity: melding, exploding, blending. *Educational Action Research*, **14** (2), 239–266.

Melton, J., Forsyth, K., & Freeth, D. (2011) The individual practice development theory: an individually focused practice development theory that helps target practice development resources. *Journal of Evaluation in Clinical Practice*. doi: 10.1111/j.1365-2753.2010.01618.x. [Epub ahead of print]

Moncrieff, J. (1999) Is strategy making a difference? *Long Range Planning Review* **32** (2), 273–276.

Morgan, G. (1997) *Images of Organisation*, 2nd edn. Sage Publications, Thousand Oaks, CA.

National Nursing Research Unit (2008) What matters to patients: the nursing contribution. *Policy Issue*, **9**, 3.

Point of Care (2009) *Are You Seeing the Person in the Patient?* King's Fund, London.

Proctor-Thomson, S.B. (2008) *Developing Leadership Practices: Constellations or Stars? What is Being Developed in Leadership Development?* Lancaster University Management School, Centre for Excellence in Leadership (CEL), Lancaster.

Revans, R. (1983) *The ABC of Action Learning*. Republished 1998. Lemos & Crane, London.

Rolfe, G. (2011) Fast food for thought: how to survive and thrive in the corporate university. 22nd International Networking Education in Healthcare Conference, September 6–8, Cambridge University, Cambridge.

Roosevelt, Eleanor (1884–1962) http://www.brainyquote.com/quotes/authors/e/eleanor_roosevelt_2.html# ixzz1niKFuH67 (Accessed 14 March 2012).

Seligman, M.E.P. (2011) *Flourish: A New Understanding of Happiness and Well-Being – and How to Achieve Them*. Nicholas Brealey, London.

Senge, P. (1990) *The Fifth Discipline*. Century Books, London.

Shaw, T., Dewing, J., Young, R., Devlin, M., Boomer, C. & Legius, M. (2008) Enabling practice development: delving into the concept of facilitation from a practitioner perspective. In: *International Practice Development in Nursing and Healthcare* (eds K. Manley, B. McCormack & V. Wilson), pp. 147–169. Blackwell Publishing Ltd., Oxford.

Solman, A. & Fitzgerald, M. (2008) Leadership support. In: *International Practice Development in Nursing and Healthcare* (eds K. Manley, B. McCormack & V. Wilson), pp. 261–262. Blackwell Publishing Ltd., Oxford.

Thompson, D. & Watson, R. (2008) Asymmetrical professors – unbalanced or misunderstood? Response to Rolfe, G. (2007) Nursing scholarship and the asymmetrical professor [Nurse Education in Practice, **7** (3) pp. 123–127]. *Nurse Education in Practice*, **8** (2), 73–75.

Titchen, A. (2011) Creating a rose garden: showing links between cause and effect in practice development evaluation. *International Practice Development Journal*, **1** (1). http://www.fons.org/library/journal/volume1-issue1/article6 (Accessed 3 March 2012).

Toffler, A. (1970) *Future Shock*. Bantom Books, New York.

Warner, J.R. & Burton, D.A. (2009) The policy and politics of emerging academic-service partnerships. *Journal of Professional Nursing*, **25** (6), 329–334.

Webster, J. & Dewing, J. (2007) Growing a practice development strategy for community hospitals. *Practice Development in Healthcare*, **6** (2), 97–106.

Wheatley, M.J. (1999) *Leadership and the New Science: Discovering Order in a Chaotic World*. Berrett-Koehler Publishers, San Francisco, CA.

Wheatley, M.J. (2007) *Finding Our Way Leadership For Uncertain Times*. Berrett-Koehler, San Francisco, CA.

13 The Use of Action Hypotheses to Demonstrate Practice Development Strategies in Action

Kim Manley[1], Randal Parlour[2] and Joan Yalden[3]

[1]Canterbury Christ Church University, Canterbury, UK
[2]St. Conal's Hospital, Letterkenny, Ireland
[3]Practice Development Facilitator, Melbourne, Australia

INTRODUCTION AND OVERVIEW

This chapter aims to show how key strategies in practice development (PD) achieve similar outcomes and impact across different organisational contexts. This will be achieved by sharing the journeys and the transferable insights we have gained from working with PD principles across three diverse settings: (1) a community setting, from the perspective of introducing an evidence-based approach to continence care in Ireland; (2) an acute National Health Service (NHS) Trust working initially with specialist nurses and midwives in England; and finally, (3) an acute stroke unit in a public health care organisation in Australia involving the development of a dysphagia screening tool with a multi-disciplinary team. Not only were the contexts and countries very different, but also the time frames, client groups and the primary purpose of the PD journeys experienced by both ourselves and the project participants.

We use the metaphor of a journey to describe the inquiry adventure we embarked on together to illustrate:

- how as facilitators of PD and research, we used the principles of collaboration, inclusion and participation (CIP) across our different projects;
- the journeys experienced, from their starting points – the triggers and issues experienced in practice – through to the use and refinement of strategies implemented to address these triggers, and ultimately the outcomes achieved; and
- how as authors we have worked together to make sense of our very different projects using a framework to tease out the commonalities and differences in our approaches across three common themes that are often experienced in PD work: (1) achieving a shared vision; (2) developing effective workplace cultures and (3) getting evidence used in practice.

To enable us to theorise about the strategies that consistently appear to demonstrate similar outcomes, we have used a framework termed as 'action hypothesis' (AH). This framework is used to illustrate the theories we have developed from our collaborative inquiry across our three projects. We have worked with and identified: three common triggers/starting points; the goals we set out to achieve; the strategies we used to achieve the goals and whether our goals were achieved and finally, the evidence that demonstrated outcomes.

Practice Development in Nursing and Healthcare, Second Edition. Edited by Brendan McCormack, Kim Manley and Angie Titchen.
© 2013 John Wiley & Sons, Ltd. Published 2013 by John Wiley & Sons, Ltd.

This framework originally developed by Binnie and Titchen (1999) has further been refined in a project with consultant nurses (CNs) and aspiring consultant nurses (ACNs) to identify transferable insights about PD and the facilitation processes that transcend the scope and variation in different contexts (Manley & Titchen, 2012).

Sharing our AHs will enable others to try the strategies out in response to similar triggers within their own contexts, as well as contribute to ongoing refinement of both the theories resulting and the strategies used.

We start then with our three different contexts and also explain how we planned to use the CIP principles, underpinning PD as a complex intervention to achieve our intended purposes (see Chapters 1 and 3). We then construct and present the three AHs about: (1) developing a shared vision, (2) creating effective cultures and (3) enabling evidence to be used in practice. Our chapter concludes with our own reflections on the role of AH as a framework for making more explicit the relationship between PD as a complex intervention, its processes and outcomes, the similarities and differences arising and our next steps for implementing our own learning.

OUR JOURNEY AND THE CIP PRINCIPLES

Three different contexts, three different purposes!

Although, our different projects were undertaken in three different settings and countries – (1) a publicly funded community hospital in Ireland, (2) a large NHS acute provider in England and (3) an acute stroke unit in Australia – there are common drivers present in the descriptions of the following contexts:

- Major health care reform, unprecedented change and austerity measures.
- Need to improve the quality of care locally and address health care failures nationally.
- Need to demonstrate impact of change on patient outcomes and/or develop the evidence base.
- Focus on nursing, other roles and innovation, as well as health care team effectiveness.

Context 1

Randal's research study was situated within a publicly funded community hospital, within Ireland, where in the past there has existed a comparatively weak evidence base for practice among nursing staff. This study examines the implementation of a PD programme with practitioners who work with older people and the impact of the interventions used with the aim of transforming practice around continence care.

In recent times, nursing practitioners across the Irish Health Service Executive (HSE) have experienced unprecedented levels of change as a 'managerialist' ideology continues to dominate the health services landscape and reform programme. This has included repeated modification to the macro structures and processes within which these organisations and practitioners operate; a turbulent strategic policy context within which there exist competing professional and organisational priorities and the impact of the political and economic crisis within Ireland adds further pressures that challenge both the personal and professional values of nursing practitioners and other care workers.

No robust evaluation of the impact of the HSE reform programme and Department of Health rationalisation measures upon patient outcomes within Ireland had previously taken place. There was, however, both anecdotal and tangible evidence (HSE, 2010) of the severe impact these drivers were exerting upon both clinical practice and nursing working environments.

For nurses working within rural community hospital settings, this has entailed a change of focus towards preventive and health-promotion-based programmes for which many are ill-prepared. It has also necessitated a change in nursing roles to facilitate a primary-care-driven service. Although challenging, this in itself is not necessarily viewed as negative, as it provides an opportunity to deliver innovative nursing care. However, as noted by Mahnken (2001), personnel and educational restrictions pose a constraint to this potential. Juxtaposed with the micro context of the participating unit within this study, this provides an overarching contextual backdrop within which a collaborative facilitation framework for changing practice was implemented. Previously, the potential of PD in enabling the attainment of this objective had been under-utilised within the Irish health system (DoH&C, 2010).

Context 2

An acute health care provider comprising three large district general hospitals with its partner university in England commissioned a 3-month project to develop a framework for nursing and midwifery specialist practice.

Kim's project was undertaken within a national context characterised by uncertainty over national health service restructure; implementation of austerity measures across the health economy; national concern about health care failures around the delivery of essential nursing care and the maintenance of patients and service users' human rights; media publicity around the role of specialists; and concern that many nursing titles in particular are unrecognisable by patients.

Policy drivers around quality, quality assurance, patient safety and measurement had become a priority for organisations and practitioners alike. The *Principles of Nursing Practice* (RCN, 2010), modernising nursing careers (DH, 2006), and advanced practice initiatives (DH, 2010) identify the need to streamline career structure, aligning it with the national career framework, and the role of nursing and midwifery at all levels in improving quality, implementing innovation and improving productivity.

A recent organisational restructure within the organisation aimed to strengthen professional leadership and management across all sites to achieve the Trust's mission for and with its local population.

Specialist nurses, midwives and advanced practitioners across the Trust worked under different titles with variation in the purpose of roles and little consistency. 'Specialist nurses' included a range of nurses working within different specialisms and others, such as educators, research nurses, clinical site managers, practice developers, as well as ward managers.

The purpose of the first phase of the project (reported here) was to develop a framework that reflected the contribution of all these practitioners to person-centred, safe and effective care and a culture that continues to sustain this across the organisation, hence explicitly addressing both the policy agenda and the purposes of PD.

Specific objectives included: developing a career structure and framework; scoping the number, range and contribution of roles across the organisation; making recommendations for implementation and education commissioning; identifying the contribution of specialist, advanced practitioners and CNs to quality improvement, innovation and productivity agenda; identifying the specific skill set required by clinical leaders to develop effective workplace cultures, including system change; making recommendations for the roll-out in phase 2, including identifying the resources required and informing university curricula. Practice development was the project's underpinning approach.

Context 3

Joan's research was conducted and reported several years ago (Yalden et al., 2005) in response to initiatives by nurse researchers from the University School of Nursing and Midwifery and the nurse unit manager (NUM) in the multi-disciplinary team of the specialist stroke unit in an outer metropolitan public hospital network in Australia. The aim of the study was to improve the quality of care for patients with dysphagia admitted to the acute care stroke unit.

Early screening of patients for swallowing difficulties following admission to the acute stroke unit was a requirement of the Australian hospital stroke clinical pathway. Screening for early detection of dysphagia is an intervention to prevent aspiration pneumonia and delayed nutritional support. Patients arriving on an acute stroke unit required screening for swallowing difficulties by a speech pathologist in order to formulate appropriate care plans. There was a shared concern among clinicians about existing practice protocols and also the implementation of the clinical pathway due to the unavailability of a speech pathologist after normal business hours and at weekends. In the absence of formalised bedside dysphagia screening during these times, patients assessed 'at risk' were often placed on 'nil oral' for extended periods of time. Concerns were expressed by staff about the need to improve the quality of care following admission to the unit, particularly with regard to screening patients at risk of difficulties in eating and drinking.

Following an approach by the university-based researchers to collaborate in developing practice and education programmes with nurses in practice, early discussions with the NUM evolved into early planning with the multi-disciplinary stroke care team to extend their work on the recently completed stroke clinical pathway. A 3-year action research study followed. The collaborative study included nurses, allied health members of the stroke care team and university nurse researchers who facilitated the project with the NUM.

Using the CIP principles

The intention of all three projects was to use PD, described as a complex intervention that integrates the systematic development of practice with empowerment of practitioners, and cultural change that sustains outcomes in practice. For Kim, the underpinning approach to her project was PD, for Joan and Randal, realistic evaluation and participatory action research (PAR), respectively, were specific research approaches used with PD principles.

The three CIP principles – (1) collaboration, (2) participation and (3) inclusion – underpin PD approaches and guide ways of working with participants and stakeholders. How these principles were used in each project is now explained.

A contracted purpose!

For Kim, the purpose of the project and the project deliverables were agreed in advance with the commissioner. PD as an intervention in its own right was the agreed approach for achieving the purpose, which was specifically to develop a framework that focused on providing person-centred, safe and effective care and workplace cultures to sustain these outcomes. The commissioned purpose therefore matched the purpose of PD (see Chapter 3). PD also encompasses systematic evaluation and is underpinned theoretically by critical social science and critical creativity (see Chapter 4). This theory includes identifying and working with everyday assumptions and the barriers to action through enabling participants to become first enlightened (self-aware) about the barriers, both within themselves and the external environment; becoming motivated to want to act due to this self-awareness (empowered); and then implementing these actions in their everyday practice within a culture of ongoing critique and learning (emancipation).

The purpose of the project was to develop a 'shared purpose framework' for person-centred, safe and effective care and developing cultures of effectiveness in the workplace that makes clear expectations at different levels of the career framework. Role clarity and clear expectations are prerequisites to effectiveness (Manley et al., 2011a). The CIP principles were used to guide the project processes, primarily through using active learning (a form of supported learning based on practice described in Chapter 6). Up to 400 different specialist nurses and midwives across the organisation were provided with the opportunity to attend up to 6 active learning sessions from a choice of 65 pre-arranged sessions. Sessions were organised across different sites and times, including evening sessions, over a 3-month period to enable both accessibility and inclusivity. A set of common ground rules were developed collaboratively, based on participants' perspectives of the factors that would enable them to experience a safe environment for learning, support and safe challenge. These ground rules were used consistently across all sets, as the combination of participants attending any one set were not the same each time.

In the active learning sets, participants were supported to begin their own journeys of cultural change (although they did not recognise this at the time) through being exposed to ways of working that reflected the CIP principles. The focus of the active learning sets was self-assessment against six frameworks to help participants develop their own insights about where they were across a number of continua and where they wanted to be. The frameworks included: person-centredness, effectiveness and innovation; leadership; facilitating learning and development in the workplace; consultancy practice; research and scholarly inquiry; and PD. This was followed by an opportunity to undertake a qualitative 360-degree feedback and a reflective review. These activities were used to collaboratively construct the shared purpose framework for the organisation.

Clinical leaders were simultaneously supported through shorter sessions and these focused on identifying issues that were important to them in their daily work as well as helping them to work together to support and challenge each other. The CIP principles were therefore used at two levels: firstly, as the principle ways of facilitating the project, and secondly, to support participants with using these principles with their own teams, patients and stake-holders. In all groups it was clear that practitioners were not used to working collaboratively outside of their own immediate silos, with many feeling isolated and unsupported as well as sceptical about the organisations intention for developing the framework. Systematic process evaluation was undertaken across all active learning sets with both individual and collective opportunities for learning. The framework and project recommendations resulting were constructed from practitioners' own self-assessment data and exposed to critique through consultation processes.

How the CIP principles were integrated into Randal's and Joan's research is now explained together with their specific research approach.

Blending emancipatory practice development and realistic evaluation methodologies

The aim of Randal's study was to generate new insights into the effectiveness of specific facilitation strategies in developing practice within an older person setting and the implementation of evidence into practice around continence. In doing so, this would illuminate the specific components of context, relating to the practice environment or setting, that exert an influence on the mechanisms used to successfully implement and sustain evidence in practice. This purpose was agreed at the outset, including collaborative principles for joint working between the researcher, the service and the participative and inclusive involvement of managers.

The methodology employed within this study was based upon an emancipatory PD approach (see Chapter 4) set within a realistic evaluation framework. Realistic evaluation recognises the significance of context in understanding why interventions work (e.g. action learning), for whom, how and in what circumstances. The logical argument for realistic evaluation is that programmes are effective (have successful outcomes – O) only insofar as they initiate suitable ideas and opportunities (mechanisms – M) to groups in the appropriate social, cultural and discursive conditions (contexts – C) (Rycroft-Malone et al., 2009). Thus, context refers to the settings within which a programme is situated and the factors outside the control of the researcher (people's motivation, educational background, leadership qualities, macro-political events, etc.). Mechanisms are the elements and interventions within a programme that bring about an effect or outcome and are the pivotal components around which realist research revolves (Pawson & Tilley, 1997; see Chapter 9). The purpose of realistic evaluation is to establish which contexts are most effective in activating the mechanisms that deliver the intended programme outcomes.

The study centred on five PD cycles that included contextual assessment/re-assessment measures, development of 'AHs' and design and implementation of a collaborative facilitation framework. In a realistic approach to evaluation, the main implications from the literature, together with practitioners' knowledge, are used to propose 'AHs'. These 'AHs' informed the action cycles within this study, that is, testing the effectiveness of facilitation methods in implementing evidence-based and person-centred continence practice.

At the outset of the study, participants discussed available facilitation options and chose to commence with an action learning approach, as they felt that this intervention would promote collaborative working among staff, provide a safe forum for support and challenge, would allow for exploration of issues relevant to practice and would promote sustainable change. Issues of wider stakeholder inclusion (staff disciplines and grades) were addressed within this process. Central to this approach were reflective processes employed as programme mechanisms that stimulated processes of reflexivity, through which study participants explored contradictions, dilemmas and possibilities relating to their own practice context. Through this mechanism, participants became more aware (enlightened) concerning their roles as 'actors' within their work context with the ability to influence changes and outcomes to that context (empowerment). This, by definition, opens up a space within which 'emancipation' may take place. This evidence of engagement and involvement are very much the foundation of PD facilitation as participants achieved a state of raised consciousness through engaging in reflection and critical dialogue, and as evidenced in this study, took action to transform their work practices based upon these findings.

A participative and collaborative approach to data collection and analysis was implemented throughout and, arising from this, 'AHs' resulted. Subsequently, these were tested out and the findings were fed back into the action learning groups to promote further reflection, discussion and refinement of the facilitation model. During the phases of action learning, sub-mechanisms were collaboratively reviewed and agreed with participants as enablers. The sub-mechanisms were generated following negotiation with participants, were directly linked to the AHs and had capacity for change. Each mechanism interacted with the particular context into which it was introduced in order to transform that context. In turn, this helped to create new understandings about the culture and context within which practice was situated and interventions that enable the development of practice.

Participatory action research

PAR is a critical, self-reflexive cycle of inquiry that engages people as co-equal participants in investigating their social world and relationships within it in order to transform it (Kemmis & McTaggart, 2008). It is an approach to research conducted in a democratic spirit that originated in the work of Kurt Lewin (1947). Lewin introduced action research as an embedded element in a broad suite of theories that emphasised context and the dynamics and processes of planned change (Lewin, 1947). It has been carried forward in modern critical social theory with an emancipatory intent that begins by including key stakeholders in the processes of inquiry and transformative action. This means that in health care practice, action research aims to enable practitioners and researchers to explore problems in practice and develop strategies and implement innovations to improve services and patient care (Hart & Bond, 1995).

Evaluation is inherent in PAR because it involves participants in a systematic process of inquiry that uses both qualitative and quantitative methods (Hart & Bond, 1995; see Chapter 9). The inquiry process uses theory and emergent data to inform decisions and to drive actions. The inquiry proceeds through a spiral of inter-related steps that unfold as iterative cycles of data collection, analysis and review, planning, action and critical reflection on action. Research questions focus on 'what' and 'how' and enable reflexive analysis of differences between theory, data and practice. Further, action research supports the integration of evidence in practice (Waterman et al., 1995) and the generation or extension of theory from practice (Kemmis & McTaggart, 2008).

The processes used by the three of us as project facilitators to enable CIP, therefore, included:

- collaborative problem identification and joint identification of issues;
- negotiating agreed focus for project work;
- facilitated action or active learning;
- enabling self- and/or collective assessment of practice/culture;
- co-creation of frameworks, action cycles and action plans;
- collaborative process evaluation.

ACTION HYPOTHESIS – A FRAMEWORK FOR THEORISING FROM PRACTICE

We decided to use the 'AH' framework to share our common understanding and insights across our different settings and experiences. Following a mapping exercise, we identified three starting points that were common to us all, the strategies we used to address these starting points and their impact. We hope that this approach will help those new to PD to focus on the key practical strategies necessary for achieving successful person-centred outcomes in any setting regardless of the client groups involved or the size of the project.

The AH framework is a tool that enables theory development from practice to be made explicit. The framework derives from an action research study in which it was developed to capture and develop theory from a PD project (Binnie & Titchen, 1999), it is also an integral part of realistic evaluation as previously explained by Randal.

In a research project with CNs and ACNs (Manley & Titchen, 2012), the framework was further refined for the purpose of helping participants to understand how exploration and analysis of their own practice could contribute to theory, as well as to capture similarities and differences arising from three different research cohort groups across England. The main process used in the CN study was active learning (see Chapter 12), comprising action learning and other workshop activities relevant to learning in and from work. Forty critical incidents were presented in action learning by participants and later linked to emerging themes from the project's meta-analysis. At subsequent meetings, presenters of critical incidents reported back their findings relating to the action they had taken, the impact of the action and how effective it had been. Cohort group members, using verified notes captured by the research assistant, undertook a joint analysis of each action learning presentation (Prideaux, 1995), and revisited this over time in relation to achievement of stated action points, recording the sources of evidence for each aspect (e.g. the triggers, goals, achievements, etc.). Through the action learning process and across all the cohorts, a number of strategies were identified that were documented, tried and refined in practice over a period of time. The outcomes resulting from implementing the strategies were also identified. For each stage of the framework, evidence was collated from a number of different sources that substantiated the issue, the strategies used and the outcomes achieved. In tandem, consideration was given to the theoretical principles in the literature to either strengthen understanding of the issue or to challenge theory in relation to actual practical experience.

AH led to the identification, from different stories and contexts, of strategies or interventions that CNs could use in their practice. These strategies have been generalised from incidents involving different CNs who identified similar triggers in different contexts but achieved similar outcomes.

Figure 13.1 provides one illustration of the AH framework in relation to the trigger labelled 'turf wars' over bed use, experienced by a new CN in the area of intermediate care. 'Turf wars' is characterised by a number of descriptors on the left hand side that included the existence of no single referral systems. The strategies used and refined over time are identified as practical strategies that enabled the outcomes to be achieved as reflected by a number of indicators.

The AH framework, therefore, enabled links to be made between: the incidents and triggers that challenged CNs and ACNs in their everyday work; the strategies they were trying out in practice to address the triggers; and the outcomes achieved. Part of the process of theorisation is developing a tentative statement about the proposed relationship between concepts, often called a hypothesis. In this case, the hypothesis is about actions in the workplace. The AH identifies potential actions/strategies to address particular triggers to achieve particular endpoints. With practitioners researching this relationship in their own practice and across a number of communities of practice (practice cohorts), the AH can be transferred to other contexts and settings. The strategies therefore identified can be shared with others to help them in their roles to address similar triggers.

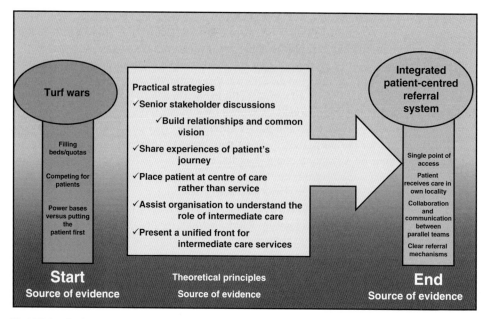

Fig. 13.1 Turf wars.

This AH framework also enables theorising from practice to contribute new insights about social impact through illustrating the inter-relationship between inputs, actions, outputs, outcomes and impact.

In this chapter, we plan to build on the use of this framework to make explicit the relationships between key issues in our three different projects, the strategies we used, as well as the outcome and impact. Such a process to enable transferability (which is determined by the reader) across diverse PD projects has not previously been undertaken. It is hoped that through our reflections on the process, we may be able to inform the core data sets that may need to be captured to contribute to international activity that could enable systematic capture of the impact of PD as a complex intervention (Manley et al., 2011b).

STARTING POINTS AND GOALS

The overarching aims and contexts of our projects have been described earlier. Through mapping and analysing local drivers across our projects, we identified three significant drivers to inform the development of our AHs. These following local drivers are often the starting points in many PD projects (see Chapter 3):

1. Lack of common shared purpose/vision in relation to the project focus (trigger 1).
2. Unreceptive/underdeveloped workplace cultures, characterised by factors such as lack of feedback processes/systems/evaluation/professional networks, support and challenge (trigger 2).
3. Issues with getting evidence into practice or using evidence to demonstrate impact (trigger 3).

The first two triggers are closely linked as effective workplace cultures are characterised by a shared purpose and vision and the implementation of shared values in practice (Manley et al., 2011a; see Chapter 8). For this reason, triggers 1 and 2 will be explored together.

Triggers 1 and 2: lack of a common shared purpose and an unreceptive/underdeveloped workplace culture

Box 13.1 shows the inter-relatedness of the first two triggers in Randal's starting point but starts with describing how the triggers were identified by systematically measuring the workplace context and culture at the beginning of the project.

Box 13.1: Starting point – no shared vision and underdeveloped workplace culture in context 1

A combination of qualitative and quantitative methods of data collection were used to distinguish the key features of existing care. Four data collection measures (context assessment index (CAI); McCormack et al., 2009); observations of practice (Wright et al., 2007); continence audit (DH, 2003); and focus groups were employed during a baseline evaluation that was undertaken collaboratively between the participants and the researcher. Using a variety of data sources helped both the researcher and the participants to generate a more meaningful understanding of the practice context. This phase of evaluation is referred to as realistic cumulation (Pawson & Tilley, 1997) whereby emergent theories, in the form of AHs, are continuously improved upon through processes of generalisation and specification until a point is reached where theory becomes focused and fine-tuned. This complexity is both represented and interpreted by means of conjectured and observed outcomes within the AHs and, once again, arises as a consequence of collaborative working between the researcher and participant groups.

This approach proved invaluable as it helped to uncover, among other things, the presence of conflict between both individuals and staff groups. Contradictions in practice were also manifested, demonstrating variation between actual and espoused practice values. It was theorised that these conditions were due to a lack of shared sense of purpose, lack of trust, practice not questioned, traditional values and poor sense of belonging, and that this could be addressed through the introduction of PD strategies, such as action learning, values clarification and leadership development.

The first two triggers were also inter-related in Kim's starting point. The commissioning and contracting process for the project made clear the project's purpose, which was to develop a framework that made explicit the contribution of nursing and midwifery to four outcomes: (1) person-centred care, (2) effective care, (3) safe care and (4) effective workplace cultures. The relevance of these outcomes to both the organisation and practitioners was linked to the national policy that consistently echoed messages around the need to improve the patient experience, patient safety, effectiveness, nurture innovation and productivity. However, the lack of shared purpose in Kim's context was more about what these words meant in everyday practice to practitioners and what values and beliefs, activities and behaviours would be expected to achieve these outcomes. Whilst the purpose of the intended framework was articulated as words and goals at the organisational level, there was little shared understanding about what this would mean for actions at the frontline by specialist nurses and midwives, clinical leaders and other niche roles. As no explicit framework previously existed across the Trust, there was therefore no shared vision about the activities expected to be undertaken by practitioners to deliver on these outcomes across the organisation. The second trigger, the need to develop an effective workplace culture to embed core values and ways of working, had been identified in a recent re-organisation. The need to address organisational culture so as to deliver better services using an affordable model of service delivery was highlighted following extensive staff interviews. In particular, there was recognition of the need to: work collaboratively with staff as a key resource for improving quality, enable staff to contribute to the future success of the organisation, help staff take responsibility for their actions and develop leadership capability if the organisation's vision was to be achieved. It was recognised at executive level that leadership and cultural change skills were required to implement and sustain a shared purpose within and across mixed staff teams and pathways. Cultural change needed to address barriers such as silo working, duplication of effort, lack of shared purpose, invisibility of impact, enhancing staff creativity, leadership and learning to create workplaces where everyone could flourish, as well as enabling patients and service users to consistently experience person-centredness and contribute to its evaluation. At the workplace culture level, many practitioners were cynical of the organisational motives, felt demoralised, demotivated and 'done to' when the project was initiated. The project therefore began by including all specialist practitioners who wished to be involved, enabled active participation through active learning and its activities and modelled and nurtured collaboration between and within different groups: practitioners, clinical leaders, different specialists, patients and service users, other clinical team members and higher education providers.

In relation to Joan's stating point and trigger 1, there was a shared recognition by different health care team members that a problem existed when caring for people following stroke admitted to an acute stroke unit. The problem was broadly defined as a lack of timeliness, safety and effectiveness of swallowing assessments performed regularly by nursing staff on stroke patients admitted overnight or during the weekend, and in the absence of a speech-language pathologist. There was shared recognition of the problem and a shared desire to do something about the problem across the health care team. However, there was no shared understanding of different professional roles or purpose regarding how such patients were to be cared for, the responsibilities of each team member, how the team should be working together to reduce gaps in the service and achieve improvement in dysphagia management or how to improve practice and continuity more generally. Trigger 1 was further augmented by a non-enabling workplace culture (trigger 2):

- where many people were expected to be told what to do rather than thinking through for themselves – using peer support, reflection, critical debate and patients experience when using evidence in practice – and, taking responsibility for this;
- that did not embrace shared values, goals or processes for collaborative development and improvement of this aspect of practice, mutual learning in and through practice and giving and receiving feedback as a multi-professional group.

Trigger 3: issues with using evidence in practice

Trigger 3, the third common trigger experienced across our three contexts, comprised an 'unclear evidence base for practice'. For Randal, this trigger emerged from the baseline recordings in relation to continence care for older people provided by registered nurses and health care assistants. Following a robust diagnosis of context at the outset, it was clearly indicated from the data sets, utilising PARIHS (Promoting Action on Research Implementation in the Health Services – see Chapter 7) as an underpinning framework, that the organisation did not represent what would be understood as a receptive context for practice change and the implementation of best evidence around continence care. The PARIHS framework further endorsed that the context and culture did not support evidence use, demonstrated through the presence of staff conflict, low levels of effective teamwork and lack of constructive feedback.

For Joan likewise, there was a shared concern that the lack of a formalised, evidence-based bedside assessment tool for swallowing put patients at risk of being placed on inappropriate care plans for eating and drinking. This problem was impacting on the patients' ability to eat and drink and the goals of maximising rehabilitation potential.

A stroke clinical pathway was designed and developed by the multi-disciplinary team with the aim of providing standardised, pre-scheduled, sequential interdisciplinary care to achieve improved health care outcomes for patients. However, on implementation of the clinical pathway it was revealed that some disparities existed between the clinical pathway schedules of care and the needs of some patients with swallowing or potential swallowing difficulties. The identification of these disparities was the outcome of discussions over several months between the NUM, the nurse researchers and the speech language pathologist. These disparities were later elaborated and re-defined within focused group work inclusive of most members of the stroke care team through the first and subsequent iterations of the action research cycle.

For Kim, from the self-assessments undertaken by practitioners, it was clear that most participants in the project were very aware of, and were using, the National Institute of Clinical Excellence (NICE) guidelines within their interdisciplinary teams and everyday practice, where such guidelines existed for patients or specific client groups. The challenges around unclear evidence for practice related not so much to clinical evidence, but evidence about whether person-centred care was experienced and how to help others to become more effective. This evidence base fell into the following three areas:

1. How clinical leaders and expert practitioners could help others (more generally) to implement clinical evidence-based standards across the organisation consistently – the evidence base that was lacking here was around how to facilitate learning, development and evidence utilisation in the workplace, the processes of PD.
2. How to demonstrate the contribution and impact that practitioners were having on patient experience and outcomes – the evidence base that was lacking here was around how to comprehensively and systematically evaluate their impact in a way that is politically informed.
3. How to systematically gather and use patient experience data to show whether care was experienced as person-centred or to identify what aspects needed to be improved. Other than national patient surveys, no evaluation date around the patient's experience was formally captured.

We have shown that although the focus of our PD projects and contexts may have been very different, common triggers acted as starting points for our PD journeys. Recognising and evidencing these triggers is the first step to developing our AHs. The next step is to identify the strategies we used, experimented with, reviewed and refined that were helpful in achieving the goals we aimed for.

THE STRATEGIES USED TO ADDRESS TRIGGERS

The strategies we intentionally used in practice to address identified triggers and/or to achieve collaborative goals included the use of the CIP principles and ourselves as facilitators, as well as, how we helped others to learn in and from practice and use processes and tools to achieve the purposes of our PD projects. Some strategies addressed a number of triggers either simultaneously or sequentially, others focused on single triggers. Tables 13.1–13.3 identify some of the key overarching strategies and sub-strategies used in each of our contexts in relation to each trigger. In addition, the process outcomes resulting from using the strategies are also identified.

How the strategies achieve their outcomes through increasing self-awareness and reflective ability

Within Tables 13.1 and 13.2, strategies used by Kim and Joan aimed to achieve changes in practice based on developing shared values and a shared purpose; and then embedding these values in practice, by supporting practitioners individually and collectively, to critically reflect on and challenge the barriers, behaviours, social norms and attitudes that work against their implementation. Shared values are not just about specific areas of practice that teams are trying to improve for patients and service users, but also about how practitioners work with each other, patients and stakeholders to achieve patient outcomes, improve the patient's experience and improve workplaces so that everyone can flourish (see Chapter 8).

Joan captures the impact of these strategies from analysis of data derived from synthesising various reflections:

> *An empowering experience? Action research, an unconventional methodology at that time was met with a mixture of curiosity and scepticism by key stakeholders and practitioners. As subsequent evaluation of the group processes indicated, some of the participants were more familiar with a directed research program, prescribed aims and objectives to work with. The project was facilitated by the researchers to maximise collaboration, inclusiveness and participation of a health care team in a project that from a practice development perspective could be aligned with a technical approach but with an emancipatory intent. There were challenges in creating the conditions for 'safe' and open dialogue given the multi-professional group and limitation on time available for discussion and development within the daily routine of the stroke unit. Tensions in the early stages of study gave way to sustained commitment and enthusiastic collegial working relationships within the main group.*

Within Randal's use of realistic evaluation, strategies were also used to identify shared values, develop a common vision and develop a culture that reflected these values in practice (Table 13.3).

PD strategies that raise awareness as the impetus for implementing evidence or changing behaviours and social norms are not based on 'giving people' the most up-to-date evidence/national standards about something and asking them to implement these. Whilst, it is important 'to know' what evidence and national standards exist, PD strategies help practitioners develop their own self-awareness about their own practice and to become self-critical through experiencing support and challenge. This self-awareness leads to the emergence of an internal motivation that drives practice and behaviour change, recognised in practitioners by increasing self-direction and wanting to do things differently. Practitioners become

Table 13.1   Strategies used by Joan to address triggers 1–3, linked to the process outcomes resulting.

Triggers (T)	Strategies to address triggers	Process outcomes

Joan T1, T2, T3	1. Raising awareness of staff at different organisational levels and within/across different stakeholder groups by:
	  a. providing feedback/data from observations of care and literature reviews to engage staff in a critical dialogue.
	2. Providing opportunities for:
	  a. multi-professional critical reflection, dialogue and learning;
	  b. identifying claims, concerns and issues;
	  c. making sense of data; and
	  d. participating in action cycles, action plans, implementation and evaluation.
	3. Values clarification to identify shared values and beliefs.
	4. Critical reflection around own practice and literature.
		• Raised awareness of the need for innovation around:
		  ○ information for patients and families, bedside illustrations for correct positioning for eating and drinking;
		  ○ flow-charts to guide changes to diet and monitor eating and drinking;
		  ○ acquisition of resources such as up-to-date cutlery and crockery assistive devices;
		  ○ incremental changes to ward and clinical policy; and
		  ○ the development of a specific education programme.
		• High level of motivation to engage in learning and inquiry.
		• Self-esteem and achievement as members of the multi-disciplinary team.

T3	5. Reviewing existing practice in relation to the evidence base underpinning best practice by:
	  a. focused review of the literature;
	  b. reviewing existing protocols for managing patients locally;
	  c. surveying tools used in other hospitals;
	  d. critical appraisal of evidence supporting different indicators.
		• A single tool with validated indicators for screening patients for dysphagia following stroke developed.
		• Screening tool tested, indicating high level of agreement between nurses and speech pathologist diagnoses.
		• Tool integrated into the hospital stroke clinical pathway.
		• Network development for acute stroke care.

T1, T2	6. Developing a culture of learning, inquiry and collaboration by:
	  a. critical reflection and review of learning needs to address dysphagia screening and bedside care;
	  b. facilitated group processes with an ethic of valuing contributions from all members;
	  c. challenge and support, recording and sharing critical incidents from practice;
	  d. sharing learning and knowledge with others;
	  e. evaluation of practice and learning outcomes using quantitative and qualitative inquiry methods, review of literature and group feedback processes;
	  f. recognition and celebration of achievements.
		• Increased individual and team learning and effectiveness.
		• Development of a framework for the construction and delivery of a short dysphagia education programme for nurses.
		• Participation in hospital seminars and professional conferences through presentations of outcomes and experiences by participants.
		• Others began to use the tool.
		• Sustained engagement in critical reflective and review group processes despite staff turnover and normal attrition on the ward.
		• Joint award from the university and health care organisation presented to participants for completion of the short dysphagia education course.

Table 13.2 Strategies used by Kim to address triggers 1–3, linked to the process outcomes resulting.

Trigger (T)	Strategies to address triggers	Process outcomes

Kim T1, T2	1. Active learning to support practitioners with:
	  a. self-assessment;
	  b. critical reflection;
	  c. mutual support and challenge;
	  d. celebrating achievements;
	  e. evaluation;
	  f. qualitative analysis of data;
	  g. role clarity; and
	  h. understanding the political context.
		• Practitioners begin to work together, support and challenge each other.
		• Skills in collaborative analysis developed.
		• Clinical leaders set up forums for own peer support and review.
		• Clinical leaders feel less isolated and take responsibility for their actions.
		• Practitioners feel less isolated and more enthused about practice.
		• Role clarity.
		• Practitioners identify areas for increasing individual and team effectiveness.
		• Networks begin to develop for sharing best practice.

T2, T3	2. Qualitative 360-degree feedback to enable practitioners to:
	  a. access evidence about patient experience and other sources of evidence to inform practice change;
	  b. give and receive feedback to each other openly; and
	  c. build effective relationships with multi-disciplinary team members and develop effective team cultures.
		• A formal trust protocol that enables practitioners to obtain feedback about their practice from patients and careers.
		• Practitioners more confident in giving and receiving open feedback to/from each other.
		• Practitioners feel more confident about their contributions because of the feedback received.
		• Practitioners begin to identify common themes from feedback they can work on together as a team.

T1, T2, T3	3. Co-creation of framework and project recommendations using the CIP principles through working with practitioners.	• A Trust-wide framework that makes explicit how person-centred safe and effective care and effective workplace culture would be recognised, with plans to embed in job descriptions and appraisals.

motivated to act on this self-knowledge, and challenge and dismantle the barriers that work against desired action though reflective approaches that enable self-awareness about: ones' own values, practice that has become 'taken for granted' and internal and external factors that influence practice. It is these processes that enable transformation of individuals and cultures characteristic of PD. As Randal explains in relation to his project:

> *Reflection through action learning was used as a strategy within this context. The intention within this mechanism was to engage staff in critical dialogue around the foundations of their practice, i.e. working with older people and providing evidence-based and person-centred continence care. It was also to examine the meaning of evidence as this related to their practice.*
>
> *This process was implemented through the action learning set with the focus on challenging both themselves and each another to confront the realities of practice as it existed, with that which was espoused as desirable following critical dialogue.*

Active and/or action learning provide the formal opportunities and methods for developing skills in relation to learning in and from work but also provide ongoing support and challenge

Table 13.3 Strategies used by Randal to address triggers 1–3, linked to the process outcomes resulting.

Trigger (T)	Strategies to address triggers	Process outcomes
Randal T2, T3	1. Raising awareness of role and context through: a. action learning that included reflective accounts and critical dialogue on own practice and practice context.	• More aware of own role and potential for influence. • Promotion of collaborative working among staff. • A safe forum for support and challenge. • Enabled sustainable change.
T1, T2	2. Developing shared values through: a. values clarification.	• Contradictions between espoused values and actual practice identified. • Cultural shift towards more person-centred approaches.
T2, T3	3. Implementing evidence into practice through: a. action learning, critical dialogue and reflective practice.	• Evidence-based policies and guidelines developed to support continence care. • Previous accepted practice challenged. • Improved skills in policy and guideline development. • Improved practitioner confidence.
T3	4. Providing support for staff through: a. action learning and enabling critical reflection.	• Transformation in practice culture.

to sustain this approach in day-to-day work to help embed changes into everyday culture. Active and/or action learning sets are, therefore, frequently used in PD projects. Alternatively, in PAR or other approaches to action research, collaborative and cooperative groups work together through reflective and critical spirals of activity to achieve similar ends, supported by a research facilitator.

Kim identifies the impact on participants of using active learning as a growing reflective ability and increased self-awareness, as well as increasing ability to self-assess in relation to complex drivers in the workplace and becoming self-critical. The following haikus (Zen poems) generated by different participant groups in her project as an evaluation and closure strategy at the end of different active learning sessions substantiate this claim:

'Nervous and inspired
Overwhelming. Challenging
Seeing the way forward'

'Reflective hard work
A thought provoking headache
Challenge, reassuring'

'Honest, uplifting
.Supporting, understanding.
Not a waste of time!'

'Challenging, inspired
Thought provoking, emotive
Insightful, Timely'

Strategies involving the use of tools, frameworks and evidence

A lack of shared sense of purpose and an underdeveloped/unreceptive culture characterised by lack of trust, practice not being questioned, traditional values and poor sense of belonging described triggers that could be addressed by the use of specific tools. Randal used a values clarification process within his context to establish an agreed set of values that practitioners cherished about working with older people. These values were then translated into a values statement for all staff within the unit. This was the first outcome and tangible evidence of a shift in thinking and provided a foundation for transforming practice. Consistencies across three of the data collection instruments affirmed the presence of this strengthening PD culture with improved communication among staff.

Observations of practice, a specific development tool, also highlighted participant engagement with strategies advocated by the PARIHS framework that enabled staff to assess their practice context. Focus group participants were positive in their feedback regarding the use of the PARIHS framework for informing practice (see Chapter 7 for how practice developers use PARIHS). Outcomes observed as a result of these interventions included evidence of an intimate and caring approach; less focus on carrying out 'routine duties'; increased awareness and comprehension of PARIHS components; and the implementation of PD tools associated with PARIHS.

In Joan's project, the review of multiple sources of evidence enabled the structure and selection of indicators for recognising dysphagia to be included in the screening instrument through collaborative effort. Facilitating strategies for raising awareness provided a values base from which to focus the parameters of the review, the process of critically appraising the evidence and questioning the existing evidence base for practice. The outcome enabled the group to design a compact, three-stage dysphagia screening tool that was successfully developed and tested over several iterations of the action research cycles (Yalden et al., 2005).

The collaborative development and completion of the supporting education programme, test screenings and bedside innovations to practice demonstrated a high level of motivation, effort and commitment from the whole group. The combined strategies contributed to the creation of conditions conducive to critical review and dialogue, sharing knowledge, learning and outcomes, collaborative inquiry and informed actions for improving dysphagia care for stroke patients. These strategies helped to address triggers 1, 2 and 3.

Having unpicked key strategies that were intentionally used to address the triggers identified, and linking these to the process outcomes resulting across the three projects, the chapter moves to highlighting outcomes, impact and consequences. Tables 13.1–13.3 identify the process outcomes achieved. These are the outcomes that resulted directly from using the strategies and were captured through a range of evidence that included evaluations, reflections, reviews, action plans, interviews, observations, claims, concerns and issues. It has been argued that such process outcomes arise from enabling effective workplace cultures that then are influential in achieving other key outcomes and impact (Manley et al., 2011b).

OUTCOMES, CONSEQUENCES AND IMPACT

In this section, we explore whether the overall intended outcomes of each project were met, how these outcomes were evidenced and whether there were other consequences and impact. Table 13.4 captures the relationships between purpose, outcomes and impact, identifying the associated evidence. This table enables us to then build our tentative AHs to link the three triggers, intentional strategies, to outcomes and impact.

Table 13.4 Purpose, outcomes, evidence and impact in the three practice development projects.

Context and purpose	Outcome and impact	Evidence
Randal's project purpose To generate new insights into the effectiveness of specific facilitation strategies in developing practice within an older person setting and the implementation of evidence into practice. *Specific objectives* To increase experience of managing complex change, strategic documents and plans influenced by core person-centred values, receptive practice development culture, evaluation culture developed, self-help infrastructure developed and available to patients and practitioners.	This study has depicted a philosophical model of emancipatory practice development underpinned by the principles of realistic evaluation. It has demonstrated the efficacy of this approach in explicating underlying mechanisms within the practice context and how these impact upon practice. *Impact* • Improved patient care. • Transformed cultures and contexts of care. • Changes in practice effected via a systematic approach. • Refinement of facilitation methods.	• The data collected across the three cycles of evaluation indicated overwhelming support for a positive transformation in practice culture and context. • Evidence of transformation of culture and context was demonstrated through implementation of espoused values in practice, development of positive staff relationships and conflict resolution and the attainment of standards of person-centred practice in continence care. • Actions related to continence care detail the improvements in patient care. • Development of a practice development framework established methodological coherency between emancipatory practice development and realistic evaluation and enabled the attainment of evidence-informed and person-centred cultures within practice.
Kim's project purpose To develop a framework that reflected the contribution of specialist nurses/midwives to person-centred, safe and effective care and a culture that sustains this across the Trust. *Specific objectives* To develop a career structure and framework; scope the number, range and contribution of roles across the organisation; make recommendations for implementation and education commissioning; identify the contribution of specialist, advanced practitioners and consultant nurses to quality improvement, innovation and productivity agenda; identify the specific skill set required by clinical leaders to develop effective workplace cultures, including system change; make recommendations for the roll-out in phase 2.	*Outcome* Project purpose and objectives all achieved *Impact* • Board sign up for roll-out of framework across all staff groups. • Key recommendation for organisation around practice and practice development to be taken forward in five work streams. • Establishment of a faculty of practice. • Integration of recommendations with organisational development and quality strategies. • Development of an interdisciplinary leadership programme for changing culture. • Interest in framework from other health care providers.	• Project report and resulting career and competence framework provided tangible evidence that demonstrated achievement of the purpose and objectives. • The organisation's steering group provided the governance and sign-off that project objectives were achieved and the outputs delivered.

(continued)

Table 13.4   (Continued)

Context and purpose	Outcome and impact	Evidence
Joan's project purpose To improve the quality of care for patients with dysphagia admitted to the acute care stroke unit through university and health care collaboration. *Specific objectives* To develop a dysphagia screening tool for use by nurses; clarify the evidence base for indicators and structure of the tool; develop supporting interventions and resources to support safe eating and drinking for patients at mealtimes; develop and implement a supporting education programme for nurse; test and use of the tool by nurses on the unit; and establish processes for critical review, learning, feedback and development.	*Outcome* Project purpose and all objectives achieved. *Impact* • Tool used by others. • Screening tool adopted as a component of a larger multi-site study of the clinical stroke pathway and subsequently refined. • Sustained practice development active learning on the stroke unit. • Re-focus of work on person-centred bedside dysphagia management. • A sense of achievement.	*Evidence* • Dysphagia screening tool developed, tested and approved for use with the hospital Stroke Clinical Pathway. • Twenty-seven nurses completed the dysphagia education course. • Permission granted to nurse unit manager (NUM) of the hospital's emergency department for use of tool by the study steering group. • Material evidence of the refined version of the tool in current use as an integrated component of the evidence-based Clinical Stroke Pathway. • Observation and verbal report from NUM of continued reflective group processes on the ward at time of writing. • Qualitative evaluation data related to theme of 'feedback and learning'.

Achievement of project purposes are evidenced through a variety of data sources that range from re-assessing baseline data as in Randal's study, undertaking semi-structured interviews with the multi-disciplinary team in Joan's study (Box 13.2) or demonstrating achievement of objectives to the satisfaction of governance groups in Kim's project. The development of tangible products and the movement towards cultural transformation in all three contexts with evidence of more effective care to patients and service users and also positive impact on the staff's experience has to be balanced against the further evidence required to demonstrate positive impact on the patient's experience.

Box 13.2: Data illustrating impact in Joan's study

'. . . (differences) at times were openly discussed . . . you came to agreements . . . '
'. . . I found it a great learning experience . . . team-building was part of it too . . . '
'In terms of working with patients . . . yeah, I felt more knowledgeable, more confident.'
'I could relate to them being nil by mouth (NBM) and became more aware of their needs'
'. . . it made a difference to the way I thought about everyday practice'

In summary, from the analysis of our journeys across all three projects, we believe we can populate three AHs frameworks around the common themes that were central to our PD projects, even though their purposes and contexts were very different. The themes lack of common vision, underdeveloped/unreceptive cultures and issues with evidence use in practice were the common triggers around which a range of strategies was implemented and used. The strategies in each context were very similar, with the exception of qualitative

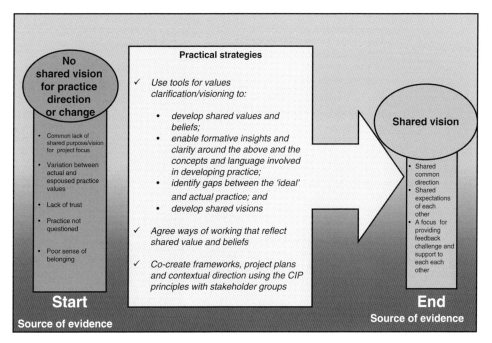

Fig. 13.2   Developing a shared vision for practice direction/change.

360-degree feedback, which was only used in one context. We have analysed our personal variations in the use of these strategies to synthesise the key descriptors of each part of the AH framework. We are able to propose that in relation to the triggers identified, and through using specific strategies, those similar outcomes can be achieved in other PD projects and contexts. The AH for each of the three triggers is outlined in Figures 13.2–13.4. We hope that by making explicit our AHs, we will foster further critique and critical dialogue in the PD community as well as contribute to both understanding and articulating the impact of PD.

REFLECTIONS ON USING ACTION HYPOTHESES

Within Randal's realistic evaluation approach, the development of AHs was a key part of the process unlike the other two projects presented in this chapter. Our reflections therefore focus on how we have used AHs across our three studies and its potential for demonstrating the impact of PD. Whilst AHs have occasionally been used within single studies to achieve insights into specific aspects of PD with different practitioners (Binnie & Titchen, 1999; Manley & Titchen, 2012), this is the first time to our knowledge that it has been used across different studies and contexts to synthesise common insights. Titchen (2011) refers to the reluctance of practice developers, up to this point, in using AHs. Titchen observes that when practice developers really experience using AHs and give new meaning to the language, they experience how powerful a tool it can be for theory development. We believe therefore that we are amongst the first to experiment with this approach in PD.

Reflecting on how we used the CIP principles across our different contexts has provided ways of thinking and working with others that uses democratic, humanitarian values to support actions and interaction. Specifically, through thinking about collaboration, we identified our rationale for using reciprocal processes and formalising/theorising the rationale for

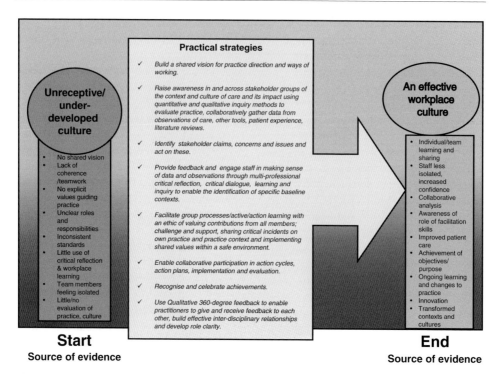

Fig. 13.3 Developing a culture of effectiveness.

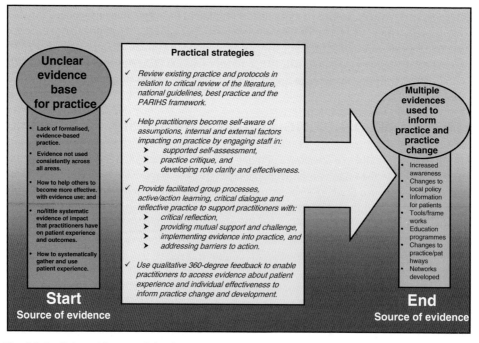

Fig. 13.4 Using evidence and developing evidence.

mutually agreed working relationships. Collaboration has guided facilitation processes in terms of negotiating, motivating, organising, communicating within and across sectors and groups and levels of the organisations.

Through reflecting on inclusiveness, we recognise that we have been guided to think about the need to include key stakeholders at different levels of the organisation to ground our work within the context and culture, establish a shared vision, common and specific goals and ensure support and resources. It has also enabled us to think about inclusiveness of different sources of data and evidence to inform both inquiry and transformative processes.

Reflecting on participation has enabled us to provide opportunities for key stakeholders/participants to engage in planning, action, reflection and evaluation and critical dialogue about their practice context and potential strategies to be introduced. It has also highlighted the need to accommodate different levels of engagement of team members across the clinical practice and management settings because of different roles, responsibilities and constraints.

We believe we have begun to demonstrate evidence of the application of the CIP principles in our three contexts and fundamental similarities in our PD processes related to similar outcomes. These similarities, despite differences in tools and methods, begin to make possible the identification of inclusion criteria that would discriminate PD from other interventions.

The combined CIP principles and the AH framework has helped us to break down distinctions between methodology and methods, underpinned by processes of critical reflection, by making visible the multiplicity of theoretical and assessment frameworks, inquiry methods and tools used to achieve outcomes across the three different contexts. Through identifying common triggers, AHs have helped to pinpoint the critical components of the macro and micro contexts, which require consideration within the contextual assessment process.

The systematic AH framework has made explicit how PD processes and strategies enabled transformative action in our studies. We believe the AH framework has the potential to demonstrate the robustness of PD processes in environments of rapid change and knowledge development through sustaining critical reflection and dialogue in clinical practice. The interdependent components of the AH framework has helped to validate the practical, scientific and emancipatory nature of the main strategies used to enable transformation in our three contexts. Through working with our common trigger points we have begun to realise that the three we selected to include in this chapter are probably the most common starting points for many practice development projects, regardless of the focus of the project. Through AHs, we have begun to identify potential data sets that could be captured to demonstrate the outcomes and impact of PD, specifically its influence on attaining culture shift and enabling changes in practice. It has clarified our thinking and helped us make the connections between contexts, strategies, outcomes and impact. Our closing reflection endorses this:

Using the action hypothesis framework has been a journey of moving from scepticism and misconceptions related to terms more commonly associated with experimental inquiry and deductive reasoning to gradual understanding of how action hypothesis has paved the way to unfolding the complexity of practice development through the systematic and logical sequence. It has enabled the translation of the CIP principles for ways of working and achieving mutual goals.

ACKNOWLEDGEMENT

Contributions by Joan Yalden are based on examples from practice development research completed when previously a senior lecturer and student at Monash University, School of Nursing & Midwifery, Melbourne, Australia.

REFERENCES

Binnie, A. & Titchen, A. (1999) *Freedom to Practise: The Development of Patient-Centred Nursing.* Butterworth Heinemann, Oxford.

Department of Health (DH) (2006) Modernising nursing careers: setting the direction. http://www.dh.gov.uk/en/Publicationsandstatistics/Publications/PublicationsPolicyAndGuidance/DH_4138756 (Accessed 27 July 2011).

Department of Health (DH) (2010) *Advanced Level Nursing: A Position Statement.* http://www.dh.gov.uk/prod_consum_dh/groups/dh_digitalassets/@dh/@en/@ps/documents/digitalasset/dh_121738.pdf (Accessed 16 February 2011).

Department of Health (DH) (2003) *Essence of Care. Patient-focused Benchmarking for Health Care Practitioners.* HMSO, London.

Department of Health and Children (DoH&C) (2010) *Review of Practice Development in Nursing and Midwifery in the Republic of Ireland and Development of a Strategic Framework.* Stationery Office, Dublin.

Hart, E. & Bond, M. (1995). *Action Research in Health and Social Care: Guide to Practice.* Open University Press, Buckingham.

Health Service Executive (2010) *Impact of the Health Service Recruitment and Promotions Moratorium on the Provision of Nursing and Midwifery Services.* Final report. Health Services Executive, Dublin.

Kemmis, S. & McTaggart, R. (2008) Paricipatory action research, communicative action and the public sphere. In: *Strategies of Qualitative Inquiry* (eds Norman Denzin & Yvonne Lincoln), 3rd edn, pp. 271–330. Sage Publications, Los Angeles, CA.

Lewin, K. (1947). *Field Theory in Social Science: Selected Theoretical Papers* (ed. Cartwright, D. (1951)). Harper & Row Publishers, New York.

Mahnken, J.E. (2001) Rural nursing and health care reforms: building a social model of health. *Rural and Remote Health,* **1**. http://www.regional.org.au/au/rrh/2001/011214_104.htm (Accessed 18 November 2012).

Manley, K. & Titchen, A. (2012) *Being and Becoming a Consultant Nurse: Towards Greater Effectiveness through a Programme of Support.* Royal College of Nursing, London.

Manley, K., Sanders, K., Cardiff, S. & Webster, J. (2011a) Effective workplace culture: the attributes, enabling factors and consequences of a new concept. *International Practice Development Journal,* **1** (2). Article 1.

Manley, K., Crisp, J. & Moss, C. (2011b) Advancing the practice development outcomes agenda within multiple contexts. *International Practice Development Journal,* **1** (1). Article 4.

McCormack, B., McCarthy, G., Wright, J., Slater, P. & Coffey, A. (2009) Development and testing of the context assessment index (CAI). *Worldviews on Evidence-Based Nursing,* **6** (1), 27–35.

Pawson, R. & Tilley, N. (1997). *Realistic Evaluation.* Sage Publications, London.

Prideaux, D. (1995) Beyond facilitation: action research as self-research and self-evaluation. *Evaluation Journal of Australasia,* **7** (1), 3–13.

RCN (2010) *Principles of Nursing Practice.* Royal College of Nursing, London.

Rycroft-Malone, J., Fontenla, M., Seers, K. & Bick, D. (2009). Protocol-based care: the standardisation of decision-making? *Journal of Clinical Nursing,* **18**, 1490–1500.

Titchen, A. (2011) Creating a rose garden: showing links between cause and effect in practice development evaluation. *International Practice Development Journal,* **1** (1), Article 6. http://www.fons.org/library/journal.aspx (Accessed 1 October 2012).

Waterman, H. Webb, C. & Williams, A. (1995) Parallels and contradictions in the theory and practice of action research and nursing. *Journal of Advanced Nursing,* **22**, 779–784.

Wright, J., McCormack, B., Coffey, A. & McCarthy, G. (2007). Evaluating the context within which continence care is provided in rehabilitation units for older people. *International Journal of Older People Nursing,* **2** (1), 9–19.

Yalden, B.J., Lack, H., Stojkovski, M. & Sellick, K. (2005). Developing a Nurse Dysphagia Screening Tool: an action research approach. Unpublished paper, Monash University, School of Nursing & Midwifery, Melbourne, Australia.

14 The Contextual Web of Practice Development

Brendan McCormack[1], Angie Titchen[2] and Kim Manley[3]

[1]University of Ulster, Newtownabbey, UK
[2]Fontys University of Applied Sciences, Eindhoven, The Netherlands
[3]Canterbury Christ Church University, Canterbury, UK

So we have come to the end (for now!) of this journey through the theory, methodology and methods of practice development. In this journey we have experienced different ways of expressing the meaning of practice development, different but complementary approaches to its facilitation and a range of personal reflections from experienced practice developers. We have reflected on and critiqued methodologies and methods, and have introduced new ideas that could help us to make the case for practice development being an integral part of an organisation's DNA. However, we are not naïve, and after more than 25 years of effort, we are well aware that the nature of practice development means that it is not something that can be easily packaged into a glossy toolkit and promoted as an answer to the ills of health and social care provision. The intricately bound relationship between the 'self' or being of the practice developer and the tools of practice development means that it is always going to be something that needs to be promoted and articulated by individuals who have a passion for making the health care experience more person-centred for all.

So, where does that leave us now? We have evolved our methodologies, we have continually improved, refined and innovated methods, we have demonstrated the effectiveness of the processes in achieving important person-centred outcomes and we have articulated individual experiences of the journey so far. However, our work is not done! The very nature of practice development means that it is in a continuous state of evolution, development and transformation. Many of the contributors to this book are experienced practice developers, practitioner researchers and expert practitioners/managers/leaders, yet it is obvious from our writing that we are still learning and developing and in the process, and continue to evolve the methodologies of practice development. This evolution illustrates the importance of not viewing practice development as a 'thing' that can be turned on and off, but instead highlights the need to see it as an integral, integrated and ongoing part of the culture of an effective workplace. In other words, practice development becomes a way of life or, put differently, a way of knowing, doing, being and becoming as an individual, a team or an organisation.

So in this final chapter, we will reflect on what has gone before and argue that our ultimate purpose as practice developers is to facilitate 'human flourishing'. We will reflect on the previous chapters, identify what they contribute to this agenda and the contribution that practice development makes to the creation of workplaces that enable people to flourish.

Practice Development in Nursing and Healthcare, Second Edition. Edited by Brendan McCormack, Kim Manley and Angie Titchen.
© 2013 John Wiley & Sons, Ltd. Published 2013 by John Wiley & Sons, Ltd.

FROM TECHNICAL CHANGE TO PERSON-CENTRED CULTURES

You've Been Framed
He thinks it's serious
It's all set up
The roles are established
He can't cop out
He identifies the plan
He takes on the role
He tries to make sense of it
He knows the score

He approaches the work with a fixed mind
He fills the space with careful intent
He can't make it work, it's all a mess
He tries to fix it but nothing works
He changes the space and fills it again
and again and again and again and again
He changes the colours, the texture, the flow
The drums keep on beating but he can't let it go

He focuses on the rhythm and moves with the beat
His mind is confused and recognises defeat
He needs to let go and go with the beat
He suddenly needs to get out of the heat
The cameras are rolling, they come into view
He sees it all false and not the real you
He notices the pattern, the plot that repeats
He needs to break it, it's not defeat

He abandons the imposter and goes with the flow
He listens to the drums and what they know
He moves, he shakes, he dances with grace
The paint breaks the frame and finds a new space
He releases his passion, he sees it all now
He enters the colour with all that it holds

The frame falls away
The drum beat is strong
The picture's complete
The cameras are gone
The lessons are learnt
Don't limit the view
Release your colour
and be the real you

(McCormack, 2001)

When reflecting on the chapters in this book, we revisited the poem written by one of us (Brendan) as he struggled to find his 'place' in practice development, an experience all three of us shared. The poem captures the internal 'fight' between the cognitive and rational desire to be effective through a technical systematic approach to practice development and the need to be creative and authentic. Many practice developers will resonate with the essence of the poem and will 'feel' the internal struggle that we each experience in being authentic as practice developers whilst simultaneously ensuring that we are effective and achieve outcomes.

When edition 1 of *Practice Development in Nursing* was published, we knew that practice development was poorly understood, had little conceptual clarity and was under scrutiny from decision-makers in terms of the reality of what it actually achieved in improving patient care. At that time, many organisations routinely employed 'Practice Development Nurses' without having any real vision for the role and what it could achieve, without any significant infrastructure to support the role and its effectiveness and without any real understanding of practice development. Since then, whilst most of these roles have been disbanded, a lot has been learned about practice development in organisations and how it is best integrated into the health and social care system. A key part of this learning and the evolution of practice development has been a greater recognition of practice development as being 'everyone's business' and not dependent on the existence of specific or particular practice development roles, as shown so clearly by Jan Dewing and colleagues in Chapter 12.

Of most significance is the focus away from linear models of technical change to models that recognise the need for environments that enable all persons to flourish. As the methodologies of practice development have evolved, a clearer understanding of person-centred cultures has been articulated and a broader and more inclusive understanding of person-centredness has developed. Central to this recognition has been the evidence accrued that shows the incongruity of promoting person-centred care for patients without considering how the same person-centred values can imbue the way staff in the organisation work with each other, whatever role they hold or contribution they make. In Chapter 10 of this book, for example, the work of Jill Maben and colleagues is described, with its focus on how cultures are created that enable staff to experience nurturing, caring and growth. This work is one example of evidence that shows a direct connection between staff well-being and person-centred patient outcomes. Similar work by Binnie and Titchen (1999), McCormack and McCance (2010) and Manley et al. (2011) are also highlighted in the chapters of this book, and together they represent a powerful body of evidence that should not be ignored by managers and policy makers. The key message is of course that if we want practice environments that enable patients to flourish and achieve the best possible outcomes, then we need to create practice cultures that nurture staff and enable them to achieve their potential. At a time when health care is under particular economic scrutiny and resources are few, organisations struggle to place value on 'staff empowerment' strategies and indeed, continuing education and development programmes are often the first to be cut when money is short.

However, at the same time there is an increased emphasis on the importance of 'environments that enable persons to flourish'. Our work in practice development has been instrumental in promoting this agenda (see, e.g., Stephens et al., 2004; McCormack & Titchen, 2006; Titchen & McCormack, 2010). A good example of this emphasis is the growing movement in the Republic of Ireland that is redeveloping residential continuing care from a predominantly medical and institutionalised model, to one that is focused on a social model of care and community integration. See, for example 'Places to Flourish' – a resource guide and support programme for developing practice in residential continuing care settings (http://www.placestoflourish.org/). The resource emphasises the need to change patterns of care in nursing homes as a means of changing the culture of practice. The 'My Home Life Programme' in the United Kingdom is also an example of the growing emphasis on positively enabling people to flourish in their lives (http://myhomelifemovement.org/).

HUMAN FLOURISHING FOR ALL – THE ULTIMATE PURPOSE OF PRACTICE DEVELOPMENT

So when we talk about human flourishing, what do we mean?

The term 'human flourishing' can be traced back to Aristotle who suggested that *human flourishing occurs when a person is concurrently doing what he [sic] ought to do and doing what he wants to do*. What Aristotle suggests here is a moral perspective on our being as agents in the world and which should resonate with us as health care practitioners. The argument being that we are effective as a person when the actions we actually take are the same as those we ought to be taking as a moral agent. To do this requires an understanding of what is required of us as practitioners (the evidence that informs our practice), whilst at the same time being in a position to want to do what is the right thing and to enjoy doing it. Whilst it is commonplace these days to be highly critical of nursing and health care practice, as evidenced by the continuous media profiling of poor practice and poor health care experiences, Aristotle's view of flourishing should give us a pause for reflection. It is easy to 'blame' poor practice on individual practitioners and their lack of care, compassion and competence. However, if we bear in mind Aristotle's view, then we also need to ask more significant questions about the context in which practitioners work. The chapters in this book highlight the importance of different and complementary forms of 'evidence' in practice development work and this evidence provides a basis for understanding how person-centred practice 'ought' to be provided. This same evidence, however, also highlights the multiplicity of the challenges that exist in practice settings and that hinder the practice that ought to be provided. So if this is the case, can nurses and health care practitioners practise in the way that they want to, if our values are that all nurses and health care practitioners 'want to' do the right thing for patients? Well the answer is surely not, as without the best possible context, how practice ought to be undertaken and how practitioners want to deliver it can never be combined as one.

McCormack and Titchen (2006) and Titchen and McCormack (2010) have argued that human flourishing is both the end (outcome) and the means (processes) of transformational practice development. They argue that practice development is transformational when the creative energies of different forms of knowledge and intelligences are blended and used to enable growthful experiences for all. For example Kate Sanders, Jo Odell and Jonathon Webster (Chapter 2) show their blending of propositional emanicipatory knowledge (from critical social science) with their personal knowledge (craft knowledge or practical know-how accrued through their experience of practice development, their lives and their reflexivity). These knowledges are 'danced' by emotional intelligence (being attuned to the emotions and using them wisely) and embodied intelligence (listening to the wisdom of the body). These intelligences, amongst others, seem to have enabled them to better understand themselves and think about their thinking as they develop their practice development expertise. Their chapter bubbles with the energy this mix has created.

McCormack and Titchen further argue in the two papers above that engaging in these human flourishing processes enables human flourishing to be experienced as an outcome, that is, being able to simultaneously do what I want and ought to do.

Many of the chapters in this book have highlighted the characteristics of care environments that enable persons to flourish, including:

- respect for all persons;
- cultures that value feedback, challenge and support;

- commitment to transformational learning;
- leaders who possess the skills of enabling facilitation;
- organisations with a person-centred vision;
- strategic plans that support person-centred and evidence-informed cultures of practice;
- continuous evaluation of effectiveness;
- equal valuing of all knowledge and wisdom.

However, whilst having an environment that enables persons to flourish is critical, being attuned to our personal attributes as persons and how we use these to our advantage is equally important. In her recent work, Maureen Gaffney (2011, p. 6) focuses on this issue and identifies four essential elements of flourishing persons:

1. *Challenge*: Some call or demand for you to do something, to get over an obstacle, to engage with some life task, to make something happen.
2. *Connectivity*: Being attuned to what is happening inside you and outside you. Connectivity orientates you to the challenge and gets you ready to deal with it.
3. *Autonomy*: Feeling free to move and to act in pursuit of the challenge. This gives you the energy to get going and sets the direction of travel.
4. *Using your valued competencies*: The experience of using your talents, especially the strengths you most value in yourself, to the full.

These four essential elements provide a deceptively simple framework for understanding what it means to flourish as a person. Gaffney argues that the best kind of challenge is one that we 'own'. That does not mean that we have to identify the challenge willingly ourselves as sometimes we can find ourselves being challenged, not of our choice but because of a context we are in. In the context of practice development, we have identified these as 'critical moments' when we have a choice to grow, develop and transform or not. However, irrespective of the challenge and where it comes from, Gaffney further argues that flourishing requires 'connectivity' or 'psychological attunement' (p. 8). Essentially, this element is similar to that of reflexivity, that is our need to be aware of what is happening inside ourselves (our feelings, emotions, desires, etc.) in order to feel connected, and to interact effectively, with others. There is ample evidence to suggest that strong connections between team members, between team members and the values and goals of an organisation and between the organisation and the personal values of employees, create effective workplaces and indeed environments that flourish (e.g. see Chapters 8 and 10). There is equally strong evidence to illustrate the impact of what are termed 'psychologically unsafe' environments, that is, environments that are disrespectful of persons. Recent work by Donna Brown (see Brown & McCormack, 2011 for details), an expert acute pain management nurse, demonstrates the impact of psychologically unsafe environments on staff well-being, patient experience and patient outcome. However, Donna's work also illustrates how these same environments can be made more psychologically safe through a systematic programme of practice development. Gaffney suggests that persons need to be able to survive emotionally in order to be able to flourish. To do so, they need to be in a context that is psychologically safe, where they are able to feel good about themselves and where there are close connections between individuals and groups that are important to them – all characteristics of an effective person-centred culture and a central focus of emancipatory and transformational practice development activities.

But no matter how connected we may feel, we also need a sense of 'autonomy', as Gaffney (2011, p. 10) says:

> *To flourish you need to have a feeling of autonomy in your life. That means feeling that you can use your free will to set the direction of your life; that you have sufficient elbow room to act; that your opinions count for something. So autonomy is closely connected to feeling that you matter and that what you do matters. Unless you feel like that, there is no real sense of ownership over what you do, no felt responsibility for what happens – good or bad. If you don't feel you are autonomous, you won't be happy in your relationships or satisfied in your work.*

This assertion by Gaffney highlights the importance of individual freedom to 'act', to express one's creativity, to engage in a relationship with others that nurtures our personhood and that makes us feel valued. It is not a co-incidence that Binnie and Titchen's (1999) action research about developing person-centred care was called, 'Freedom to Practise'. This was a strong reference to the seminal work of Carl Rogers and his book, 'Freedom to Learn' (Rogers, 1983).

As practice development has evolved, grown and developed, it has brought with it its critics who have questioned its legitimacy – particularly its legitimacy as an academic pursuit (e.g. Thompson et al., 2008). Those of us committed to practice development have defended it using many of the arguments and conceptual positions articulated throughout this book. For example Tanya McCance's work clarifying 'the "D" of R&D' (see Chapter 9) is a good example of a systematic and rigorous strategic approach to legitimising practice development within a broader context of knowledge generation, translation, implementation and use. However, the importance of autonomy as asserted by Gaffney provides the clearest rationale of all as to why practice development is important and why policy makers need to take note. Whilst health care practice is increasingly criticised for its ineffectiveness and in particular its lack of care and compassion, more and more top-down solutions are being imposed on practitioners and clinical teams that are not owned by them and that increasingly alienate them from their own motivations and feelings. So, unless the increasing resources that are spent on providing solutions are implemented in partnership with practitioners and clinical teams, there will be no *felt* ownership of these solutions and practice will not change. Practice development has always adopted the principles of collaboration, inclusion and participation (CIP) as its primary methodological position, and as such is a key strategy for improving health care and how it is experienced by staff and patients.

The fourth element for flourishing identified by Gaffney (2011, p. 11) is that of 'using your valued competencies'. Quite simply, this means '. . . doing what you were put into the world to do'. Titchen et al. (2007) and Titchen (2009) have identified the importance of 'multiple intelligences' (see Gardner, 1983) in caring, development and research processes that are transformational. Intelligences are the capacity to quickly grasp or apprehend something. We have already introduced the more well-known emotional and embodied intelligences, but there are others that come into play within these transformational processes. These are artistic intelligence (the capacity to engage in aesthetically satisfying care, development and research, and to create, perform and appreciate artistic expression) and spiritual intelligence (the capacity to address and solve problems of meaning and value, and place our lives and journeys within wider, richer meaning-giving contexts). Spiritual intelligence is essential for being creative and working at the edge of what we know. Both these intelligences are palpable in Kate Sanders, Jo Odell and Jonathon Webster's reflections (Chapter 2), but note that they do not mention them. This may be because they are often tacit, inexpressible or deeply buried within us. In transformational practice development, these intelligences are nurtured intentionally by facilitators who help people bring them to the surface, often through the use of creative imagination and expression and working in and with nature. When we become aware of our intelligences and the significant role they play in practice development, then we can further develop them through reflection and critique, alone and with others. So, it is the blending of different knowledges, ways of knowing and these intelligences (amongst other things) that gives us the capacity to improvise and act quickly in the moment and enable effective helping relationships. What we are talking about here is the professional artistry of care, practice development and research.

Being competent is an essential element of person-centredness and a key concept in the person-centred practice framework of McCormack and McCance (2010). This notion of competence goes way beyond any notion of technical competence. It focuses instead on how technical competence is blended with life experience, wisdom, intelligences and knowledge in order to maximise our potential to positively manage uncertainty whilst making wise decisions. So, it is therefore essential that as practice developers we utilise a variety of strategies that can help persons access their hidden talents, their creativity, their wisdom and their intelligences and thus develop their professional artistry. Many of these strategies have been illustrated in the various chapters of this book.

AS PRACTICE DEVELOPERS, HOW DO WE HELP PERSONS TO FLOURISH?

In the development of their framework of 'critical creativity', Titchen and McCormack (2010) articulated methodological principles for helping persons to flourish. We use these principles to summarise the key themes arising from the chapters of this book and to propose a future agenda for practice development, so that it can be the methodology of choice for enabling all persons to flourish.

Spiralling through turbulence: authentic facilitation that is consistent with the shared values and beliefs of co-participants and that results in human flourishing

Whilst specific chapters in this book deal with facilitation methods and approaches (Chapters 5, 6, 11 and 13), throughout the book we have identified facilitation tools, methods and processes. The metaphor of *spiralling through turbulence* challenges us as practice developers to recognise and acknowledge that bringing about transformational change between different stakeholders and in practices themselves is challenging and turbulent (Figure 14.1). However, such turbulence is necessary for real and enduring change to happen, as shown so vividly in Chapter 2 and in participants' experiences of active learning in Chapter 5. This is best illustrated by the work of Senge et al. (2005) and their work on 'presencing'.

Senge et al. propose that we can learn from the future (that which is yet to unfold) and discovering our role in bringing that future into being. In times of profound change, Senge et al. argue that learning from the past alone is an inadequate guide to the future. They propose that when demanding and complex issues require in-depth understanding, commitment and sustained change, a different process is necessary. Senge et al. argue that through a future-orientated learning process, different levels of perceiving reality and action

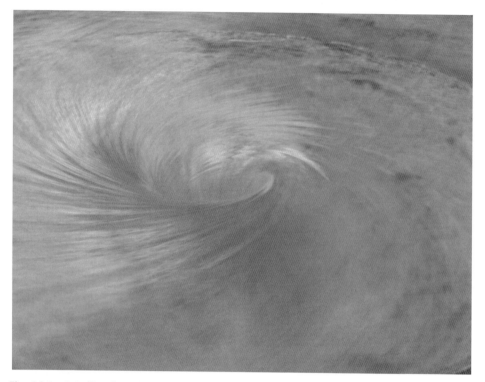

Fig. 14.1 Spiralling through turbulence.

that can follow from it are realised. The three levels proposed are (1) *sensing*, (2) *presencing* and (3) *realising*. *Sensing* incorporates gathering information to gain insight into that which is occurring (e.g. through using picture cards, observations of practice, 360-degree feedback, patient stories). *Presencing* is the deep reflection stage, where individuals or groups try to reach a state of clarity, a complete connection with what is occurring and a state of 'inner knowing' (understanding; e.g. the use of claims, concerns and issues to reach consensus, the engagement with creative processes such as reflective walks and the use of metaphors (see Chapter 11) or group analysis of practice observations). *Realising* is the action phase where individuals or teams bring something new into reality (e.g. agreeing shared team values, agreeing to use high challenge/high support to address team relationships, developing mealtimes practice with patients). The depth of *sensing* and *presenting* holds the key to the success of *realising* or spiralling through turbulence.

Brown and McCormack (2011) identified that the essence of psychological safety is to create an environment where people feel able to focus on underlying issues without the threat of loss of self-identity or integrity. Discouragement and fear prevent us from changing the systems in which we are embedded. So, a facilitator who is spiralling through turbulence helps others to remove tensions arising from fear (of change), build trust, enable people to feel less vulnerable and thus build capacity for cooperation and collaboration. Thence people are able to spiral *through* the tough times, rather than get sucked into a vortex or down the proverbial plug hole. We see these approaches evidenced in Chapter 12, for example, whereby Jan Dewing worked with the values of the new health Trust and used a whole range of existing strategies and visions as a starting point.

Circles of connection: co-construction of a shared reality and spiralling awareness and understanding that has no beginning and no end

The three frameworks underpinning this book (the conceptual framework for practice development, the person-centred practice framework and the framework for holding on to the whole practice development journey), introduced in Chapter 1 and operationalised throughout this book, highlight the importance of shared values as a key foundation for practice development. Developing shared values as a team and holding these values as a 'rudder' to guide the development of practice, enables circles of connection to be created expressed symbolically in Figure 14.2. These connections are formed through discussion, collaboration and the development of a culture that values 'high challenge and high support. Ultimately, what is needed is the creation of meaningful critically reflective conversations that lead to support for, and engagement with, the changes that the teams initiate as a result of active learning. This is not a one-off process, but something that is embedded in team processes,

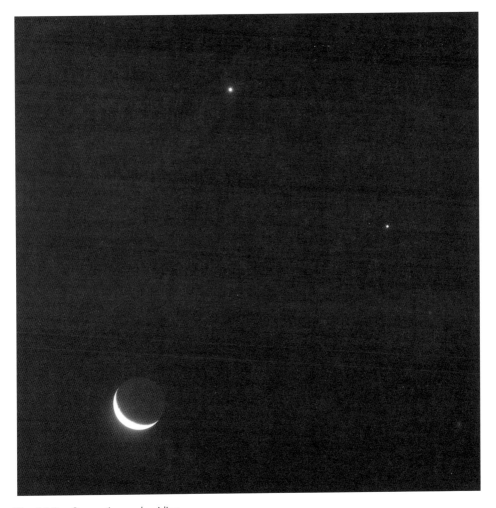

Fig. 14.2 Connecting and guiding.

with each new learning and the resulting change leading to even deeper conversations and ongoing change. We see something of this in Story 8.1 of ward managers using the CIP principles in practice and the outcomes accrued. It also seems to us that the authors of several chapters in this book created circles of connection as they talked, discussed and emailed ideas about their chapter and came to spiralling awareness and deeper understandings. Perhaps, Kate Sanders, Jo Odell and Jonathon Webster in Chapters 2 and Kim Manley, Randal Parlour and Joan Yalden in Chapter 13 show this co-construction most overtly because they include reflections on their experiences over time as well as in the process of preparing for and writing their chapters.

Creative effectiveness: through blending, improvisation, synchronicity, attunement and balance

Throughout this book, examples of blending, improvisation, synchronicity, attunement and balance have been presented. The blending of different forms of knowledge/evidence is the *raison dêtre* of practice developers. In Chapter 7, Jo Rycroft-Malone showed how evidence is blended in the PARIHS framework and how this blending thus needs to be facilitated in order to make evidence-informed decisions. These different forms of evidence need to be balanced with none taking precedence over the other, rather the importance and significance of each type of evidence is determined by the practice context. So, for example, when Donna Brown (Brown & McCormack, 2011) was trying to change how pain management was practised, she needed some of the time to privilege the empirical evidence of effective pain management (upon which there is a lot to draw). However at other times, she needed to use the local information provided by staff discussions, reflections, patient feedback and observations of care to show to the teams the issues that were hindering the empirical evidence from being used/applied. This balance was important in Donna's facilitation work and ultimately was significant in achieving outcomes. Similarly, within the Expertise in Practice Project, facilitators called critical companions (see Titchen, 2004; Hardy et al., 2009) explicitly showed how they blended different kinds of knowledge as they helped nurses with expertise to research and demonstrate their expertise and effectiveness in their work with patients, families and colleagues. Increased insights and growing understanding of professional artistry enabled them to work more effectively with future patients and colleagues. In Chapter 5 of this book, Brendan McCormack and Jan Dewing show how they, with the co-researchers/facilitators, blended different forms of knowledge and knowing in order to make explicit the connections between the facilitation processes used and the outcomes achieved through the programme of work. The explicit commitment to CIP enabled the co-researchers to be attuned to different forms of knowledge and to balance them in determining outcomes for different stakeholders and to ensure that all voices are heard.

However, Donna Brown, and the fictional characters Abbie and Mike in Chapter 6, like all of us, needed to improvise. One reflection you might have on reading the individual chapters, and the book as a whole, is that experienced practice developers have it 'all worked out' when engaging in facilitation work. As Abbie and Mike showed, the contrary is more the reality. Whilst experienced practice developers are deliberate and intentional in their actions, expert facilitation requires the facilitator to improvise according to the context of the practice development work and the needs of individuals and groups. Kate Sanders, Jo Odell and Jonathan Webster illustrate in Chapter 2 how important it is to learn how to improvise. Learning to become an effective facilitator is not just about knowing what tool, method or process to use in a given situation, it is also about being attuned to co-participants (through multiple intelligences) and responding to expressed or anticipated need in a meaningful and person-centred way. Sometimes this means abandoning established plans, working instead with individuals and groups to create a new plan and blending different approaches to achieve a particular outcome.

However, being strategic in these decisions is important. In Chapter 12, Jan Dewing describes her work with Alice Webster in which they demonstrate improvising, synchronising, being attuned to the unfolding strategic development in the new health Trust and as such accommodated complexity and chaos in the situation. This requires embodied knowing and the recognition of patterns in complexity and chaos. Practice development at a strategic level needs to be multi-faceted as shown in Chapters 12 and 13 and yet, relatively simple to survive in complex cultures. In the short term, it feels like being part of a web or constellation where complexity is escalating, where many of the existing enterprises are not equipped to cope with this complexity. Because of this, being creative in the workplace and making use of the learning that comes from being creative is becoming the single most important survival competency in the nursing and midwifery workforce. Tied into this is the ability to be resilient. As we move towards becoming more simplified and effective, we will become more of a learning organisation.

Along with blending and improvisation, synchronicity, attunement and balance are all aspects of professional artistry. Professional artistry is the hallmark of expertise of any kind of practice including the giving of patient care and practice development facilitation. It involves the blending, interplay, synthesis, balancing and synchronising of diverse but interconnected dimensions, as already touched on. Professional artistry is essentially the process that puts the dimensions together to create the dance of fluent and seamless practice. Such practice has an elegant simplicity that seems easy to the onlooker, but is enormously complex and skilled (Titchen, 2009).

Movement in stillness: the stillness of reflection, contemplation and emptying the mind creates a movement that enables future meaningful, ethical action and understanding to occur

Energy mixed fast
Speeding through body soul
Stop, change sources

The above Haiku was written by Brendan and Angie, and arose from reflection on a shared authentic movement to explore facilitation effectiveness and our 'being' as facilitators. The third line (*stop, change sources*) captures the essence of the metaphor 'movement in stillness'. Have you ever found yourself in a situation as a facilitator whereby the activity/co-participant/group are 'stuck' and you keep on trying to fix the situation (just like Brendan in his earlier poem)? Nothing seems to work and you try and try again! Similarly, a practice development programme of work may be in progress, but you feel that after a lot of input, nothing has changed and sustaining commitment to the programme is too challenging.

It is our contention that contexts such as these require what the philosopher Heidegger (1990) referred to as 'distanciation', that is the creation of distance. An example of creating distance is shown in Chapter 11 by Angie Titchen and Ann McMahon's walk in silence in the park and their using their body senses and imagination to come to new understandings

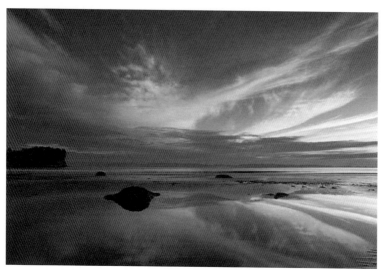

Fig. 14.3 Distanciation.

about the nature of creativity and innovation in practice development. McCormack (2001) suggested that distanciation was an essential concept in being person-centred as connected relationships can sometimes be overpowering, and space for reflection is needed. The more we try to 'fix' the problem, the more problematic it becomes. Creating distance and engaging in reflection enables a different perspective on the issue to emerge and be realised (Figure 14.3).

Being reflective (evaluating the effectiveness of my doing and being as a facilitator) and having reflexivity (learning from reflecting on my doing and being, turning that into meaningful action and engaging in further reflection for future action) are essential skills in enabling flourishing.

The fictional characters in Chapter 6, for example, demonstrate the artistry of reflection in their engagement with each other, with co-learners and with the context within which they work. Whilst there is a range of structured facilitation tools available in the literature for the practice developer to draw upon, it is our reflective experience that sometimes these structured tools can get in the way of authentic reflective engagement with the context of practice. There are numerous illustrations of this authentic engagement throughout this book, but using environmental stimuli, engaging in facilitated critical dialogue and using arts and creativity as reflective processes can be seen in particular in Chapters 2, 6 and 11.

However, reflection may not be enough and sometimes 'being still' and becoming sensitive to our ways of being is also important. This practice, also known as *mindfulness* focuses on becoming aware of our 'automatic patterns'. Siegel (2007, pp. 134–135) suggests that being mindful is about 'waking up from a life on automatic'. Our brains become wired to respond in a particular way in particular contexts through years of similar responses to similar situations, and so our mind tells us to respond in particular ways. Becoming mindful is like 'looking in on ourselves' and actively using our mind to change established patterns. Gaffney highlights two strategies for becoming more mindful – (1) practising meditation and (2) thinking in more flexible ways. Whilst practice development facilitation does not usually extend to meditation (although engaging in quiet listening, being still, relaxation, guided imagery and contemplative/meditative walks as described in Chapters 2 and 11, e.g., are becoming more commonplace in our work as a means of working with turbulence), a key attribute of a practice development facilitator is that of helping others to think in more flexible ways. The posing of reflective questions, using appreciative inquiry techniques (Cooperrider & Whitney, 2005; Dewar & Mackay, 2010), engaging emotionally with a situation such as through the use of 'emotional touchpoints' (Dewar et al., 2010), the use of actionable hypotheses (see Chapter 13) and engaging in creative reflection (see Chapter 11) are all strategies for enabling thinking in more flexible ways and the identification of new possibilities.

Embodied knowing: connection with the environment through an internalisation of its culture(s) or the culture is enacted and seen through a person's body/being in the world

Our work increasingly identifies the importance and significance of engaging our whole selves in practice development work. As already suggested earlier, there is an inextricable relationship between the being of a practice development facilitator and the doing of practice development. This relationship can be seen in this beautiful painting, 'The Healing Touch' by Michele Petroni (Figure 14.4) and could equally be symbolic of person-centred connections between colleagues. Thence, it is never enough to just know how to use particular tools, methods or processes. However, such work is challenging and requires practice development facilitators to have a deep knowledge and awareness of 'self' and/or being in the world. This can come about through previously identified processes such as movement in stillness and creating circles of connection – all of which enable reflection, mindfulness and creative thinking.

The need to be aware of our whole-selves is consistent with the philosophy of Merleau-Ponty and his position that the person 'is the body' and thus our mind and body are one. Mental and physical properties are inseparable, each intertwined with the other creating a seamless whole (Edwards, 2001). Dewing (2007) (drawing on the work of Merleau-Ponty)

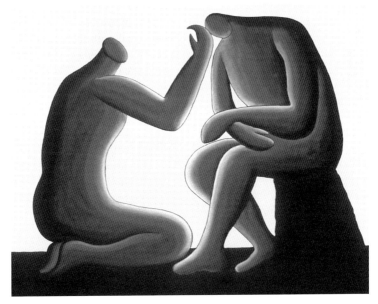

Fig. 14.4 Embodied knowing. Painting by Michele Pietroni. Courtesy of the MAP Foundation (www.mapfoundation.org).

argues and demonstrates that there are four fundamental life-world themes (or existentials) that constitute experience as persons. She calls these 'discovery guides' for reflecting on personhood and lived experiences. The four existentials are (1) lived body (corporeality), (2) lived human relation (relationality), (3) lived space (spatiality) and (4) lived time (temporality). By implication of Merleau-Ponty's idea of them being existentials, they cannot be separated from each other and each existential is embedded and interwoven with the other. Merleau-Ponty's ideas on embodiment offer a radically different and even hopeful construction of the body as an agent that is trying to act appropriately based on perception. So the practice development facilitator (who draws on these 'discovery guides') is conscious, deliberate and intentional in their reflections on the body as an essential tool for effective engagement with others. So paying attention to the messages we carry (and give off to others) in our body, our relationships with others, and, the way we are influenced by space and time are all critical foci for reflection and for our development as facilitators.

In Chapter 11, Angie Titchen and Ann McMahon have shown how connecting with the environment enables a bodily knowing that transcends cognitive and rational processes of analysis (see Vignette 3 in Chapter 11). A key difference between emancipatory and transformational practice development is that of 'connection with nature/the natural environment'. It is this connection that facilitates thinking differently, the release of untapped internal resources and the finding of creative solutions in moments of crisis. What this means is that essentially we can know something through our bodies before we come to know it in our brain. In Chapter 11, the natural environment plays a significant role in shaping the reflections and activities of the authors. There is a connection between the participants being in the world and the environment and this connection is held through the body and articulated through movement, artistry, metaphor, poetry and prose. Similarly, in Chapter 8, we can see how transformational leaders and facilitators carry person-centred cultures in their bodies as they role-model and articulate embodied knowing. This embodied role-modelling is enabled through reflexivity as discussed earlier. However, capturing such embodied knowing is important in the articulation of person-centred outcomes, as otherwise demonstrating the outcomes arising from the development of person-centred cultures and practices is reduced to evidence of technical change. In Chapter 10, Brendan McCormack, Tanya McCance and Jill Maben provide a framework for outcome evaluation that enables equal importance to be placed on 'embodied outcomes' (such as engagement, well-being, effective interpersonal relationships) and technical outcomes (such as safe patient care). The chapter highlights the importance of practice developers engaging in holistic evaluation and using creative approaches to the collection of evidence.

Energising forces: transformation occurs through moments of 'crisis' that trigger a need for change. Creative expression at moments of crisis generates energy from a new ability to express feelings, experiences, spirituality, ethical concerns, embodied and tacit ways of knowing

> *Water crashing down*
> *Magnificent energy*
> *Holding on and letting come*

The literature on 'change management' is largely predicated on a rational, logical perspective of a need for change. What we mean is that it is often assumed that when people are presented with evidence of a need for change that they will understand that need and be willing to change. However, rarely do any of us willingly change without an 'emotional stimulus'. The philosopher Brian Fay (1987) identified the theory of 'crisis' as a critical factor in bringing about social change. Whilst in many major social changes in the world, 'crisis' occurs when there is a stimulus driven by uprising, for example uprising against dictatorial power and control and movement towards greater democracy. Fay suggests that it is through our body that we recognise crisis. Think about major historical and political changes – for example in Berlin, 'the wall' did not just fall, instead it was brought down by the sheer force of feeling amongst individuals that drove the population of East Berlin to knock down the wall and free themselves. It was the strength of emotional feeling driven by ethical, moral and social justice concerns and emotions that enabled the mass expression of feelings that were embodied through an energy that was unstoppable, just as the surge of energy in a waterfall is inexorable (Figure 14.5). At that moment of crisis, there was no option but to take action, express the embodied energy of an oppressed population and set themselves free. As we write, we see the same energising forces at work in the Arab Spring bringing about momentous changes in political systems previously thought unassailable. The philosopher Margaret Mead (1955) highlighted that nothing brings about significant change as effectively as small groups of highly committed, highly driven individuals. In many ways, this is the essence of practice development as illustrated in this book. Practice development is predicated on capturing the concerns of individuals and teams regarding the need to be more effective in aspects of person-centredness. Whilst sometimes this may be driven by a corporate agenda, without the existence of highly committed practitioners in practice settings, no such change will happen.

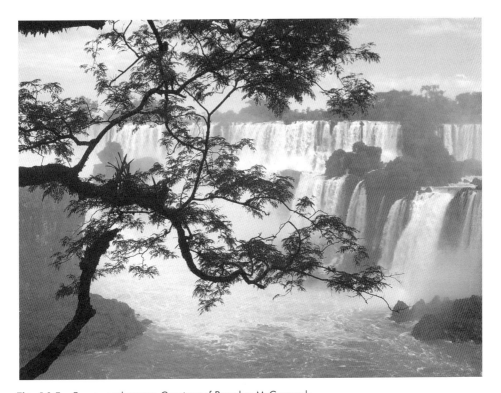

Fig. 14.5   Energy and power. Courtesy of Brendan McCormack.

Whilst the fall of the Berlin Wall might seem like a dramatic example to use, the principles underpinning major social change such as this apply in the context of changing practice. In various chapters of this book, it has been identified time and time again, that through the accumulation of evidence, feelings of crisis became the powerhouse for individual, team and organisational change. We see this best illustrated in Chapter 12 in the Cambridge Health Trust case study. The practice development facilitator role was ended with the potential loss of achievements gained over many years. However, instead of fighting against this change the facilitators and senior leaders worked within the new and emerging strategic framework that has ultimately led to a more sophisticated development framework. The new framework has enabled deeper and more sustained developments in patient involvement in care/services provision, the development of a work-based learning culture, facilitation skills development, and continuous evaluation of care and services.

However, Mezirow (1981) suggests that to bring about emancipatory change requires 'perspective transformation', that is the changing of how we view the world or the part of the world (no matter how small) over which we can have some influence and control. To be person-centred in our ways of being, requires us to pay attention to the values that drive our practice, to have a deep respect for others and to feel a sense of control over our own destiny as a person. These principles and values act as driving forces for small steps to be taken in changing how we view practice and ourselves as practitioners. At times such as this, the work of a facilitator is largely about working with energy, releasing, drawing out, re-directing, creating or transforming energy flows. Without working with energy, the danger is that we shut down the crisis or replace it with something 'safe'. The use of creativity acts as a means of opening up the crisis; living it through the body (we have to find a way to express it) and using metaphor rather than words to 'name' it enables the crisis to become visible and tangible and something that potential creative solutions can be identified and explored. With creative expressions of crisis, for example, positive energy for change is released through catharsis or emerges from a new ability to express the previously inexpressible. This principle (along with others here) connects with Marshall and Reason's (2008, p. 79) notion of 'dancing in beauty rather than fighting ugliness'.

Openness to all ways of being: practitioner researchers need to be open to and appreciative of different world views

This principle is probably blatantly obvious to all practice developers and is well-illustrated in this book. The nature of practice development work means that it is not possible to focus on one particular view of the world. What we mean by 'world view' in the context of practice development is the perspective we adopt, based on our beliefs and values, that shapes our ways of engaging and behaving with others and in particular contexts. So, for example if I believe that there is a 'right' way to do something (and no other way), then my role as a practice developer will be to ensure that as many people as possible also practice in this way. I am probably able to source evidence to support my particular view of the world and my purpose as a practice developer is to convince others about the merits of this evidence and why it should be adopted in practice. There are many examples (especially in clinical practice) where this stance is appropriate (e.g. implementing the most current evidence about good practice in pressure damage prevention) and there is a need to ensure that all practitioners practice in a way that is reflective of the best available evidence. However, not all evidence will be as clear as that of (say) pressure damage prevention, particularly when

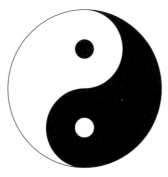

Fig. 14.6   Balance and being able to flow between different ways of being.

we are focusing on more 'relational' aspects of practice. So, for example if we are concerned about the person-centred outcome of 'patients experience of good care' (see Chapter 10 for details) then it is unlikely that the same evidence (as that of pressure damage prevention) will be available or relevant. So, whilst a practice developer may have identified appropriate evidence, such evidence is always conditional, and so the role of the practice development facilitator is to reach consensus with key stakeholders about the best approach to practice. However, as shown in Chapter 7 by Jo Rycroft-Malone, context is everything(!) and so even the 'best' evidence is always conditional on the context in which it is to be used. This means that a practice development facilitator needs to be able to adopt different and complementary approaches to their facilitation, their engagement with others, the methods they use for implementing a change and the approaches to evaluation they adopt.

We have also argued throughout this chapter for practice development facilitators to focus on both their being and doing as facilitators. In the context of 'openness to all ways of being', this is also important. We have illustrated and argued for the importance of being creative and using creative ways of engaging with others. A further argument for creativity is its unifying impact on different world views, that is, if we start from the position of 'what is my essential purpose as a facilitator in this particular context?', then we will maximise our potential to be authentic in our being as facilitators (we go with the shared world view of key stakeholders) and choose methods appropriate to the desired purpose, focus and outcomes (the doing) (see Figure 14.6).

Flowing with turbulence: working with turbulence requires the use of emotional and spiritual intelligences

Realising or transforming crisis into positive action is deeply connected with being able to act with flow and be truly present in the moment. Working with turbulence is often scary and painful because we are working well beyond our comfort zones in unknown conditions where things often seem beyond our control. We feel afraid, exposed, inadequate and vulnerable. These feelings get in the way of flow and being present. To act with flow, we need to be able to stay connected with our authentic selves and be truly present with the whole of ourselves. We can do this by transforming negative emotions and this is where our emotional and spiritual intelligences (as discussed earlier) come in. As we refine these intelligences, we are more able to be present wherever and whatever we are doing. This flowing with turbulence is illustrated in many chapters in this book. For example in Chapter 8, the transformational leaders and facilitators' use of emotional intelligence to put a negative emotion on one side to help others deal with the situation without that emotion. Similarly in Chapter 12, Jan Dewing recognised that 'chaos is part of order in systems and can also indicate a time and space for new ordering to emerge'.

The following poem by Angie captures the essence of her trip to the Red Centre of Australia and the profound effect it had on her. It shows the different energies of flow and turbulence as well as the emotional and spiritual intelligences needed to be present in the moment.

> *Vast plained Uluru*
> *Snake warriors into Rock*
> *Create sacred space*
>
> *Kata Tjuta Sun*
> *Red-rising three sailed shadow*
> *Breathless, takes my breath*
>
> *Red-staired climb to sky*
> *Dips to waterhole palm fringed*
> *Andy-baked-fruit-cake*
>
> *Cliff-hung Helen's Glen*
> *Cold stars Milky Way arched*
> *Mouse says bring a cat!!*
>
> *Washing up laughter*
> *Campfire warms frozen fingers*
> *Gentle group circling*
>
> *Dry walk river bed*
> *Gouged waterhole beach-rock tumbled*
> *Ledged wallabies*
>
> *Aboriginal*
> *Tooth-missed Ken shares mystery*
> *Rock circles, spirals*
>
> *Ancient palms grow tall*
> *Hidden water seeps through stone*
> *Canyon round echoes*
>
> *Ancestral symbols*
> *Repeat fathomless message*
> *Return to my source*

FUTURE AGENDA

So we have reached the end of this particular journey, or maybe it is just the beginning of a new journey for many readers of this book! Whether you are new to practice development or an experienced practice development facilitator, we hope there is something in this book for you. The collection of works in this book is a real and tangible illustration of the expertise that exists amongst colleagues who are committed to developing practice and helping to change the life-world of practice that patients/service users experience every day. The collection is merely a snapshot, though of the exciting and high-quality work that is happening around the world and that is helping to make health care a better experience for all. The passion for their craft that contributors to this book demonstrate is tangible and we hope that as a reader, you are able to embody this passion into your own being and doing as a practice developer. The future agenda for all practice developers, irrespective of our individual world views is to ensure that we make a contribution to creating health care experiences that enable all persons to flourish. We believe this book makes real, the complexity of practice development, whilst at the same time offering particular approaches and insights that can help to deal with this complexity. Whether you are at the beginning of a journey with practice development or challenging your thinking as an experienced practice developer, we hope that this book provides some help, insights, tools, methods and reflections on your effectiveness and your onward movement.

It seems appropriate to conclude with a piece of creative writing undertaken by 14 practice development facilitators at the conclusion of a facilitator development programme. These facilitators captured their reflections on being a facilitator of practice development through this narrative that expressed their collective experience of being a facilitator and what practice development means:

> *The sun is shining, the Daffodils are blooming. The air is clear, Le Chèile[1] forever. This place is buzzing today. Small parcel, big product. We are open to challenging practice. We will take the rough with the smooth. Each individual voice has a valuable story to tell. Don't be afraid to be different. Learning to analyse abstract, but risk taking doesn't have to be bad. Take small steps and keep going. Don't be afraid to take a risk. Support effective decision making, small ideas, big changes. Inspire your colleagues by embracing and valuing creativity. Face the challenges as challenge isn't always a bad thing. Rocky roads can develop into easy ones, so have courage. Shine a light on the power in numbers. Look to the future, be happy as it will be so much better when we are old. Embrace new people and new ideas. Don't get lost in the fog and recognise accomplishments. Reward freely and with gratitude. Appreciate the little things and remember it is always a team effort. Nobody is alone.*

REFERENCES

Binnie, A. & Titchen, A. (1999) *Freedom to Practise: The Development of Patient-Centred Nursing*. Butterworth Heinemann, Oxford.

Brown, D. & McCormack, B. (2011) Developing the practice context to enable more effective pain management with older people: an action research approach. *Implementation Science*, **6** (9), 1–14.

Cooperrider, D. & Whitney, D. (2005) *Appreciative Inquiry – a Positive Revolution in Change*. Berrett-Koehler Publishers, San Francisco, CA.

Dewar, B., Mackay, R., Smith, S., Pullin, S. & Tocher, R. (2010) Use of emotional touchpoints as a method of taping into the experience of receiving compassionate care in a hospital setting. *Journal of Research in Nursing*, **15** (1), 29–41.

Dewar, B. & Mackay, R. (2010) Appreciating and developing compassionate care in an acute hospital setting caring for older people. *International Journal of Older People Nursing*, **5**, 299–308.

---

[1] Le Chèile is Gaelic [Irish] for 'together'.

Dewing, J. (2007) *An Exploration of Wandering in Older Persons with a Dementia through Radical Reflection and Participation*. PhD thesis, University of Manchester.

Edwards, S.D. (2001) *Philosophy of Nursing: An Introduction*. Palgrave, Basingstoke.

Fay, B. (1987) *Critical Social Science: Liberation and Its Limits*. Polity Press, Cambridge.

Gaffney, M. (2011) *Flourishing: How to Achieve a Deeper Sense of Well-being, Meaning and Purpose – Even when Facing Diversity*. Penguin Ireland, Dublin.

Gardner, H, (1983) *Multiple Intelligences: The Theory in Practice*. Basic Books, New York.

Hardy, S., Manley, K., Titchen, A. & McCormack, B. (eds) (2009) *Revealing Nursing Expertise through Practitioner Enquiry*. Wiley-Blackwell Publishing, Oxford.

Heidegger, M. (1990) *Being and Time*. Basil Blackwell, Oxford.

Manley, K., Sanders, K., Cardiff, S. & Webster, J. (2011) Effective workplace culture: the attributes, enabling factors and consequences of a new concept. *International Practice Development Journal*, **1** (2), 1–29. http://www.fons.org/library/journal.aspx (Accessed 17 November 2012).

Mead, M. (1955) *Cultural Patterns and Technical Change*. The New American Library, New York.

Mezirow, J. (1981) A critical theory of adult learning and education. *Adult Education*, **32** (1), 3–24.

McCormack, B. (2001) *Negotiating Partnerships with Older People – A Person-Centred Approach*. Ashgate, Basingstoke.

McCormack, B. & McCance, T. (2010) *Person-centred Nursing: Theory, Models and Methods*. Blackwell Publishing Ltd., Oxford.

McCormack, B. & Titchen, A. (2006) Critical creativity: melding, exploding, blending. *Educational Action Research: An International Journal*, **14** (2), 239–266.

Rogers, C. (1983) *Freedom to Learn for the 80s*. Charles E. Merrill, London.

Senge, P., Scharmer, C.O., Jaworski, J. & Flowers, B. 2005. *Presence: Exploring Profound Change in People, Organisations and Society*. Nicholas Brealey Publishing, London.

Siegel, D.J. (2007) *The Mindful Brain: Reflection and Attunement in the Cultivation of Well-being*. WW Norton & Company, New York.

Stephens, G., Titchen, A., McCormack, B., Odell-Miller, H., Sarginson, A., Hoffman, C., Francis, S., Petrone, M.A., Manley, K., Philipp, R., Naidoo, M., McLoughlin, C. (2004) *Creative Arts and Humanities in Healthcare: Swallows to Other Continents*. The Nuffield Trust, London.

Thompson, D.R., Watson, R., Quinn, T., Worrall-Carter, L. & O'Connell, B. (2008) Practice development: what is it and why should we be doing it? *Nurse Education in Practice*, **8** (4), 221–222.

Titchen, A. & McCormack, B. (2010) Dancing with stones: critical creativity as methodology for human flourishing. *Educational Action Research: An International Journal*, **18** (4), 531–554.

Titchen, A., Higgs, J. & Horsfall, D. (2007) Research artistry: dancing the praxis spiral in critical-creative qualitative research. In: *Being Critical and Creative in Qualitative Research* (eds J. Higgs, A. Titchen, D. Horsfall & H.B. Armstrong), pp. 282–297. Hampden Press, Sydney.

Titchen, A. (2009) Developing expertise through nurturing professional artistry in the workplace. In: *Revealing Nursing Expertise through Practitioner Inquiry* (eds S. Hardy, A. Titchen, B. McCormack & K. Manley), pp. 219–243. Wiley-Blackwell, Oxford.

Titchen, A. (2004) Helping relationships for practice development: critical companionship. In: *Practice Development in Nursing* (eds B. McCormack, K. Manley & R. Garbett), pp. 148–174. Blackwell Publishing Ltd., Oxford.

Index

Note: Page number followed by b, f and t indicates text in box, figure and table respectively.

Practice Development in Nursing and Healthcare, Second Edition. Edited by Brendan McCormack, Kim Manley and Angie Titchen.
© 2013 John Wiley & Sons, Ltd. Published 2013 by John Wiley & Sons, Ltd.

Keep up with critical fields

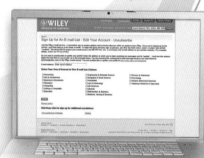

Would you like to receive up-to-date information on our books, journals and databases in the areas that interest you, direct to your mailbox?

Join the **Wiley e-mail service** - a convenient way to receive updates and exclusive discount offers on products from us.

Simply visit **www.wiley.com/email** and register online

We won't bombard you with emails and we'll only email you with information that's relevant to you. We will ALWAYS respect your e-mail privacy and NEVER sell, rent, or exchange your e-mail address to any outside company. Full details on our privacy policy can be found online.

WILEY-BLACKWELL

www.wiley.com/email

17841